D1576443

Gamete and Embryo Micromanipulation in Human Reproduction

Edited by

Simon Fishel
and
Malcolm Symonds

Nottingham University Research and Treatment
Unit in Reproduction (NURTURE),
Queen's Medical Centre

Edward Arnold
A division of Hodder & Stoughton
LONDON   BOSTON   MELBOURNE   AUCKLAND

© 1993 Simon Fishel and Malcolm Symonds

First published in Great Britain 1993

Distributed in the Americas by Little, Brown and Company,
34 Beacon Street, Boston, MA 02108

British Library Cataloguing in Publication Data

Gamete and Embryo Micromanipulation in Human Reproduction
  I. Fishel, S.   II. Symonds, E.M.
  612.6

  ISBN 0–340–57370–8

All rights reserved. No part of this publication may be reproduced
or transmitted in any form or by any means, electronically or
mechanically, including photocopying, recording or any information
storage or retrieval system, without either prior permission in writing
from the publisher or a licence permitting restricted copying. In the
United Kingdom such licences are issued by the Copyright Licensing
Agency, 90 Tottenham Court Road, London W1P 9HE.

Whilst the advice and information in this book is believed to be true
and accurate at the date of going to press, neither the author nor
the publisher can accept any legal responsibility or liability for any
errors or omissions that may be made. In particular (but without
limiting the generality of the preceding disclaimer) every effort has
been made to check drug dosages; however, it is still possible that errors
have been missed. Furthermore, dosage schedules are constantly being
revised and new side effects recognised. For these reasons the reader is
strongly urged to consult the drug companies' printed instructions
before administering any of the drugs recommended in this book.

Typeset in 10/12 pt. Baskerville by Anneset, Weston-super-Mare, Avon.
Printed and bound in Great Britain for Edward Arnold, a division of
Hodder and Stoughton Limited, Mill Road, Dunton Green, Sevenoaks,
Kent TN13 2YA by Butler and Tanner Limited, Frome and London.

SHEFFIELD
UNIVERSITY
LIBRARY

Preface

Has the eighth decade of the 20th century marked a major turning point in the study of human reproduction? As the use of extracorporeal fertilisation has become widespread throughout the world, remedying childlessness for many thousands of couples, we have also witnessed the micromanipulation of human gametes and embryos; the former being micromanipulation primarily for the procurement of conception in vitro, the latter for pre-implantation diagnosis of sex-linked and autosomally-inherited disorders. Even in the few years since our first book, in 1986, there has been the introduction into clinical practice of procedures which were then considered 'futuristic'. It is, however, too early to evaluate many of these procedures, the technologies themselves must still be explored and developed to greater levels of efficiency.

In an attempt to assess current developments, we organised a gathering of representatives of the major centres involved with gamete and embryo micromanipulation. This meeting took place between 14th and 15th December 1990, in the beautiful city of Rome. Cognizant of the fundamental role of animal research for human studies we were fortunate that Professor Godke was able to present to us the exciting work in current use on the micromanipulation of animal embryos for procreating livestock. Whether much, or any, of their 'simple' techniques will be applicable to the human remains to be seen. However, this book represents 'the state of the art' at that time, an analysis of the current situation worldwide and an update on the value of these procedures in the global concern for infertility and inheritable disorders.

New science brings new ethical dilemmas. The sheer complexities of the procedures in micromanipulation and pre-implantation diagnosis result in unexpected choices for the future. Pre-implantation diagnosis with the use of single blastomeres will lead to a choice of embryos free of a wide range of human diseases, but where should one draw the line in defining acceptable diseases? So often the animal models of the past have been absorbed into human practice despite species differences. Progress is occurring at a breathtaking pace. It will require great vision and wisdom to capitalise on the benefits that can accrue from this technology without losing sight of the ethical implications.

We recognise that many of our colleagues have different names and different acronyms for the same technique, for example, MIST (micro-injection sperm transfer) by the group in Singapore, SZI (sub-zonal insertion) by the group in New York for what we call SUZI (subzonal insemination). Some refer to micro-injection only when referring to the injection of a spermatozoon directly into the oocyte, and microfertilisation when into the perivitelline space only. Others use micro-injection for all techniques, and most use the terms interchangeably. We have opted for a reasonable degree of consistency in the text, have often chosen the editors' prerogative, and we beg the forgiveness of our colleagues!

S B Fishel and E M Symonds
1992

Acknowledgements

We are indebted to Dr. Severino Antinori whose great energy and persistence enabled RAPRU (RICERCATORI ASSOCIATI PER LA RIPRODUZIONE UMANA, Rome, Italy) to provide the funding for the International meeting on Gamete and Embryo Micromanipulation in Human Reproduction.

A very special debt of gratitude must go to Barbara Gallimore, without whose support, patience and expertise, this book would probably never have been completed.

We also thank Jenny Hull for the provision of some of her recent data on sperm morphology, but particularly for the use of Table 7.1. We are most grateful also to our publisher, Edward Arnold, for agreeing to take on this work and deliver the book as rapidly as possible; and, most important, to all our contributors for their patience with us and, after all, without whom the text would be nothing!

Contents

List of contributors

Mina Alikani
Dept of Biology
Rollins Research Center
1510 Clifton Road
Emery University
Atlanta
Georgia 30322
USA

Z Ben-Rafael
Department of Obstetrics & Gynaecology
Chaim Sheba Medical School
Tel Hashomer 52621
Israel

I Ben-Shloma
Department of Obstetrics & Gynaecology
Chaim Sheba Medical School
Tel Hashomer 52621
Israel

M W Berns
Beckman Laser Institute
Dept of Obstetrics & Gynaecology
University of California
Irvine
California 92715
USA

D Bider
Department of Obstetrics & Gynaecology
Chaim Sheba Medical School
Tel Hashomer 52621
Israel

Ariff T Bongso
Dept of Obstetrics & Gynaecology
National University Hospital
Lower Kent Ridge Road
Singapore 0511

Judge Christian Byk
Formerly Special Adviser for Bioethics
Secretariat General, Council of Europe
67000 Strassbourg
France

Gloria Calderon
Dept of Obstetrics & Gynaecology
Instituto Dexeus
Paseo-Bonanova 67
Barcelona
Spain

Jaques Cohen
Dept of Biology
Rollins Research Center
1510 Clifton Road
Emery University
Atlanta
Georgia 30322
USA

Joy Delhanty
The Galton Laboratory
Department of Genetics and Biometry
University College London
4 Stephenson Way
London NW1 2HE

J Dor
Dept of Obstetrics & Gynaecology
Chaim Sheba Medical Centre
Tel Hashomer 52621
Israel

G R Dunstan
Department of Theology
The University of Exeter
Exeter
Devon EX4 4QH

B Fisch
The Unit for Assisted
Reproductive Technologies
Beilinson Medical Centre
Saculer School of Medicine
Tel-Aviv University
Israel

Simon Fishel
NURTURE
Dept of Obstetrics & Gynaecology
Queen's Medical Centre
Nottingham

Robert Godke
Department of Animal Science
Louisiana State University
Baton Rouge
Louisiana 70803
USA

Jamie Grifo
Dept of Biology
Rollins Research Center
1510 Clifton Road
Emery University
Atlanta
Georgia 30322
USA

Alan H Handyside
Human Embryology Laboratory
Institute of Obstetrics & Gynaecology
Hammersmith Hospital
Du Cane Road
London
W12 0NN

A Kuranty
Dept of Obstetrics & Gynaecology
University of Kiel
MichaelisstraBe 16
D 2300 Kiel 1
Germany

Orly Lacham-Kaplan
Centre for Early Human Development
Monash Medical Centre
Monash University
246 Clayton Road
Clayton, Victoria
Australia

Franco Lisi
NURTURE
Dept of Obstetrics & Gynaecology
Queen's Medical Centre
Nottingham

S L Liow
Dept of Obstetrics & Gynaecology
National University Hospital
Lower Kent Ridge Road
Singapore 0511

Henry Malter
Dept of Biology
Rollins Research Center
1510 Clifton Road
Emery University
Atlanta
Georgia 30322
USA

Shlomo Mashiach
Dept of Obstetrics & Gynaecology
Chaim Sheba Medical Centre
Tel Hashomer 52621
Israel

Liselotte Mettler
Dept. of Obstetrics and Gynaecology
University of Kiel
Michaelisstrasse 16
Kiel
Germany

M Montag
Dept of Obstetrics & Gynaecology
National University Hospital
Lower Kent Ridge Road
Singapore 0511

David Mortimer
Sydney IVF
187 Macquarie Street
Sydney NSW 2000
Australia

S Chyne Ng
Dept of Obstetrics & Gynaecology
National University Hospital
Lower Kent Ridge Road
Singapore 0511

S S Ratnam
Dept of Obstetrics & Gynaecology
National University Hospital
Lower Kent Ridge Road
Singapore 0511

L Rinaldi
NURTURE
Dept of Obstetrics & Gynaecology
Queen's Medical Centre
Nottingham

R W Rorie
Department of Animal Science
Louisiana State University
Baton Rouge
Louisiana 70803
USA

Z Rosenwaks
Dept of Biology
Rollins Research Center
1510 Clifton Road
Emery University
Atlanta
Georgia 30322
USA

A Henry Sathananthan
Lincoln School of Health Sciences
La Trobe University
Locked Bag 12
Carlton South IC 3053
Australia

A Simon
Dept of Obstetrics & Gynaecology
Hadassah University Hospital
P O Box 1200
Jerusalem 91120
Israel

Y Tadir
Dept of Obstetrics & Gynaecology
University of California
Irvine
California 92715
USA

Beth E Talansky
Dept of Biology
Rollins Research Center
1510 Clifton Road
Emery University
Atlanta
Georgia 30322
USA

J Timson
Dept of Obstetrics & Gynaecology
University of Nottingham
Queen's Medical Centre
Nottingham

V Tok
Dept of Obstetrics & Gynaecology
National University Hospital
Lower Kent Ridge Road
Singapore 0511

A O Trounson
Centre for Early Human Development
Monash Medical Centre
Monash University
246 Clayton Road
Clayton
Victoria
Australia

A Veiga
Dept of Obstetrics and Gynaecology
Instituto Dexeus
Paseo-Bonanova 67
Barcelona
Spain

L Wilton
Institute of Zoology
Regents Park
London

R M L Winston
Royal Postgraduate Medical School
Hammersmith Hospital
London W12

J Younis
Hadassah University Hospital
Dept of Obstetrics & Gynaecology
P O Box 1200
Jerusalem 91120
Israel

Section I
Introduction

Chapter 1

Historical overview of the use of micromanipulation

Simon Fishel

Historical context

Until the beginning of the nineteenth century, investigators used magnifying lenses to reveal tiny, anatomical structures; cells were actually depicted during the seventeenth and eighteenth centuries, but the significance of these delicate structures was not realised. Few experimenters gave their attention to the diminutive cells. One early method used by a few researchers was to exert gentle pressure on the cellular tissue placed between a slide and cover slip and to note the effect of partially crushing the cells – not too dissimilar to some current methods for observing the penetration of hamster eggs by human sperm. These early experiments were done on free living cells, Protozoa.

At this stage it may be worth a brief historical note on the earliest deductions about the living cell. Felix Dujardin (1801–60), using the partial squashing technique of free living cells, determined the fluid nature of protoplasm, which he called Sarcode. He observed that when the cell wall was ruptured the interior would exude without being destroyed. In one experiment he used a chance cotton fibre which lay across a Paramecium, and by pressing the preparation he caused a bulging mass of the 'Sarcode', or protoplasm, to be completely pinched off. The resulting fragment rounded up and the beating cilia, still active on its surface, carried it away.

A few months ago, while performing the partial zona dissection procedure on a human oocyte, I observed the remarkable 'individualness' of a small amount of extruded ooplasm. A part of the ooplasm was damaged, such that a small amount was 'pinched off', but still attached to the outside of the zona pellucida. The oocyte and extruded cytoplasm seemed to maintain their integrity and were placed in the suspension of spermatozoa. Eighteen hours later, the main body of the oocyte had two pronuclei, and what appeared to be a single pronucleus was observed in the extruded cytoplasm. Synchronously with the oocyte, the extra zonal cytoplasm underwent cleavage over the following 48 hours (Figure 1.1).

Karl Nageli (1817–91) – who introduced into botany the concept of meristem, and demonstrated the importance of the sequence of cell divisions in plant formation – experimented on crushing plant cells and found that the interior of the cell could be extruded and separated off as viable masses or bodies. Three important deductions were drawn from these early experiments:

1. An isolated portion of protoplasm from a living cell may exhibit properties of 'life'.

3

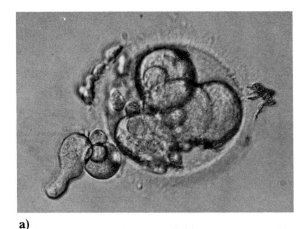

a)

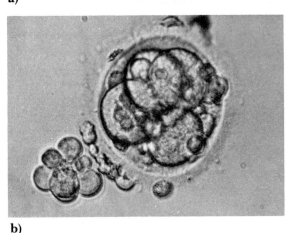

b)

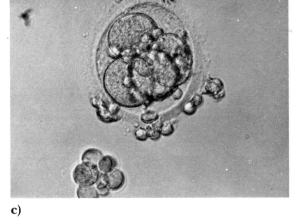

c)

Figure 1.1a Four cell human embryo 44 hours after damaging the ooplasm during PZD, resulting in extra-zonal ooplasm. The embryo has a few cytoplasmic fragments. The extrazonal cytoplasm is progressing through cleavage. The embryo *per se* had two pronuclei and the extrazonal cytoplasm had what appeared to be a single pronucleus after 18 hours insemination

Figure 1.1b Four hours later the extrazonal ooplasm has divided into four 'cells' with some fragmentation.

Figure 1.1c Six hours later one of the cells of the extrazonal ooplasm has divided further and the whole has separated from the zona pellucida

2. The manner in which the internal material flows out of the cell and rounds up indicates the fluid nature of protoplasm.

3. The persistence of a sharply defined boundary between the exuding protoplasm and the medium demonstrated either that the proto-plasm is non-miscible with water, or is able to reconstitute a membrane about itself.

Wilhelm Pfeffer (1845–1920) – whose work on osmotic pressure made him a pioneer in the study of modern plant physiology, and to whom is cred-ited the term 'plasma membrane' – was convinced that the exuded material maintained its integrity by the formation of a precipitation membrane about it. In one of Pfeffer's papers he actually proposed the possibility of building a mechanical contrivance for

moving minute glass needles and pipettes to permit operations on living cells.

The invention of the microscope permitted all sorts of microdissections carried out in the micro-scopic field, but it was the invention of mechanical devices which guide the operating tools proper that heralded the advent of micromanipulators (see Chapter 2).

A paper, which is often overlooked, was pub-lished by W. H. Ransom in the *Philosophical Transactions of London* in 1867. In this study on fish eggs, Ransom extracted nuclei and demonstrated that in certain media they need not lose their struc-tural integrity when removed from the cell. Nuclei became excellent material for micromanipulation.[1] One of the first researchers reported to have used a microscope dissector for the dissection of tis-

4

sues was H. D. Schmidt in 1895.[2] During the ensuing years, biological microdissection, which was termed micrurgy by Peterfi in 1923[3] (see Chapter 2), proved of great importance in experimental cytology, bacteriology, cellular physiology and embryology.

It was the bacteriologists who inspired the use of micromanipulative techniques to the microdissection of living cells. George Lester Kite delivered a lecture (never published) in 1911 in which he astonished his audience by describing the interposition of the tip of a microneedle between the male and female pronuclei of a recently fertilised toxopneustes egg.

By the 1940s micromanipulation was devoted to three general procedures: the dissection of cells and cell aggregates, the removal of materials from within cells, and the injection of solutions into cells. The role of the nucleus in certain cells was studied. It was demonstrated that the nucleus was essential, not only genetically, but also for the continued existence of the cell.[4,5]

The application of micrurgical techniques to the study of cell differentiation and regulation of genetic activities commenced in the early 1950s with the use of relatively large somatic or germ cells. Examples are the studies of Hammerling[6] on acetabularia, various experiments using amphibian embryos[7,8], or Chironomid larval glands.[9]

It was between the two decades of the 1940s and 1950s that the microsurgical or micromanipulation techniques were first used to study the living eggs of the rat[10], the human[11], the mouse[12] and the rabbit.[13]

Developmental studies in mammalian embryology

During the late 1950s and into the 1960s, interest in mammalian experimental embryology was increasing. A major influence during this period was T. P. Lin, who performed numerous studies on the technical and experimental nature of egg micrurgy.[14,15] Lin demonstrated the two essential steps to a successful micro-injection technique, penetration and withdrawal. The zona pellucida,

which is elastic, and the ooplasm, which is watery, required different care. Lin also noted that the zona pellucida of the fertilised pronucleate egg was less elastic and the vitellus substance was more viscous: thus micro-injection is smoother at the pronuclear stage compared to the unfertilised egg. Lin used hyaluronidase to soften the membranes of the unfertilised egg, and observed the importance of injecting into the ooplasm smoothly and slowly – sudden penetration caused disruption of the oolemma – in contrast to the zona pellucida which requires a thrust of the microneedle. Lin and co-workers also studied the effect of microsuction and the removal of small amounts of the egg cytoplasm: they observed that the eggs remained intact with half the cytoplasm aspirated. Lin also performed the earliest experiments involving the transfer to foster mothers of micromanipulated eggs. By micromanipulation the eggs were radiolabelled prior to transfer and the developing fetuses could be identified not only by fetal eye pigment – and coat colour after birth – but also the presence of radio-activity in the fetus.[16] Lin also demonstrated the survival of eggs that had been micro-injected with various solutions, such as citrate-Locke's or DNase into pronuclear eggs, and compared them with punctured but uninjected eggs. The data demonstrated that 15 per cent of the eggs injected with citrate-Locke's solution developed into living fetuses which appeared normal when analysed at day 17 of gestation. By observing the volume of fluid that could be injected into the ooplasm from $180 \pm 8u^3 - 270 \pm 57u^3$ a range of survival was predicted. Lin and co-workers demonstrated the viability of many other techniques which eventually permitted studies on cytochemical and embryological mapping and differentiation, and the early experiments involving the transplantation of minute subnuclear structures, such as a chromosome[18], into mammalian oocytes.

The microsurgical approaches to the study of early mammalian development progressed with the advance of the use of exogenous gonadotrophins to increase the number of oocytes ovulated.[19] This technique made available large numbers of oocytes or pre-implantation embryos for experimental manipulation. The most extensively studied animals were the mouse and rabbit. One striking observation in 1968, by Moore et al.[20], was the production of live young from a single blastomere of an eight-cell rabbit embryo in which the remaining clastomeres had been destroyed.

During the past 30 years a fascinating array of manipulations have been carried out on the pre-implantation embryo. The majority of these experiments have involved the addition or removal of cells, or the transplantation of nuclei. More recently the introduction of exogenous DNA into the zygote or early embryo has been done to study the function of gene products and the regulation of gene expression. This technique has combined the skills of embryologists and molecular biologists, resulting in the generation of transgenic animals.

Various microsurgical experiments were devised to study the fate of the early differentiating embryo, to study the contributions of cells from the inner cell mass (ICM) and trophectoderm cells, and the time of X-chromosome inactivation in the fetal lineage. Much of the early pioneering work was done by Professor Richard Gardner, who initially utilised microscalpels made by gluing small pieces of the sharp edge of safety razor blades onto microneedles. The generation of chimaerism by mixing and swapping cells of embryos gave important insight into the developmental potential of individual blastomeres within a cleaving embryo.

The first successful report of chimaera production was by Tarkowski in 1961[21], following an unconfirmed report in the rat by Nicholas and Hall in 1942.[10] Between the early 1960s and 1980s, various techniques were used to aggregate either whole embryos or individual blastomeres of free dissociated cleavage stages. Techniques using simply temperature[22,23], phytohaemagglutinin[24], or a polyclonal anti-mouse serum[25] were used to facilitate the initial adherence of the cells. Some experiments were used to create blastocysts formed by the aggregation of as many as five to nine individual embryos, which were then transferred to foster mothers to yield normal offspring.[26] However, not all the cells of such giant embryos contribute to the resulting offspring, and to date the maximum number of embryos aggregated in which the cells contribute to the offspring is four.[27] Using these techniques of aggregating embryos at different stages, it was possible to study the distribution

of chimaerism[28,29] to demonstrate that the more advanced cells in these heterochronic combinations contribute a disproportionately large cellular component to the ICM, with the less advanced cells contributing proportionally more cells to the trophectoderm. Techniques using fully dissociated blastomeres at the different cleavage stages and of a different genotype were utilised by Kelly[30,31], and provided the most conclusive information on the developmental potential of blastomeres of the mouse embryo. The aggregation procedure was also utilised for the incorporation of embryonal carcinoma cells into the pre-implantation embryo in a not very successful attempt to encourage these cells to participate in normal embryogenesis.[32,33] However, despite the disappointing generation of embryonal cells by this technique, chimaeric offspring were obtained.

In 1968 Gardner[32] generated chimaeras by injecting cells into the blastocyst stage. Despite the early difficulties of micromanipulation[33], subsequent simplified versions of the technique utilising dissociated cells rather than pieces of tissue were successfully transplanted.[34,35] While the blastocyst injection technique was used for the transplantation of the malignant embryonal carcinoma cells[36–38], it was initially utilised to investigate the fate of ICM and trophectoderm cells and the stage of X-chromosome inactivation.[39,40] A later development, using embryonic stem cells derived from blastocyst outgrowths *in vitro*[41–44], was used in the early 1980s, yielding adequate rates of germline colonisation[45], and extensive somatic chimaerism.[46]

Using these micromanipulation techniques, elegant studies by two groups of researchers in 1987 resulted in the production of mice which it was hoped would provide the animal model for the Lesch-Nyhan syndrome of humans. The approach which introduced novel mutations into the laboratory mouse utilised embryonic stem cells that had mutated spontaneously *in vitro* and were deficient in hypoxanthine phosphoribosyl transferase (HPRT) activity.[47] The other approach utilised cells in which mutation was induced by insertion of a retrovirus into the gene.[48] In both groups the HPRT deficient mice were obtained after colonisation of the germline of wild type mice with the mutant embryonal stem cells injected into blastocysts. The potential value of this animal model for studying the Lesch-Nyhan syndrome is discussed in Chapter 17.

Apart from the discussion about intraspecific chimaeras, a number of workers studied the formation of chimaeras from embryos belonging to different species of mammal. Such studies were able to provide information on the introduction of trophectoderm and ICM[49,50–52], early embryogenesis[53–55] and implantation.[56,57]

A variation on the interspecific chimaeras has been the injection of Mus Caroli ICMs into Mus Musculus blastocysts or trophectoderm vesicles[58–60], with the use of the latter species as uterine foster mothers. Variations on these techniques have enabled the development of an embryo from one species within the placenta of the same species of the uterine foster mother, with subsequent delivery of viable postnatal chimaeras between the sheep and goat[61,62] (see Chapter 15). These experiments, particularly those of M. Musculus and M. Caroli, provide important information on materno-fetal relations[60,63], as well as being a useful *in vitro* cell marker for lineage analysis.[64]

Another form of manipulation associated with these studies is blastocyst reconstitution. This technique developed from microsurgical isolation of ICMs. The latter were injected into trophoblastic vesicles which were generated from short term culture of mural trophectoderm which had been separated from other blastocysts by the use of a microscalpel as described by Gardner in the early 1970s.[65,66] The more simplified approach utilises immunosurgery which causes specific destruction of the trophectoderm cells generating isolated ICMs.[67] These experiments were initially important for studying the interaction between the ICM and polar (overlying) trophectoderm[66], and, more recently, to investigate cell lineage relationships in the chorio-allantoic placenta[68], the role of the trophoblast in maintenance of pregnancy[60] and the evaluation of genomic implanting and lineage specificity.[69]

Apart from mixing and combining cells, the other microsurgical approaches involved the removal of blastomeres to study partial embryos. Early workers studied the extent to which the cleaving embryo could compensate for the loss of blasto-

meres, [10,70–72] to the remarkable production of live young from the work of Moore et al. 1968.[20] More recent studies with an obvious implication envisaged for human embryology were the removal of blastomeres for typing embryos for sex and other genotypic diagnosis.[73–75] Further studies in the 1980s utilised separating blastomeres to produce genetically identical twins, triplets or quadruplets.[76,77] The success of these manipulations in different mammals depended upon the number of cells in the embryo at the time of blastulation. If the cell number is high at that stage, individual blastomeres isolated at the four- or eight-cell stage were shown to develop normally to term.[20,76] In those species, such as the mouse, in which the cell number at blastulation is lower, development at term has been obtained only with blastomeres from two-cell embryos.[77]

These techniques have obvious implications, not only in agriculture where successful sexing of embryos and the production of two or more from one would be of enormous cost benefit to the farmer, but also in humans. Should it be desirable, proven genetically defective human embryos may be aborted *in vitro*, or, conversely, two or possibly three embryos could be created to increase the chances of implantation when only one embryo exists.[78] The possible use of individual blastomeres from human cleaving embryos for pre-implantation diagnosis is the subject of Chapters 16–19.

Another arm of the micromanipulation procedures which has received somewhat infamous attention over the years has been that of nuclear transplantation, or cloning. The early attempts of transplanting nuclei into enucleated eggs in amphibia were to determine whether cellular diversification during embryogenesis was accompanied by stable alterations in the genome.[79,80] Attention of this technique was turned to the mammalian egg in a belief that cloning may benefit animal husbandry. More recent studies, however, have centred on the failed development of diploid parthenogenetic embryos beyond mid-gestation. Various techniques were tried to successfully fuse nuclei or cells with other cells of the early embryo. However, the most significant micromanipulative procedure was developed in the mouse by McGrath and Solter in 1983.[81]

This procedure used a micropipette which did not actually penetrate the plasma membrane of the oocyte but deformed the surface of the egg while applying suction to entrap one or both pronuclei which are removed from the oolemma at the same time the latter seals as the pipette is withdrawn. Karyoplasts or donor cells which had been exposed to inactivated Sendai virus to promote fusion with the egg were then injected inside the zona pellucida. This technique was used successfully to transplant pronuclei.[81–83] Using a modification by Tsunoda et al.[84] of slitting the zona pellucida of the eggs prior to the removal of the pronuclei enabled enucleation to be done with a smooth-tipped pipette, reducing possible damage to the oocyte.

These techniques provided information on the developmental requirements of the maternal and paternal genome, and the capacity of nuclei to support the development of enucleated eggs. Diploid gynogenetic and androgenetic embryos were studied, the former closely resembling diploid parthenogenomes. These, quite astonishingly, progress to fairly advanced fetal development. Diploid androgenetic embryos, although showing an early demise with failure of growth of the fetus, still showed some advanced development of the membranes.[83] This work resulted in the findings that suggested the inhibition of development of parthenogenomes was a result of their pronuclear rather than cytoplasmic constitution.[85]

The use of embryonic nuclei for nuclear transplantation experiments has been disappointing. They appear to lose the capacity to substitute for the zygote nucleus well before the end of cleavage in the mouse. However, pronuclear transplantation appears to be a powerful tool to study the onset of activation of the embryonic genome in relation to the expression of maternal rather than paternal alleles[86], and the fundamentals of parental effect mutations.[87,88]

A recent and most powerful micromanipulation tool is involved in the generation of transgenic animals. By transferring genes to cells in culture, only a restricted number of cell types may be propagated while retaining their tissue-specific characteristics. Cell culture systems often do not provide the necessary complex interactive systems present in complete organisms which may be necessary to study the complete effects of gene products. The need to study genes, for example those directly involved in tumour induction, is a powerful reason for the need to introduce genes into all cells of a mammalian organism. This can now be achieved by gene transfer into pre-implantation embryos.

Currently there are three major procedures for transferring genes, and this depends upon the target cell used. This can be achieved by micro-injection, DNA transfection, and infection using retroviral vector systems.

The most efficient procedure to generate transgenic mice – up to approximately 30 per cent of the animals born – is direct micro-injection of DNA into one pronucleus, preferentially the male, of the zygote.[89,90] These techniques use approximately 100 linear DNA molecules in a volume of one picolitre. Accordingly the DNA is integrated into the chromosomal DNA during the early cleavage stages and the genetic trait is transmitted to the offspring according to Mendelian computation. Genes which have been shown to be expressed in a developmental and tissue-specific fashion include elastase, insulin, α-fetoprotein, albumin, myocin, crystalin, immunoglobulin, MHC class 1, T-cell receptor, collagen, beta- and alpha-globin, vimentin, and others.[89,90]

Another route for infecting the pre-implantation embryo is to use retroviruses which have been manipulated so that they serve as a carrier for specific genetic information. At the blastocyst stage the virus or virus-producing cells are injected into the blastocoele, from which they will infect the inner cell mass cells and be incorporated into the embryo. This technique generally results in the offspring being mosaic for the transgene as incorporation usually arises in a subset of the mucosa embryonic cells. Quite remarkably it has been observed that these transgenes are generally expressed in the correct development and tissue-specific fashion at levels close to the endogenous cognate gene. Therefore, the endogenous chromosomal DNA is flexible enough to incorporate and permit the correct expression of large pieces of exogenous DNA. These experiments have also shown that these results are applicable even if the transgene has been derived from another species.

Aside from the obvious potential advantages of

these techniques in the production of new pharmaceuticals, alteration of animal products for use in humans and the alteration of the resistance of livestock against disease, there remains the potential for this technique to be used for gene therapy in humans in the future. However, risks have been associated with the technique, especially after micro-injection insertion. This has to be considered an exciting area of fundamental research for the future.

Micro-assisted fertilisation in animals

The early investigations into the injection of sperm into eggs, which began in earnest around the mid-1960s, were primarily to investigate the early events of fertilisation, i.e. membrane fusion between homologous and heterologous gametes, activation of the ooplasm and formation of the pronuclei. Two series of early experiments by independent groups demonstrated major differences between oocytes of different species. Hiramoto[91] reported that after injecting sperm into unfertilised sea urchin eggs, the sperm nuclei did not decondense in the ooplasm. However, if the egg was inseminated after sperm injection, the injected sperm nuclei participated in the mitotic process. This demonstrated that activation of the egg cytoplasm was essential for the condensation of sperm nuclei. However, the studies of Graham[92] and Brun[93] in which frog sperm were injected into unfertilised homologous eggs and subsequently transformed into pronuclei, showed that in contrast to the sea urchin egg, the frog egg was easily activated when the egg was pricked with the microneedle.[79] Uehara and Yanigimachi[94] later demonstrated that isolated hamster nuclei could develop into pronuclei after micro-injection into homologous eggs; a similar result being obtained when freeze-dried and frozen/thawed human spermatozoa were injected into the hamster egg. These significant studies revealed that the cytoplasmic factors for controlling the transformation of sperm nuclei into the male pronucleus are not species specific. Interspecies experiments were conducted between rat and mouse[95], frog and human[96], hamster and mouse, and rabbit and

fish.[97] The results of these experiments were similar and initiated interest in heterospecific fertilisation, insemination of an oocyte of one species with the sperm of another. In 1979 Thadani[98] demonstrated that only the zona free rat oocyte was capable of fertilisation by mouse sperm, with the subsequent formation of male and female pronuclei. A further series of detailed experiments demonstrated that the interaction between the sperm and ooplasm was less species specific than the interactions at the gametes' surface membranes. In other words, during normal fertilisation specific membrane fusion events occur which can be bypassed by micro-injection without compromising the initiation of development. It was shown by Markert[99] that micro-injecting sperm heads, detached from their tails by sonication, into the ooplasm could induce the normal events of fertilisation, a result repeated using immotile and grossly defective spermatozoa. Further studies by Naish[97] demonstrated that the usual interactions associated with sperm penetration and fertilisation of an egg were not a biological prerequisite of the events subsequent to fertilisation. These events could be circumvented by direct injection. Hamster oocytes were injected with the nuclei of sperm from hamsters, mice, rabbits and fish, and hamster hepatocytes: the nuclei of each cell type transformed into pronuclei and initiated DNA synthesis.

Experiments of this kind made an enormous contribution to our understanding of the biological mechanisms of fertilisation. The processes of capacitation and acrosome reaction of sperm, surface membrane fusion between the gametes, activation of the oocyte and cytoplasmic control of the formation of pronuclei were illuminated in the course of many experiments by numerous researchers. Apart from the increase in fundamental knowledge, this work led to the appliance of techniques for animal production. For the first time it was perceived that productive and efficient use could be made of genetically valuable but biologically defective male gametes from domestic and wild animal species. Numerous individual researchers and whole units were devoted to establishing fertilisation, cleavage, pregnancies and healthy offspring from these micro-injection techniques. During the 1980s, and especially from the pioneering laboratory of Professor Iritani, enormous advances were being made in increasing the incidence of fertilisation and cleavage, with the eventual birth of live offspring in the rabbit and cow, from direct injection of spermatozoa – intact and epididymal – into oocytes.[100-107]

Despite the successes observed in the fertilisation and cleavage rate, it was becoming evident that direct injection into the ooplasm compromised the developmental rate of transferred embryos. In 1986 Gordon and Talansky[108] reported on a method by which a portion of the zona pellucida could be digested, using acidified culture medium gently released from a micropipette pushed up against the zona pellucida. By causing a permanent opening in the zona pellucida in this way, spermatozoa, defective in their ability to bind and penetrate the zona pellucida, could swim through the breach and come in direct contact with the ooplasm. This technique required the oocyte to be cultured in a suspension of motile spermatozoa after partial digestion of the zona pellucida. Although this method proved successful in the mouse, it was to prove one of the prime examples of the difficulties in extrapolating directly from animal models to the human. Despite its effectiveness in mice, the technique was to prove deleterious when applied to the human (see Chapters 6, 7 and 8).

However, the concept of zona breaching was firmly implanted in the minds of numerous researchers, and was still believed to be of clinical use, especially as direct injection into the cytoplasm had shown some success in animal studies. Further requirements to these techniques were being considered for use in human infertility, along with our own ideas in 1985 to inject the spermatozoa directly into the perivitelline space (Figure 1.2). A major aid for the injection of sperm into oocytes, directly into the cytoplasm or subzonally, and also for the zona breaching techniques was pioneered by Yang et al. in 1988.[109] To aid manipulation of the oocytes, these authors, working with rabbit eggs, suggested the shrinkage of the ooplasm using hyperosmotic sucrose. They demonstrated that the oocytes shrank to between 37–40% of their original size when incubated in 0.5 M or 1.0 M sucrose. This dramatically increased the perivitelline space, and became a major component in the techniques for micro-insemination (see Chapters 7, 8).

A series of research studies in animals concluded that fertilisation could occur in 'zona drilled' oocytes even though penetration through the zona pellucida had been blocked immunologically by the use of a monoclonal antibody against the zona pellucida sperm receptor glycoprotein.[110] Certain male mice, in which the spermatozoa carry the t^{w5}/t^{w71} genes, are infertile. This infertility is presumed to be a result of physiological or biochemical defects. Although spermatozoa from t/t mice have very poor progressive motility, compared with normal T/t carrying sperm, they are still capable of binding to the zona pellucida if inseminated *in vitro*. Sperm from $T/t^{w5/w71}$ males remain infertile as their reduction to only one t-complex decreases sperm transport, and infertility arises during normal IVF. In 1988, Depypere et al.[111] increased the incidence of fertilisation from five per cent in zona-intact oocytes to 73 per cent with 'zona drilled' oocytes. However, a recent study of Ahmad et al.[112] reported that despite fertilisation and cleavage of 'zona drilled' eggs by spermatozoa of T/t mice, t/t individuals did not achieve fertilisation.

In 1989, Lacham et al.[113] (Chapter 5) micro-injected a single sperm under the zona pellucida of mouse eggs and achieved fertilisation. Concern arose over the use of a single spermatozoon in that it would be difficult to select a capacitated and fully acrosome-reacted spermatozoon (see Chapters 5, 7). It was, therefore, becoming increasingly obvious that multiple spermatozoa should be used to increase the incidence of fertilisation.

Further refinement of these procedures, such as experiments with zona opening and subsequent insemination with various concentrations of spermatozoa, resulted in higher rates of fertilisation and cleavage, and the eventual birth of live offspring in mice.[114-19]

The use of micro-assisted fertilisation in man

Against this backdrop of essential developments in micromanipulative techniques, nearly three decades of research on the manipulation of whole, part or single cells of embryos, and almost four decades on the manipulation of animal gametes, it was a natural progression for the embryologist to utilise these techniques for the alleviation of infertility. However, it was the advent of human IVF that brought many of these procedures to the attention of the lay public who could not be expected to see the new developments in the context of micromanipulation in animals. By many it was perceived that 'half-mad' doctors bewitched with human gametes were now let loose and attempting to manipulate our own species! My own studies were prevented from progressing to clinical use because of the caution exerted by the then Interim Licensing Authority

Direct injection into ooplasm

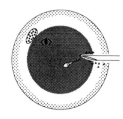

Injection into perivitelline space

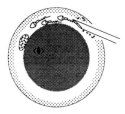

Opening the Zona pellucida

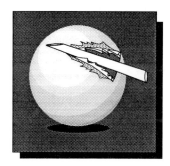
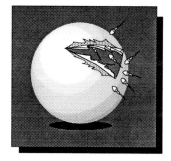

Zona drilling

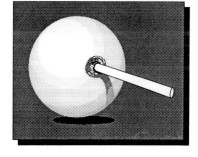
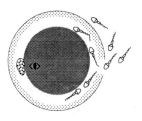

Figure 1.2 Four main approaches to micro-assisted fertilisation. Zona drilling is not recommended for use in humans (see text).

(ILA) who advised that we could proceed with this work once it was proven safe! This was a circular argument. We have learned from numerous studies on animals that, whatever animal model system is used, proof cannot be obtained without eventually working with human gametes. The development of zona drilling, using first the mouse model[108], is a good example. However, respect had to be given to the ILA guideline because, as described above, although animal data had proved it feasible, studies were not comprehensive to eliminate risk.

The clinical application of the micro-insemination techniques for procuring fertilisation *in vitro* was first reported about seven years ago, by Metka.[120] In 1987 Laws-King and co-workers[121] reported on the insertion of single sperm into the perivitelline space with subsequent fertilisation. This report used capacitated spermatozoa from donors with a normal semen profile, and sperm from donors with semen profiles of low quality, including sperm with coiled and twin tails. A number of reports were presented in 1988 suggesting different approaches to micro-assisted fertilisation. Lanzendorf et al.[122] injected sperm from infertile males directly into the ooplasm with 58 per cent of patients having an oocyte developing with a male pronucleus. Gordon and co-workers[123] used acid Tyrodes solution for 'drilling' a hole in the zona pellucida of the human oocyte before transferring them to a suspension of sperm. These tests were done using samples of semen from patients who had failed to achieve fertilisation by conventional IVF. Of 63 eggs from ten couples, 32 per cent of those zona drilled fertilised, compared with 25 per cent of the non-drilled. Although this data was not significant there was a high incidence of fertilisation considering these couples had previously failed to achieve IVF (see Chapter 8). Five diploid eggs were transferred but no pregnancies were achieved. Also in the same year, Cohen et al.[124] reported on their technique of partial zona dissection (PZD). This mechanical technique, which causes a breach in the zona pellucida by the microneedle piercing opposing ends of the zona pellucida followed by rubbing the latter up against the holding pipette until it tears (Figure 1.2, and Chapter 8), resulted in two PZD and a single control (fertilised by conventional IVF) embryo being transferred into two patients.

Both patients became pregnant, each with a set of twins. This was a turning point, and provided a degree of confidence in the clinical manipulation of human oocytes for the procurement of fertilisation.

Further work resulted in the establishment of a number of pregnancies from only micromanipulated eggs, and one patient was reported to have delivered healthy dizygotic twins. Malter and co-workers[125] applied the PZD technique to oocytes that had failed IVF. Using the previously published technique of shrinking the ooplasm by its incubation in a hypertonic concentration of sucrose[109], to enlarge the perivitelline space, this facilitated the tearing of the zona pellucida and the unfertilised oocytes were re-inseminated. Although fertilisation eventually occurred in these oocytes, a high degree of polyspermy was noted. It was reported that the high incidence of polyspermy was probably a result of aging oocytes, as these authors reported an increased polyspermy in oocytes manipulated at 25 hours after recovery, compared to those manipulated and re-inseminated between 21-24 hours after recovery. As detailed in Chapter 8 of this volume, the group of Cohen et al. went on to observe the possible benefits of PZD to the hatching of the embryo from the zona pellucida. Talansky and Gordon[116] had already noted that the effect of zona drilling resulted in a complete loss of the zona pellucida in some of the embryos, while in others blastomeres were extruded at earlier cleavage stages. About a year later Odawara and Lopata[119] also described the early hatching of mouse blastocysts after the zonae had been opened. This was apparently of no consequence in the end result as there was no significant difference in the birth rates between blastocysts with open zonae (36 per cent) and those with intact zonae (42 per cent). In the same year, 1989, Malter and Cohen[126] reported their concern that the hatching process of embryos derived from the micromanipulated oocytes may be abnormal, leading to artificial twinning or the formation of trophoblastic vesicles (see Chapter 8).

A few years earlier, in 1987, the group in Singapore[127] reported on some work in the human which followed as a result of an observation by Aitken and co-workers, published in 1983[128]. These workers demonstrated that sperm from men with immotile cilia (Kartagener) syndrome can fuse, penetrate and undergo pronuclear formation in the egg cytoplasm. Ng et al.[127] reported the fertilisation of oocytes and the formation of embryos from a patient with immotile cilia syndrome after the spermatozoa had been deposited in the perivitelline space. Continuing efforts by the Singapore group resulted in a report, in 1988, of the first human pregnancy after subzonal sperm injection[129], followed at the start of this decade with a report by this author on the birth of a set of normal, healthy twins and a singleton after subzonal insemination.[130]

Before the end of the last decade the first reports of zygote repair, or zygote microsurgery, for polypronuclei came from the group of Cohen and Malter[131] (see Chapter 8) and Gordon.[132] This work was a sequela of the high incidence of polyspermia associated with micro-assisted fertilisation techniques. The techniques were of major interest because tripronuclear zygotes are not uncommon in routine IVF. If this condition arises in one or more of only a few fertilised eggs the patient's chance of pregnancy is immediately compromised should only one embryo be available for transfer. By removing the additional male pronucleus and reverting the zygote to the normal diploid condition, clinical advantages are apparent.

These studies, which included 18 polyspermic zygotes from two intact eggs and seven from previously zona drilled oocytes, reported on the removal of supernumerary pronuclei by direct insertion of a microneedle into the ooplasm and aspiration of the pronucleus (see Chapter 8). The zygote survived and further cleavage occurred; although survival was higher from zona intact rather than PZD manipulated oocytes. Apart from the technique per se, difficulties arise in identifying the male pronucleus. However, a report by Rawlins et al. in 1988[133] suggested that viable embryos could not be obtained if tripronuclear human zygotes were 'epronuleated' to two pronuclei. Whether zygote surgery will become a viable technique in the future remains a moot point.

References

1. Duryee WR. Isolation of nuclei and non-mitotic chromosome pairs from frog eggs. *Archives of Experimental Zellforch Gewebezücht*. 1937; **19**: 171–6.
2. Schmidt HD. Minute structure of the hepatic lobules particularly with reference to the relationship between capillary blood vessels and the hepatic cells. *American Journal of Medical Science*. 1895; **37**: 13–40.
3. Peterfi T. Das mikrurgische Verfahren. *Naturwissenschaften*. 1923; **11**: 81–7.
4. Taylor, AJ, Farber D. Fatal effects of the removal of the micronucleus in euplotes. *University of California Publications in Zoology*. 1924; **26**: 131–5.
5. Chambers R, Fell HB. Micro-operations on cells in tissue cultures. *Proceedings of the Royal Society of London*. 1931; **109**: 381–92.
6. Hammerling J. Nucleo-cytoplasmic relationships in the development of Acetabularia. *International Reviews of Cytology*. 1953; **2**: 475-98.
7. King JT, Briggs R, Seril P. Transplantation of embryonic nuclei. *Cold Spring Harbour Symposia on Quantitative Biology*. 1956; **21**: 271–90.
8. Markert CL, Ursbrung H. Production of replicable persistent changes in zygote chromosomes of N *rana pipens* by injected proteins from adult liver nuclei. *Developmental Biology*. 1963; **7**: 560–77.
9. Kroger H. Microsurgery with polytene chromosomes. *Methods in Cell Physiology*. 1966; **2**: 61–92.
10. Nicholas JS, Hall BV. Experiments on developing rats. II. The development of isolated blastomeres and fused eggs. *Journal of Experimental Zoology*. 1942; **90**: 441–58.
11. Duryee WR. Microdissection studies on human ovarian eggs. *Transactions of the New York Academy of Sciences. II*. 1954; **17**: 103–8.
12. Tarkowski AK. Experimental studies on regulation in the development of isolated blastomeres of mouse eggs. *Acta Theriologica*. 1959; **3**: 191–267.
13. Seidel F. Die Entwicklungsfahigkeiten isolierter Furchungszellen aus den Ei des kaninchens *oryctolagus ciniculus*. *Archives fur Entwicklungsmech*. 1960; **152**: 43–130.
14. Lin TP. Microinjection of mouse eggs. *Science*. 1966; **151**: 33–7.
15. Lin TP. Micropipetting cytoplasm from the mouse eggs. *Nature*. 1967; **216**: 162–3.
16. Lin TP. D-L-Methionine (Sulphur-35) for labelling unfertilized mouse eggs in transplantation. *Nature*. 1956; **178**: 1175–6.
17. McClendon J. Experiments on the eggs of Chaetopterus and Asterias in which the chromatin was removed. *Biological Bulletin*. 1907; **12**: 141–5.

18. Kopak MJ. Exploring living cells by microsurgery. *Transactions of the New York Academy of Sciences. II.* 1961; **21**: 200–14.

19. Daniel JC. (ed.) *Methods in Mammalian Embryology.* San Francisco: Freeman, 1971.

20. Moore NW, Adams CE, Rosen LEA. Developmental potential of single blastomeres of the rabbit. *Journal of Reproduction and Fertility.* 1968; **17**: 527–31.

21. Tarkowski AK. Mouse chimaeras developed from fused eggs. *Nature.* 1961; **190**: 857–60.

22. Mintz B. Formation of genotypically mosaic mouse embryos. *American Zoology.* 1962; **2**: 310 (abstract).

23. Mintz B. Allophenic mice of multi-embryo origin. In: Daniel, JC (ed.) *Methods in Mammalian Embryology*, San Francisco; Freeman, 1971, pp. 186-214.

24. Mintz B, Gearhart JD, Guymont AO. Phytohemagglutinin-mediated blastomere aggregation and development of allophenic mice. *Developmental Biology.* 1973; **31**: 195–9.

25. Palmer J, Dewey MJ. Allophenic mice produced from embryos aggregated with antibody. *Experientia.* 1983; **39**: 196–8.

26. Petters RM, Mettus RV. Survival to term of chimaeric morulae produced by aggregation of five to nine embryos in the mouse, *Mus musculus.* *Theriogenology.* 1984; **22**: 167–74.

27. Petters RM, Markert CL. Production and reproductive performance of hexaparental and octaparental mice. *Journal of Heredity.* 1980; **71**: 70–4.

28. Spindle A. Cell allocation in pre-implantation mouse chimaeras. *Journal of Experimental Zoology.* 1982; **219**: 361–7.

29. Surani MAH, Barton SC. Spacial distribution of blastomeres is dependent on cell division order and interactions in mouse morulae. *Developmental Biology.* 1984; **102**: 335–43.

30. Kelly SJ. Studies of the potency of early cleavage blastomeres of the mouse. In: Balls M, Wile EA (eds.) *The Early Development of Mammals, 2nd Symposium of the British Society for Developmental Biology.* Cambridge: Cambridge University Press, 1975, pp. 97–105.

31. Kelly SJ. Studies on the developmental potential of 4- and 8- cell stage mouse blastomeres. *Journal of Experimental Zoology.* 1977; **200**: 365–76.

32. Gardner RL. Mouse chimaeras obtained by the injection of cells into the blastocyst. *Nature.* 1968; **220**: 596–7.

33. Gardner RL. Production of chimaeras by injecting cells or tissues into the blastocyst. In: Daniel JC (ed.) *Methods of Mammalian Reproduction.* New York: Academic Press, 1978, pp. 137–65.

34. Babinet C. A simplified method for mouse blastocyst injection. *Experimental Cell Research.* 1980; **130**: 15–19.

35. Bradley A. Production and analysis of chimaeric mice. In: Robertson EJ (ed.) *Teratocarcinomas and Embryonic Stem Cells: A Practical Approach.* Oxford: IRL Press, 1987: pp. 113–51.

36. Brinster RL. The effect of cells transferred into the mouse blastocyst on subsequent development. *Journal of Experimental Medicine.* 1974; **140**: 1049–56.

37. Mintz B, Illmensee K, Gearhart JD. Developmental and experimental potentialities of mouse teratocarcinoma cells from embryoid body cores. In: Sherman MI, Salter D (eds.) *Teratomas and Differentiation.* New York: Academic Press, 1975, pp. 59–82.

38. Papaioannou VE, McBurney MW, Gardner RL, Evans MJ. Fate of teratocarcinoma cells injected into early mouse embryos. *Nature.* 1975; **258**: 72–3.

39. Gardner RL, Lyon MF. X-chromosome inactivation studied by injection of a single cell into the mouse blastocyst. *Nature.* 1971; **231**: 385–6.

40. Gardner RL, Lyon MF, Evans EP, Burtenshaw MD. Clonal analysis of X-chromosome inactivation and the origin of the germline in the mouse embryo. *Journal of Embryology and Experimental Morphology.* 1985; **88**: 349–63.

41. Evans MJ, Kaufman MH. Establishment in culture of pluripotent cells from mouse embryos. *Nature.* 1981; **192**: 154–6.

42. Martin GR. Isolation of a pluripotent cell line from early mouse embryos cultured in medium condition by teratocarcinoma stem cells. *Proceedings of the National Academcy of Sciences, USA.* 1981; **78**: 7634–8.

43. Axelrod HR. Embryonic stem cell lines derived from blastocysts by a simplified technique. *Developmental Biology.* 1984; **101**: 225–8.

44. Robertson EJ. Embryo-derived stem cell lines. In: Robertson EJ (ed.) *Teratocarcinomas and Embryonic Stem Cells: A Practical Approach.* Oxford: IRL Press, 1987, pp. 71–112.

45. Bradley A, Evans M, Kaufman MH, Robertson E. Formation of germ-line chimaeras from embryo-derived teratocarcinoma cell lines. *Nature.* 1984; **309**: 255–6.

46. Robertson EJ, Bradley A. Production of permanent cell lines from early embryos and their use in studying developmental problems. In: Rossant J, Pedersen RA (eds.) *Experimental Approaches to Mammalian Embryonic Development.* Cambridge: Cambridge University Press, 1986, pp. 475–508.

47. Hooper M, Hardy K, Handyside A, Hunter S, Monk M. HPRT- deficient (Lesch-Nyhan) mouse embryos derived from germ-line colonisation by cultured cells. *Nature.* 1987; **326**: 292–5.

48. Kuehn MR, Bradley A, Robertson EJ, Evans

MJ. A potential animal model for Lesch-Nyhan Syndrome through introduction of HPRT mutation into mice. *Nature*. 1987; **326**: 295–8.

49. Mulnard J. Formation de blastocystes chimeriques par fusion d'embryons de rat et de souris au stade. VIII. *Comptes Rendus Hebdomadaires Seances de L'Academie Sceances Serie D. Sciences Naturelles (Paris)*. 1973; **276**: 379–81.

50. Stern MS. Chimaeras obtained by aggregation of mouse eggs with rat eggs. *Nature*. 1873; **243**: 472–3.

51. Zeilmaker GH. Fusion of rat and mouse morulae and formation of chimaeric blastocyts. *Nature*. 1973; **242**: 115–6.

52. Tachi S, Tachi C. Electron-microscopic studies of chimeric blastocysts experimentally produced by aggregating blastomeres of rat and mouse embryos. *Developmental Biology*. 1980; **80**: 18–27.

53. Mystkowska ET. Development of mouse-bank vole interspecific chimaeric embryos. *Journal of Embryology and Experimental Morphology*. 1975; **33**: 731–44.

54. Gardner RL, Johnson MH. Investigation of early mammalian development using interspecific chimaeras between rat and mouse. *Nature New Biology*. 1973; **246**: 86–9.

55. Gardner RL, Johnson MH. Investigation of cellular interaction and development in the early mammalian embryo using inter-specific chimaeras between the rat and the mouse. In: Porter R, Rivers J (eds.) *Cell Patterning: Ciba Foundation Symposium 29*. Amsterdam: Elsevier, 1975, pp. 183–96.

56. Tarkowski AK. Interspecific transfers of eggs between rat and mouse. *Journal of Embryology and Experimental Morphology*. 1962; **10**: 476–95.

57. Tachi S, Tachi C. Ultrastructural studies on maternal embryonic cell interaction during experimentally induced implantation of rat blastocysts to the endometrium of the mouse. *Developmental Biology*. 1979; **68**: 203–23.

58. Rossant J, Frells WI. Interspecific chimaeras in mammals: successful production of live chimaeras between *Mus musculus* and *Mus caroli*. *Science*. 1980; **208**: 419–21.

59. Rossant J, Mauro VM, Croy BA. Importance of trophoblast genotype for survival of interspecific murine chimaeras. *Journal of Embryology and Experimental Morphology*. 1982; **69**: 141–9.

60. Rossant J, Croy BA, Clark DA, Chapman VM. Interspecific hybrids and chimaeras in mice. *Journal of Experimental Zoology*. 1983; **228**: 223–33.

61. Fehilly CB, Willadsen SM, Tucker EM. Interspecific chimaerism between sheep and goat. *Nature*. 1984; **307**: 634–6.

62. Meinecke-Tillman S, Meinecke B. Experimental chimaeras – removal of reproductive barrier between sheep and goat. *Nature*. 1984; **307**: 637–8.

63. West JD, Frells WI, Papaioannou VE, Karr JR, Chapman VM. Development of interspecific hybrids of Mus. *Journal of Embryology and Experimental Morphology*. 1977; **41**: 233–43.

64. Rossant J. Interspecific cell markers and lineage in mammals. *Philosophical Transactions of the Royal Society of London B*. 1985; **312**: 91–100.

65. Gardner RL. Manipulations on the blastocyst. In: Raspe G (ed.) *Advances in the Biosciences No. 6: Schering Symposium on Intrinsic and Extrinsic Factors on Early Mammalian Development*. Oxford: Pergamon Press, 1971, pp. 279–96.

66. Gardner RL, Papaioannou VE, Barton SC. Origin of the ectoplacental cone and secondary giant cells in mouse blastocysts reconstituted from isolated trophoblast and inner cell mass. *Journal of Embryology and Experimental Morphology*. 1973; **30**: 561–72.

67. Solter D, Knowles B. Immunosurgery of mouse blastocysts. *Proceedings of the National Academy of Sciences, USA*. 1975; **72**: 5099–102.

68. Rossant J, Croy BA. Genetic identification of tissue of origin of cellular populations within the mouse placenta. *Journal of Embryology and Experimental Morphology*. 1985; **86**: 177–89.

69. Barton SC, Adams CA, Norris ML, Surani MAH. Development of gynogenetic and parthenogenetic inner cell mass and trophectoderm tissue in reconstituted blastocysts in the mouse. *Journal of Embryology and Experimental Morphology*. 1985; **90**: 267–85.

70. Seidel F. Die Entwicklungspotenzen feiner isolierten Blastomeren des Zwerizellenstadiums in Saugetieren. *Naturwissenschaften*. 1952; **39**: 355.

71. Tarkowski AK. Experiments of the development of isolated blastomeres of mouse eggs. *Nature*. 1959; **184**: 1286–7.

72. Tarkowski AK, Wroblewska J. Development of blastomeres of mouse eggs isolated at the four- and eight-cell stage. *Journal of Embryology and Experimental Morphology*. 1967; **18**: 155–80.

73. Gardner RL, Edwards RG. Control of the sex ratio at full term in the rabbit by transferring sexed blastocysts. *Nature*. 1968; **218**: 346–8.

74. Epstein CJ, Smith S, Travis B, Tucker G. Both X chromosomes function before visible X-chromosome inactivation in female mouse embryos. *Nature*. 1978; **274**: 500–3.

75. McLaren A. Prenatal diagnosis before implantation: opportunities and problems. *Prenatal Diagnosis*. 1985; **5**: 85–90.

76. Willadsen SM. The developmental capacity of blastomeres from 4-cell and 8-cell sheep embryos. *Journal of Embryology and Experimental Morphology*. 1981; **65**: 165–72.

77. Tsunoda Y, McLaren A. Effects of various procedures on the viability of mouse embryos containing half the normal number of blasto-

meres. *Journal of Reproduction and Fertility*. 1983; **69**: 315–22.

78. Fishel SB, Webster J, Faratian B, Jackson P. Establishing pregnancies after follicular stimulation for IVF with clomiphene citrate and human menopausal gonadotrophin only. *Human Reproduction*. 1991; **6**: 106–12.

79. Briggs R, King PJ. Transplantation of living nuclei from blastular cells into enucleated frogs' eggs. *Proceedings of the National Academy of Sciences, USA*. 1952; **38**: 455–63.

80. Gurdon JB. Nuclear transplantation in eggs and oocytes. *Journal of Cell Science (supplement)*. 1986; **4**: 287–318.

81. McGrath J, Solter D. Nuclear transplantation in the mouse embryo by microsurgery and cell fusion. *Science*. 1983; **220**: 1300.

82. McGrath J, Solter D. Inability of mouse blastomere nuclei transferred to enucleated zygotes to support development *in vitro*. *Science*. 1984; **226**: 1317–19.

83. Barton SC, Surani MAH, Norris ML. Role of paternal and maternal genomes in mouse development. *Nature*. 1984; **311**: 374–6.

84. Tsunoda Y, Yasuri T, Makamura K, Uchida T, Sugie T. Effect of cutting the zona pellucida on the pronuclear transplantation in mice. *Journal of Experimental Zoology*. 1986; **240**: 119–25.

85. Mann JR, Lovell-Bade RH. Inviability of parthenogenomes is determined by pronuclei not egg cytoplasm. *Nature*. 1984; **310**: 66–7.

86. Gilbert SF, Solter D. Onset of paternal and maternal Gpi-1 expression in preimplantation mouse embryos. *Developmental Biology*. 1985; **109**: 515–17.

87. McGrath J, Solter D. Maternal Thp lethality in the mouse is a nuclear, not cytoplasmic defect. *Nature*. 1984; **308**: 550–1.

88. Renard J-P, Babinet C. Identification of a paternal developmental effect on the cytoplasm of 1-cell stage mouse embryos. *Proceedings of the National Academy of Sciences, USA*. 1986; **83**: 6883–6.

89. Brinster RL, Chen HY, Trumbauer ME, Yagle MK, Palmiter RD. Factors affecting the efficiency of introducing foreign DNA into mice by microinjecting eggs. *Proceedings of the National Academcy of Sciences, USA*. 1985; **82**: 4438–42.

90. Krimpenfort P, Berns A. Gene transfer in mammalian embryos. *Human Reproduction*. 1987; **2**: 333–9.

91. Hiramoto Y. Microinjection of the live spermatozoa into sea urchin eggs. *Experimental Cell Research*. 1962; **27**: 416–26.

92. Graham CF. The regulation of DNA synthesis and mitosis in multinucleate frog eggs. *Journal of Cell Science*. 1966; **1**: 363–72.

93. Brun RB. Studies on fertilization in Xenopus laevis. *Biology of Reproduction*. 1974; **11**: 513–18.

94. Uehara T, Yanagimachi R. Microsurgical injec-

tion of spermatozoa into hamster eggs with subsequent transformation of sperm nuclei into male pronuclei. *Biology of Reproduction*. 1976; **15**: 467–70.

95. Thadani VM. A study of hetero-specific sperm-egg interactions in the rat, mouse, and deer mouse using in vitro fertilization and sperm injection. *Journal of Experimental Zoology*. 1980; **212**: 435–53.

96. Ohsumi K, Katagiri C, Yanagimachi R. Development of pronuclei from human spermatozoa injected microsurgically into (Xenopus) eggs. *Journal of Experimental Zoology*. 1986; **237**: 319–25.

97. Naish SJ, Perreault SD, Zirkin EJ. DNA synthesis following microinjection of heterologous sperm and somatic cell nuclei into hamster oocytes. *Gamete Research*. 1987; **18**: 109–20.

98. Thadani VM. Injection of sperm heads into immature rat oocytes. *Journal of Experimental Zoology*. 1979; **210**: 161–8.

99. Markert CL. Fertilization of mammalian eggs by sperm injection. *Journal of Experimental Zoology*. 1983; **228**: 195–201.

100. Iritani A, Utsumi K, Miyake M, Hosoi Y, Saeki K. In vitro fertilization by a routine method and micromanipulation. In: Jones H, Schrader C (eds.) *In Vitro Fertilization and Other Assisted Reproduction*. Annals of the New York Academy of Sciences. 1988; **541**: 583–90.

101. Iritani A, Hosoi Y. Microfertilization by various methods in mammalian species. In: Yoshinaga K, Mori T (eds.) *Development of Preimplantation Embryos and Their Environment*. New York: Allan R. Liss, 1989, pp. 145–9.

102. Hosoi Y, Miyake M, Utsumi K, Iritani A. Development of rabbit oocytes after microinjection of spermatozoa. *Proceedings of the 11th International Congress of Animal Reproduction*. 1988; **3**: Abstract No. 331.

103. Iritani A. Micromanipulation of oocytes and embryos. *Proceedings of the XIIIth World Congress on Fertility and Sterility*. 1990 (abstract).

104. Keefer CL. Fertilization by sperm injection in the rabbit. *Gamete Research*. 1989; **22**: 59–69.

105. Younis AI, Keefer CL, Brackett BG. Fertilization of bovine oocytes by sperm injection. *Theriogenology*. 1989; **31**: 276 (abstract).

106. Keefer CL, Younis AI, Brackett BG. Cleavage development of bovine oocytes fertilized by sperm injection. *Molecular Reproduction and Development*. 1990; **25**: 281–5.

107. Goto K, Kinoshita A, Takuma Y, Ogawa K. Fertilization in sperm injection in cattle. *Theriogenology*. 1990; **33**: 238 (abstract).

108. Gordon JW, Talansky BE. Assisted fertilization by zona drilling: A mouse model for correction of oligospermia. *Journal of Experimental Zoology*. 1986; **239**: 347–54.

109. Yang X, Chen J, Chen Y, Foote RH. Survival of rabbit eggs shrunken to aid sperm microinjection. *Theriogenology*. 1988; **29**: 336 (abstract).

110. Conover JC, Gwatkin RBL. Fertilization of zona-drilled mouse oocytes treated with a monoclonal antibody to the zona glycoprotein, ZP3. *Journal of Experimental Zoology*. 1988; **247**: 113–18.

111. Depypere HT, McLaughlin FJ, Seamark RF, Warnes GM, Matthews CD. Comparison of zona cutting and zona drilling as techniques for assisted fertilization in the mouse. *Journal of Reproduction and Fertility*. 1988; **84**: 205–11.

112. Ahmad T, Conover JC, Quigley MM, Collins RL, Thomas AJ, Gwatkin RBL. Failure of spermatozoa from T/t mice to fertilize in vitro is overcome by zona drilling. *Gamete Research*. 1989; **22**: 369–73.

113. Lacham O, Trounson A, Holden C, Mann J, Sathananthan H. Fertilization and development of mouse eggs injected under the zona pellucida with single spermatozoa treated to induce the acrosome reaction. *Gamete Research*. 1989; **23**: 233–43.

114. Barg PE, Wahrman MZ, Talansky BE, Gordon JW. Capacitated, acrosome reacted but immotile sperm, when microinjected under the mouse zona pellucida, will not fertilize the oocyte. *Journal of Experimental Zoology*. 1986; **237**: 365–74.

115. Mann JR. Full term development of mouse eggs fertilized by a spermatozoon microinjected under the zona pellucida. *Biology of Reproduction*. 1988; **38**: 1077–83.

116. Talansky BE, Gordon JW. Cleavage characteristics of mouse embryos inseminated and cultured after zona pellucida drilling. *Gamete Research*. 1988; **21**: 277–87.

117. Gordon JW. Use of micromanipulation for increasing the efficiency of mammalian fertilization in vitro. In: Jones H, Schrader C (eds.) *In Vitro Fertilization and Other Assisted Reproduction*. Annals of the New York Academy of Sciences. 1988; **541**: 601–13.

118. Mettler L, Yamada K, Kuranty A, Michelmann HW, Semm K. Microinjection of spermatozoa into oocytes. In: Jones H, Schrader C (eds.) *In Vitro Fertilization and Other Assisted Reproduction*. Annals of the New York Academy of Sciences. 1988; **541**: 591–600.

119. Odawara Y, Lopata A. A zona opening procedure for improving in vitro fertilization at low sperm concentrations: A mouse model. *Fertility and Sterility*. 1989; **51**: 699–704.

120. Metka M, Haromy T, Huber J, Schurz B. Artificial insemination using a micromanipulator. *Fertilitat*. 1985; **1**: 41–7.

121. Laws-King A, Trounson A, Sathananthan H, Kola I. Fertilization of human oocytes by microinjection of a single spermatozoon under the zona pellucida. *Fertility and Sterility*. 1987; **48**: 637–42.

122. Lanzendorf E, Maloney MK, Veeck LL, Slusser J, Hodgen GD, Rosenwaks Z. A preclinical evaluation of human spermatozoa into human oocytes. *Fertility and Sterility*. 1988; **49**: 835–42.

123. Gordon JW, Grunfeld J, Garrisi GJ, Talansky BE, Richards C, Laufer N. Fertilization of human oocytes by sperm from infertile males after zona pellucida drilling. *Fertility and Sterility*. 1988; **50**: 68–73.

124. Cohen J, Malter M, Fehilly C, Wright G, Elsner C, Kort H, Massey J. Implantation of embryos after partial opening of oocyte zona pellucida to facilitate sperm penetration. *Lancet*. 1988; **2**: 162.

125. Malter H, Talansky B, Gordon J, Cohen J. Monospermy and polyspermy after partial zona dissection of reinseminated human oocytes. *Gamete Research*. 1989; **23**: 377–86.

126. Malter HE, Cohen J. Blastocyst formation and hatching in vitro following zona drilling of mouse and human embryos. *Gamete Research*. 1989; **24**: 67–80.

127. Ng S-C, Sathananthan AH, Edirisinghe WR, Kum Chue JH, Wong PC, Ratnam SS, Sarla G. Fertilization of a human egg with sperm from a patient with immotile cilia syndrome: case report. In: Ratnam SS, Teoh ES, Anandakumar C (eds.) *Advances in Fertility and Sterility*. Lancaster, UK: Parthenon Publishing, 1987, vol. **4**: 71–6.

128. Aitken RJ, Ross A, Lees MM. Analysis of sperm function in Kartagener's syndrome. *Fertility and Sterility*. 1983; **40**: 696–8.

129. Ng S-C, Bongso TA, Ratnam SS, Sathananthan AH, Chan CLK, Wong PC, Hagglund L, Anandakumar C, Wong YC, Goh VHH. Pregnancy after transfer of multiple sperm under the zona. *Lancet*. 1988; **2**: 790.

130. Fishel SB, Antinori S, Jackson P, Johnson J, Lisi F, Chiariello F, Versaci C. Twin birth after subzonal insemination. *Lancet*. 1990; **2**: 722.

131. Malter HE, Cohen J. Embryonic development after microsurgical repair of polyspermic human zygotes. *Fertility and Sterility*. 1989; **52**: 373–80.

132. Gordon JW, Grunfeld L, Garrisi GJ, Navat D, Laufer N. Successful microsurgical removal of a pronuclei from tripronuclear hamster zygotes. *Fertility and Sterility*. 1989; **52**: 367–72.

133. Rawlins RG, Binor Z, Radwaska E, Dmowski WP. Microsurgical enucleation of tripronuclear human zygotes. *Fertility and Sterility*. 1988; **50**: 266–72.

Section II
Gamete micromanipulation

Chapter 2

Preparative techniques in micromanipulation

Judy Timson

Introduction

It has been my endeavour, in this chapter, to present a survey of various instruments and preparative procedures employed in micromanipulation. Although examples of applications in a variety of fields of science and technology are briefly discussed, the practical working methods presented are particular to micromanipulation as applied to micro-assisted fertilisation techniques, as this is within the authors' field of working experience. However, the descriptions given should suffice for an understanding of the processes involved and with modification varying techniques are possible for application to a wide diversity of uses.

Definition

The term 'micromanipulation' is used to include all operations performed in the microscopic field of vision with the aid of mechanical devices which guide the operating tools.

Origination of micromanipulation

It should be mentioned that microbiologists were the first to conceive and apply micromanipulative

techniques. H. D. Schmidt seems to have been the first to use a microscopic dissector which he described in 1985.[1] Since that time, micromanipulative techniques have attained a high degree of perfection. The development of the varied types of exceedingly delicate microtools went hand in hand with the development of the micromanipulators, and the significant advances in microscopy aided greatly in that direction.

Development of micro-manipulation

A clear evaluation of the advantages gained by the use of micromanipulators should first take into consideration that very delicate operations may be performed with the unaided hand, provided that the eye is assisted by optical magnification giving a distinct image of tool point and object. The use of micromanipulation, however, is also a great help for relatively simple tasks requiring only small magnification. Even a rather primitive manipulating device steadies the motion of the tool, reduces the nervous effort and increases the efficacy of the experiment.

In earlier instruments microtools had to operate between the specimen and the microscope objective, and therefore only low power objectives could be used. Between 1904 and 1914, Barber published several papers[2,3,4] describing a mechanical pipette holder and a method for isolating microscopic organisms by manipulating micropipettes in a drop hanging from the undersurface of a cover slip suspended over the moist chamber. This was a significant development since, when working in hanging drops, microtools are manipulated below the cover slip thus eliminating all obstacles between the microscope objective and the sample and permitting the use of high power and oil immersion objectives.

With the use of the inverted microscope, micromanipulative operations may be conveniently performed in lying drops on a petri dish or a microscope slide placed on the microscope stage. Because of the inversion of the microscope, the objective occupies a position under the petri dish or slide while the fluid drop lies upon it.

The operating microtools, with tips bent to a horizontal angle, approach the specimen from above. This arrangement permits the use of high magnifications since the operating tools are not between the specimen and the microscope objective. For the same reason, it also permits proper observation of the whole field of operation. In this arrangement the substage of the microscope, which usually includes both the condenser and the illuminator, lies above the moist chamber. It is possible to use the various types of illumination, including the dark field. An advantage of the inverted microscope is that the lying drop may be comparatively large and covered in paraffin oil to reduce the effects of evaporation. In addition, the specimens come to rest on the upper surface of the supporting petri dish or slide making manipulation easier.

Applications

The applications of basic micromanipulative technique may be considered within the following general categories:

1. preparation of samples of non-biological materials

2. chemical experimentation
3. working with living cells and tissues.

Within these categories are applications as diverse as nuclear research, the investigation of valuable objects of art and archaeology, studies of air pollution and artificial insemination of the queen bee.

Micromanipulation in biology

Biological microdissection, for which Péterfi[5] coined the name micrurgy, has proved of great and growing importance in experimental cytology, bacteriology, cellular physiology, embryology, as well as in other fields of the study of living cells and tissues. Various micromanipulation techniques such as subzonal insemination (SUZI), partial zona dissection (PZD) and other zona breaching techniques are now being used in clinical trials in human reproduction technology (Chapters 7, 8). Micromanipulation techniques are also being used clinically in pre-implantation diagnosis of gene and chromosome linked hereditary disorders (Chapters 16, 17)

The choice of a suitable procedure and suitable equipment is mainly dependent on the type of material and the specific problem to be investigated. The basic technique in performing operative work on living cells, tissues, and various microscopic organisms does not vary greatly.

Equipment

There are a number of commercially available micromanipulators and the choice of micromanipulator will depend on the required application.

Micromanipulators for micro-assisted fertilisation (MAF)

An Olympus IMT2 inverted microscope is used for the MAF procedures conducted in our laboratory at NURTURE (Nottingham University Research and Treatment Unit in Reproduction).

Mounted on the microscope is the TDU 0500

micromanipulator which is made by Research Instruments Ltd (Penryn, Cornwall, UK). The TDU 0500 micromanipulator has a single fine control lever which provides horizontal and vertical movement. Movement reduction is continuously variable from 100:1 up to 500:1, adjustment being carried out by raising or lowering the height of a link plate. Movement reduction is direct and without movement reversal; hand and microtool move in unison.

A coarse lever produces horizontal movement; lever reduction is 12:1. Using a tool holder vertical slide the micropipette holder can be lifted through the vertical plane and returned to the same position with a single movement.

Powerful syringes are used for the degree of control necessary during the holding of the oocyte and the aspiration into and expulsion of spermatozoa from the microneedle. The micropipette holders are joined by sterilised fine nylon tubing to the syringe. The system can be co-ordinated pneumatically or hydraulically; the preferred system at NURTURE being a simple air-based system (Figure 2.1). The MAF procedures are carried out on a heated microscope stage, enabling the full range of operative techniques to be performed at 37°C.

The micromanipulator heads and the microscope are mounted upon a heavy steel baseplate; the entire arrangement is placed on a rigid cement workbench to reduce the effects of extraneous vibration.

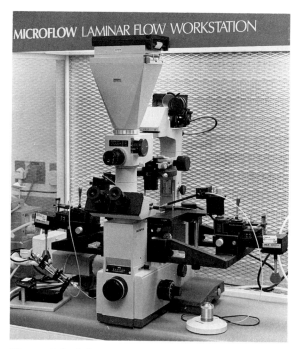

Figure 2.1 Micromanipulator, as supplied by Research Instruments Ltd, Cornwall, UK

Variations in micromanipulator equipment

While Research Instruments currently produce only mechanically operated micromanipulators, Leitz (Wetzlar, West Germany) and Narishige (Tokyo, Japan) market both electronic and mechanical micromanipulators. The electronically controlled micromanipulators can be used to assist in coarse movement and prepositioning of the microtools, while the fine movements of the micromanipulation still need to be done mechanically.

Both Narishige and Leitz produce remote control devices for operating micromanipulation fine motions. Avoiding rigid connection between the tool holder carrying the microtool and the operating tools of the instruments minimises transmission of vibration from the hand to the microtool.

The availability of remote control devices means that micromanipulation can be conducted inside controlled environment chambers for maintaining constant temperature during microscopy and manipulation of cell and tissue cultures.

With Narishige micromanipulators (as with the Research Instruments micromanipulator previously described), fine movement in three axes is controlled by a single joystick. Leitz, however, have two controls for fine movement, a joystick for horizontal movement and a control knob for vertical movement, necessitating moving the hand from one control to another.

Narishige also offer a micromanipulator (MO-204) with an extra fourth axis movement, to enable a movement to be carried out along the axis of an angled micropipette. The movement in all four axes is controlled from a single joystick control unit.

Ancillary equipment for the production and refining of microtools (injectors, microforge, pipette pullers and pipette grinders) is available from all three companies.

All the micromanipulators mentioned, and some others not discussed here, are suitable for the various micro-assisted fertilisation (MAF) procedures. The choice of micromanipulator will depend on personal preference and price. When selecting equipment for purchase it is important to consider the availability of back-up facilities such as training and the ability to communicate interactively with the manufacturer to request specific modifications and developments as required by the user. Research Instruments have been particularly helpful and responsive to requests from NURTURE scientists to modify equipment; consequently a number of changes and improvements have been made in the MAF techniques. We have found that the Research Instruments equipment adequately fulfils the requirements for the MAF techniques carried out in our laboratory, while the price is highly competitive (Figure 2.1).

Micropipettes

Microbiologists utilise a wide diversity of microtools which are carried and guided in the field by means of suitable micromanipulators. Such microtools are of different types, shapes and functions to satisfy varied requirements in different fields of practice and study of cells and tissues. In the investigation of living cells, in single cell surgery for instance, the operator can remove the nucleus or a part of it, or other cell constituents and replace them by others. To perform these tasks the operator may use microneedles, microknives, micropipettes, microforceps and a variety of other tools (Figure 2.2).

In the micromanipulation of mammalian eggs, micropipettes are required for injection, suction and egg holding. Manufacture of the microtools is the most crucial part of the entire procedure. It is important that the operator masters the techniques of preparing the microtools as they need to be replaced regularly due to their delicacy, or in the case of procedures with human cells, due to the need for sterility and avoidance of contamination.

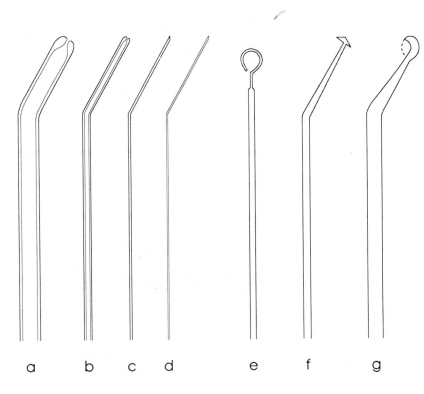

Figure 2.2 Types of microtools:

(a) holding pipette
(b) microtool for blastomere aspiration
(c) microneedle for zona breaching
(d) microneedle for subzonal insemination
(e) steadying loop
(f) microscalpel
(g) holding cup.

Microtool making equipment

Both Narishige and Research Instruments supply the pipette pullers, microforge and microgrinder needed to produce the microneedles used in MAF procedures. The important characteristic of all the manufacturing equipment is the delivery of reproducibility. Once required settings have been established, and extraneous factors remain constant, the equipment must be capable of reproducing microtools with the required precise dimensions.

The equipment described in this chapter is Research Instruments' equipment which is used in the NURTURE Unit.

For the MAF techniques (and specifically the SUZI technique), two different types of needle are required: the holding pipette and the injection pipette.

Holding pipette

The egg holder is a suction pipette, used to hold the oocyte in place while the micromanipulation is taking place.

The holding pipettes are prepared from glass capillary tubes, without filaments, of 1 mm outside diameter (available from Research Instruments and Narishige).

The procedure employed in making a holding pipette involves the following four stages:

1. pulling a capillary tube to the required external diameter of 100 microns. The tip of the holding pipette is somewhat smaller than the diameter of the human egg (120 microns)
2. breaking and squaring the end off the pipette
3. rounding and smoothing the end, as eggs can be ruptured if the blunt end is not smooth
4. putting a bend in the pipette, to allow working in a flat bottomed petri dish or slide

Equipment used to make the holding pipette

Micropipette puller

Pulling (step 1 above) is achieved by a single pull on the micropipette puller. Essentially the Research Instruments puller consists of two carriages, equipped with clamps for holding the glass tube to be pulled, a spring actuating mechanism and a heater (Figure 2.3).

A power supply unit is stabilised to ensure constant temperature of the heater and thus a high degree of reproducibility of the shape of the micropipette.

The setting that gives the required result can only be determined by experiment; the lower the temperature, the longer the pull and greater the force resulting in smaller diameter pipettes.

The pipette may be pulled as soon as the glass softens, or the pull may be delayed until after the glass has been soft for a given time, giving a larger diameter pipette – a longer softening period results in thicker walls.

The parameters may have to be changed according to room temperature and conditions, but generally the setting, once determined, can be reproduced whenever required to give the same result.

Microforge

Breaking and squaring the pipette (step 2), rounding the end (step 3) and bending (step 4) are all carried out on the microforge.

The Research Instruments microforge (Figure 2.4) consists of four main parts: an electrically heated platinum filament, a microscope, a micromanipulator for moving the microtool and a micrometer actuated positioner for positioning the filament. Movement of the micropipette in all

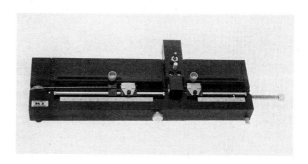

Figure 2.3 Micropipette puller, as supplied by Research Instruments Ltd, Cornwall, UK

three directions is provided by a lever operated micromanipulator which also has a rotator on its output. For ease of operation a piece of glass can be fused on to the filament to form a glass bead.

Breaking and squaring

The temperature of the filament is set so that it is just sufficient to allow the pipette to adhere to the bead when the current is switched off. The contraction of the filament during cooling then parts the

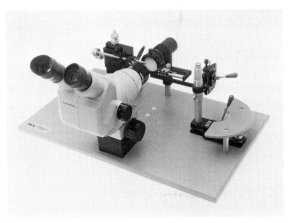

Figure 2.4 Microforge, as supplied by Research Instruments Ltd, Cornwall, UK

pipette squarely at the point of adhesion (Figure 2.5).

Rounding

Rounding or thermal polishing the blunt tip of the holding pipette is achieved by moving the tip of the pipette within close range of the heated bead (Figure 2.6). Rounding requires a high filament temperature. As the tip approaches the heat, the rounding and smoothing of the end occurs – the process is observed microscopically and the pipette moved away from the heat source when the opening is judged to be the correct size. The aperture at the tip of the holding pipette will be smaller than the oocyte to be held, but needs to be large enough to maintain a firm grip on the oocyte.

Bending

The microneedle to be bent is positioned at an angle of 60 degrees under the heated filament. The microneedle is moved towards the heat source until it starts to bend, and is held in place until it bends horizontally.

Narrowing of the holding pipette during bending is not usually a problem due to the wider diameter of the pipette. However, if the pipette does appear to narrow, the needle may be brought to the desired angle by moving the pipette along and bending in

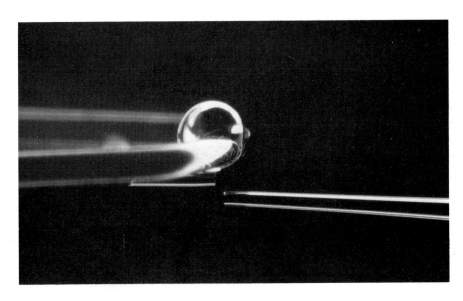

Figure 2.5 Breaking and squaring the holding pipette

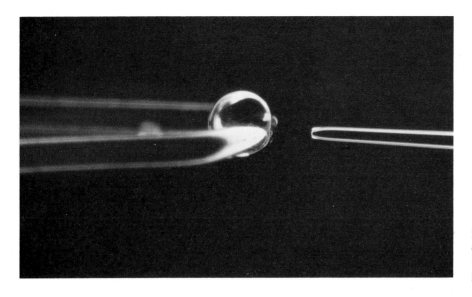

Figure 2.6 Rounding or thermal polishing the blunt tip of the holding pipette

a number of positions along the pipette, until the horizontal level is achieved (Figure 2.7). Narrowing of the pipette is more commonly a problem when bending the injection pipette, due to the smaller diameter (see below).

Cleaning and storage
The holding pipettes are placed in boxes which have been specifically designed to prevent breakage of the ends of the pipettes, and to maintain a dust-free environment (Figure 2.8).

Holding and injection pipettes are sterilised in a dry oven for 20–30 minutes at 180 degrees centigrade.

Injection micropipette

Micropipettes are used to aspirate the sperm and inject through the zona pellucida into the perivitelline space for the SUZI procedure. Simi-

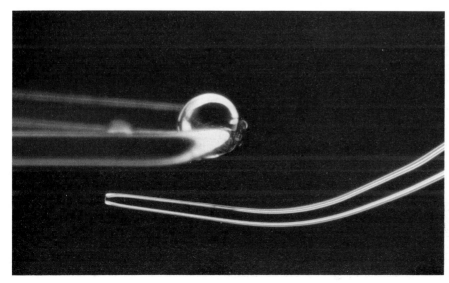

Figure 2.7 Bending a microneedle to facilitate operating in a flat-bottomed petri dish or slide

27

lar pipettes are also used to puncture, breach or dissect a portion of the zona pellucida in other MAF procedures (zona puncture and zona tearing).

Manufacture of the micropipette to the correct proportions is essential for the success of the operation. The tip must be fine enough to minimise injury to the vitellus of the egg, but of sufficient rigidity to pierce the elastic zona pellucida and vitelline membrane in the case of direct injection into the ooplasm. The bevel must be sharp and pointed, but not too long as this may cause the operator inadvertently to puncture the cytoplasm of the oocyte or to puncture the distal zona pellucida, causing a breach through which the injected spermatozoa may escape.

The internal diameter of the tip must be large enough to allow aspiration of the sperm into the needle, without blockage. Blockage of the injection micropipette is a frequent and frustrating problem and we have found the optimum inner diameter of the micropipette to be 8–10 microns. Careful sperm washing and preparation (through a Percoll gradient – see Chapter 4) is essential for the success of the operation.

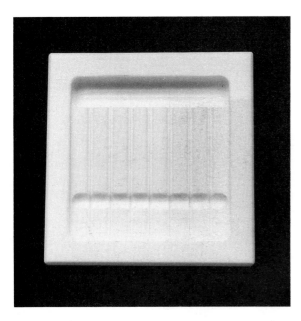

Figure 2.8 Holding boxes for sterilising microneedles while maintaining a dust-free environment

Protection against dust collection

All precautions must be taken to avoid blockage of the microneedle with dust. All equipment must be protected with dust covers when not in use. Pipettes should be protected in dust-free conditions between the various stages of manufacture. Holders have been specifically designed and built for NURTURE for standing the pipettes in a dust-free environment (Figure 2.9).

It is advisable to move directly from the grinding to the bending stage of the preparation of the microneedle. The immediate bending of the needle under heat dries it after the wet grinding, thus avoiding the collection of dust on the wet surfaces.

We have found these precautions guard sufficiently against collection of dust particles and generally it is unnecessary to sonicate the microneedles.

Stages in making the injection micro-needle

The process to make an injection microneedle involves four stages:

1. A double pull of a glass capillary tube (1 mm diameter, with a filament, supplied by Research Instruments and Narishige), to an internal diameter of 8–10 microns, external diameter 12–14 microns.

   The first pull is done to the same parameters as the holding pipette.

   To obtain the smaller diameter for the injection pipette a lower temperature, longer pull and greater force must be used for the second pull.

2. Grinding the end of the pulled pipette back to the required diameter and grinding a sharp bevel on the end.

   The microbeveller used at NURTURE is supplied by Research Instruments. Essentially the microbeveller consists of a microscope, a vertical and horizontal positioning assembly, a rotator and a lapping wheel for grinding the required pointed bevel (Figure 2.10).

A constant supply of water must be provided to the micropipette tip when microbevelling, to prevent the collection of debris. This may be

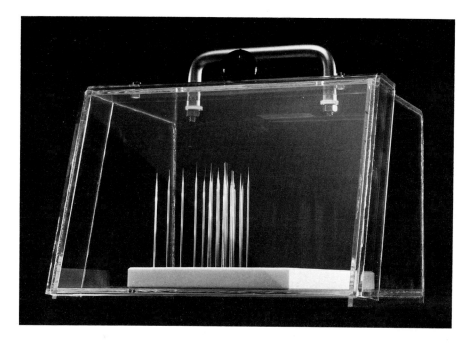

Figure 2.9 Dust protective stand designed for holding and storing micropipettes

achieved by a constant injection of water through a micrometer syringe. We have found it preferable to work with the tip immersed in water, by filling a water bath which is attached to the microbeveller and raising the bath so that the lower section of the lapping wheel is below the water level.

A more recent development is the use of a continuous jet of air through the microneedle under positive pressure. This is maintained throughout the grinding process. Although this is still being evaluated, preliminary observations indicate that this is at least as effective as immersion in water. Should this prove viable, the air process will offer an advantage as the needle will be kept dry throughout and therefore collection of dust occurring on the wet surface will be minimised.

The angle of the pipette to the grinding wheel is an important element as this affects the length of the bevel (Figure 2.11).

The sharper the angle, the longer the bevel; although a long bevel will allow easier penetration of the zona pellucida, the risk of damage to the cytoplasm, or the risk of puncturing the distal zona pellucida, is greater.

There was a significant difference in the ease of injection using a 15 μm outer bore size compared

with 19 μm, and generally there was less chance of damaging the ooplasm with the thinnest diameter. However, this had to be balanced against the ease of aspirating the spermatozoa to prevent clumping

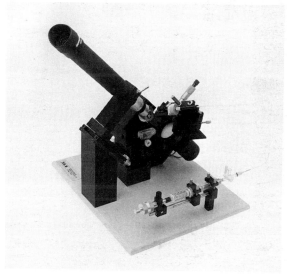

Figure 2.10 Microbeveller, as supplied by Research Instruments Ltd, Cornwall, UK

and attachment around the tip of the microneedle, and an easy passage of a single spermatozoon. The smaller diameter of the microneedle gave rise to a significant increase in both the degree of blockage and the difficulty of aspiration (see Tables 2.1, 2.2 and 2.3).

In our experience the optimum measurements for performing the SUZI technique are:

(a) Outer needle diameter = 11.3 microns (the inner needle diameter will be 8 microns)
(b) The outer length of the bevel is 16 microns (Figure 2.12).

To achieve these dimensions the pipette should be held at an angle of 45 degrees during the grinding process.

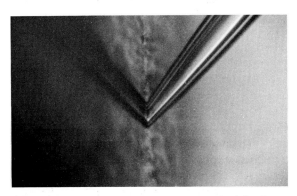

Figure 2.11 Grinding a sharp bevel on the injection micropipette.

3. Bending

Following the grinding the needle is bent to the same angle as the holding pipette (see above).

If the spermatozoa are to be aspirated into the microneedle (our preferred technique), rather than loaded through the rear end, these are often harvested from a thin film of medium under paraffin oil. For this reason we have found it efficacious to ensure that the bevel is on the lower side of the bend of the micro-injection pipette.

A collet has been specifically designed by Research Instruments, in association with NURTURE, for attachment to the microforge, to rotate the pipette so that the bevel can be reproducibly sited to any specific angle demanded of the technique.

The SUZI technique
Preparation of spermatozoa

One of the most important features for an efficient SUZI operation is the preparation of clean spermatozoa, free of debris, cells and any material which will block the microneedle and prevent aspiration or expulsion of the spermatozoa. In our laboratory we use the Percoll procedure exclusively (see Chapter 7). Only a gradient consisting of two concentrations of Percoll are used – 90 per

Table 2.1 Size of the inner diameter of the microneedle (micro-injection pipette) versus ease of penetration of the zona pellucida

| | *Subjective score* * | | | |
| | *Inner diameter of microneedle (μm)* | | | |
	19	*15*	*11*	*8*
n	12	31	17	11
$\bar{x}$	2.17†	1.32†	1.88	2.0
Standard deviation	0.72	0.6	0.7	0.89
Standard error of the mean	0.21	0.11	0.17	0.27
Min	1.0	1.0	1.0	1.0
Max	3.0	3.0	3.0	3.0

Notes: * Based on a score of 1–4: 1 = easy; 2 = moderately difficult; 3 = difficult; 4 = impossible.
† 19 μm v. 15 μm: $t = 3.874$, P < 0.001.

Table 2.2 Size of the inner diameter of the microneedle (micro-injection pipette) versus ease of aspiration of spermatozoa

| | *Subjective score** *Inner diameter of microneedle (μm)* | | | |
	19	15	11	8
n	12	13	17	11
$\bar{x}$	1.25	1.39	2.29	2.82
Standard deviation	0.62	0.56	0.92	0.87
Standard error of the mean	0.18	0.10	0.22	0.26
Min	1.0	1.0	1.0	2.0
Max	3.0	3.0	4.0	4.0

Notes: * Based on a score of 1–4: 1 = easy; 2 = moderately difficult; 3 = difficult; 4 = impossible.
19 μm v. 15 μm: N.S. 19 μm v. 11 μm: $t = 3.432$, $P < 0.002$.
19 μm v. 8 μm $t = 6.472$, $P < 0.001$. 15 μm v. 11 μm: $t = 4.267$, $P < 0.001$.

cent and 45 per cent. The force of centrifugation depends on the severity of the sample and the paucity of spermatozoa. Generally centrifugation is between 300–500g. The sedimented spermatozoa are resuspended in culture medium (Earle's balanced salt solution with 10 per cent pregnant human serum), centrifuged once more at about 300 g, and finally resuspended in a very small volume of culture medium. The volume of culture medium used for the final resuspension depends on the final concentration of sperm; if necessary the spermatozoa are sedimented in volumes as low as 0.05 ml. The suspension of spermatozoa is gassed with 5 per cent CO_2 in air and warmed to 37°C prior to SUZI. Various media and ionic concentrations have been tried to synchronise the percentage of cells undergoing the acrosome reaction, and this is described elsewhere (see Chapters 4, 7).

Preparation of oocytes

After approximately six to eight hours culture the oocyte-cumulus complex is exposed to 0.1 per cent w/v hyaluronidase (Type VIII; Sigma, Poole, UK) for a maximum of one minute. Continual pipetting of the oocyte-cumulus complex while in the solution of hyaluronidase facilitates the digestion of the

Table 2.3 Size of the inner diameter of the microneedle (micro-injection pipette) versus degree of blockage of the microneedle tip

| | *Subjective score** *Inner diameter of microneedle (μm)* | | | |
	19	15	11	8
n	12	31	17	11
$\bar{x}$	1.25	1.39	2.0	2.36
Standard deviation	0.45	0.56	0.71	0.81
Standard error of the mean	0.13	0.10	0.17	0.24
Min	1.0	1.0	1.0	1.0
Max	2.0	3.0	3.0	3.0

Notes: * Based on a score of 1–3: 1 = no blockage; 2 = blocked, but workable; 3 = blocked permanently.
19 μm v. 15 μm: N.S. 19 μm v. 11 μm: $t = 3.254$, $P < 0.003$.
19 μm v. 8 μm: $t = 4.163$, $P < 0.001$. 15 μm v. 11 μm: $t = 3.309$, $P < 0.002$.

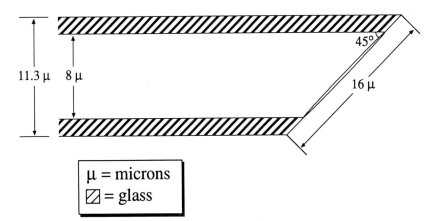

Figure 2.12
Diagrammatic illustration of the optimum measurements for the injection microneedle when performing the SUZI technique

cumulus cells in a matter of seconds. The oocytes with the attendant cumulus cells are transferred to washing droplets, which may be either Dulbecco's phosphate buffered saline with 5 per cent serum or standard culture medium. After a minimum of six washes the adhering corona radiata cells are gently removed by aspiration through a finely pulled Pasteur pipette. Each oocyte is scored for the presence of a polar body and only those oocytes in metaphase II are used for the SUZI procedure.

In earlier studies the oocytes were exposed to 0.1 M sucrose just prior to and during SUZI procedure. This facilitated shrinkage of the ooplasm and increased the size of the perivitelline space. We have abandoned the use of a hypertonic solution for increasing the perivitelline space. Almost all metaphase II oocytes that are fully mature have sufficient perivitelline space in which to perform SUZI without increasing the risk of damage to the oocyte plasma membrane. This removes an additional washing step, as the sucrose needs to be washed fully, and by saving time reduces the exposure of the oocytes to ambient conditions. Currently we have observed that there is at least no difference, but possibly an increase in the incidence of fertilisation.

Preparative stages for subzonal insemination

The following are the preparative stages immediately prior to the SUZI procedure:

1. The microscope stage is heated to 37°C (Olympus IM2-CBHP).
2. The hyaluronidase and the microwell slides (we prefer these to petri dishes) are prewarmed to 37°C.
3. A series of Pasteur pipettes are prepared, each with a different bore diameter.
4. The micropipette and microneedle are loaded into the tool holder of the micromanipulators.
5. The microneedle is lowered into a solution of Dulbecco's plus five per cent serum (the preferred medium for carrying out the SUZI procedure, for this short-term culture there is no need to maintain an ambient five per cent CO_2 atmosphere). This is an important step and time must be allowed for the medium to enter the microneedle by capillary action. When a pneumatic system is preferred to an hydraulic system it is even more important to equilibrate the microneedle before use. This allows much finer control of the aspiration/expulsion process.
6. While the microneedle is equilibrating, a microdrop of the spermatozoa solution is placed in the microwell of the slide and overlaid with light liquid paraffin. The slide is placed in the incubator. This then gives time for the motile sperm to migrate to the edge of the microdroplet at the interface between the droplet and the paraffin (Figure 2.13). The slide is maintained in an incubator providing the required ambient conditions.

7. The oocyte-cumulus complexes are transferred to the hyaluronidase and eventually metaphase II oocytes are isolated for SUZI, as described above.

8. A second microwell slide is prepared with the Dulbecco's phosphate buffered saline medium with 5 per cent serum. This is overlaid with light liquid paraffin. The oocytes are transferred to this microdrop and kept in the microwell in an incubator.

9. The slide containing the spermatozoa is presented to the microneedle on the stage of the inverted microscope.

10. The microneedle is lowered carefully into the microdrop trying to keep the tip of the microneedle towards the edge of the microdrop. Should the sample of spermatozoa still contain debris and/or many immotile cells these will congregate towards the centre of the microdrop. If the microneedle is not equilibrated fully or there is some negative pressure in the system and the tip of the microneedle is presented close to the centre of the microdrop it may inadvertently aspirate the debris/immotile cells and block the opening.

11. The spermatozoa are collected from the medium/oil interphase. The microneedle is raised out of the medium.

The subzonal insemination procedure

1. The slide with the oocyte is presented to the microscope stage and the micropipette is lowered into the microwell and culture medium and an oocyte is aspirated on to the tip of the micropipette. Care is taken not to aspirate the oocyte too forcefully causing damage to the ooplasm by 'pinching'.

2. The microneedle containing the spermatozoa is lowered into the microwell and is lined up with the zona pellucida of the oocyte. The holding pipette, oocyte and microneedle must all be in the same focal plane.

3. Our preferred approach for the microneedle is between the nine–one o'clock or ten–two o'clock position. The zona pellucida is initially prodded gently and this facilitates the largest perivitelline space to be created in the region of proposed injection. Once a clear route for injection has been created

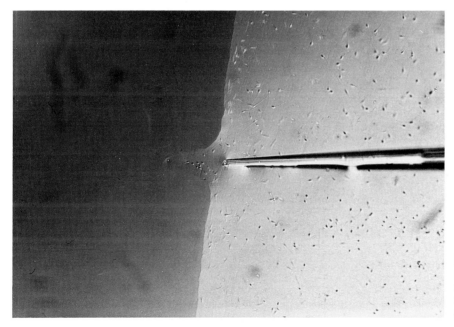

Figure 2.13 The motile sperm migrate to the edge of the microdroplet at the interface between the droplet and the paraffin

the microneedle is thrust sharply through the zona pellucida, counteracting the natural elasticity and pliability of the zona pellucida as the microneedle penetrates the perivitelline space (Figure 2.14). Care must be taken not to force the microneedle too far forward as it may penetrate the opposing zona pellucida. A second hole in the opposing zona pellucida will cause any injected spermatozoa to either swim, or under pressure be forced, out of the second hole. An aid to our approach is to use a slight movement outwards at the end of the forward thrust which slightly extends the zona pellucida but prevents the needle penetrating the opposing side.

4. Once inside the perivitelline space the tip of the microneedle is gently moved and the focus re-adjusted to observe the deposition of spermatozoa. The number of spermatozoa deposited in the perivitelline space depends upon the individual case.

5. The number of oocytes in the microdrop and injected in a single attempt depends upon the experience of the practitioner and the quality of spermatozoa. If a number of sperm are aspirated into the microneedle and can be deposited in the perivitelline space one at a time, then three, four or more eggs may be injected in one attempt. If there are so few sperm that they need to be re-aspirated after each injection, or the sample causes problems of blockage, which can be created by very 'sticky' spermatozoa adhering to the inner surface of the microneedle, it is preferable to have only a single oocyte in the microwell at each attempt. This is very much a subjective decision.

6. After the SUZI the micropipette and the microneedle are raised out of the microdrop, the oocytes are removed from the microwell into standard culture medium washed through two or three drops and cultured normally.

Another approach for loading the microneedle is to inject the solution of spermatozoa through the rear end of the microneedle before loading on to the microtool holder. Although we prefer not to use this approach, others have found it adequate for their needs.

It is preferable to keep the amount of medium deposited in the perivitelline space to a minimum. However, medium may enter the perivitelline space

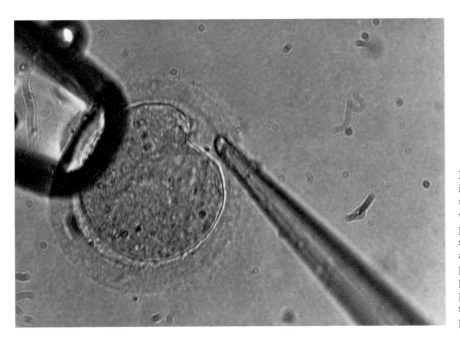

Figure 2.14 The oocyte is held in position with the holding pipette, while the injection pipette containing the spermatozoa approaches at the two o'clock position. The micropipette penetrates the zona pellucida to deposit the spermatozoa into the perivitelline space

in sufficient volume to distort the oocyte; should this occur the excess should be aspirated out to prevent creating an inordinate pressure upon the ooplasm. Under these circumstances we have not noticed a deleterious effect to the oocyte. A disadvantage of having a large volume of medium in the perivitelline space is that it will gradually seep through the hole made by the microneedle often allowing the escape of spermatozoa. If excess medium appears to be in the perivitelline space after the sperm has been deposited, the microneedle can remain in place until the motile sperm swim away from the injection site. The excess medium can then be gently aspirated without removing the spermatozoa.

References

1. Schmidt HD. Minute structure of the hepatic lobules particularly with reference to the relationship between capillary blood vessels and the hepatic cells. *American Journal of Medical Sciences*. 1859; **37**: 13–40. 13–40.
2. Barber MA, Kansas J. A method of isolating microorganisms. *Medical Society*. 1904; **4**: 489–94.
3. Barber MA. The rate of multiplication of Bacillus coli at different temperatures. *Journal of Infectious Diseases*. 1908; **5**: 379–400.
4. Barber MA. A technic for the inoculation of bacteria and other substances into living cells. *Journal of Infectious Diseases*. 1911; **8**: 348–60.
5. Péterfi T. Das mikrurgische Verfahren. *Naturwissenschaften*. 1923; **11**: 81–7.

Chapter 3

Experience with subzonal insemination in mouse and cow

Lilo Mettler and Alice Kuranty

Introduction

For over ten years the area of human *in vitro* fertilisation and embryo transfer as a treatment for human infertility has become accepted by nearly all governments. But, as discussed elsewhere in this volume, there still exist limitations in the efficacy of the IVF technique for overcoming some causes of infertility, especially those related to non-fertilisation. This may be associated with a low sperm count, reduced sperm quality or idiopathic infertility, and it represents a large number of our patients.

Attempts to overcome the barriers to achieving fertilisation *in vitro* were focused on various micro-insemination procedures (see Chapter 1). Of necessity the technique had to be evaluated using animal models to minimise any possible effects of manipulating the gametes.

In Schleswig-Holstein, Germany, to date, we have not received permission to do subzonal insemination in the human. We have examined the technique of injecting a single sperm under the zona pellucida and into the perivitelline space in both the mouse and bovine systems.

Material and methods
Mouse *in vitro* fertilisation

Figure 3.1 schematically demonstrates the 11 steps of fertilisation in the mouse. The medium used was Ham's F-10 with the addition of 1.8 mmol calcium lactate, 0.75 per cent bovine serum albumin (BSA) and 50 IU/ml of penicillin-G.

Preparation of spermatozoa

Spermatozoa were obtained from the vas deferens of male mice in the CB6/F1 generation and cultured for two hours for capacitation. Only the so-called 'swim up spermatozoa' (C-spermatozoa) were further cultured with 12 mmol dibutyryl guanosine cyclic monophosphate (dbc-GMP) and 10 mmol imidazole to complete the acrosome reaction (AR) (C+AR-spermatozoa).[1,2]

The completion of acrosome reaction was tested according to Talbot et al.[3] with slight modifications. After 20 minutes C+AR-spermatozoa were put into a drop of medium enriched with 1.5 per cent BSA on a slide adjacent to a droplet of

36

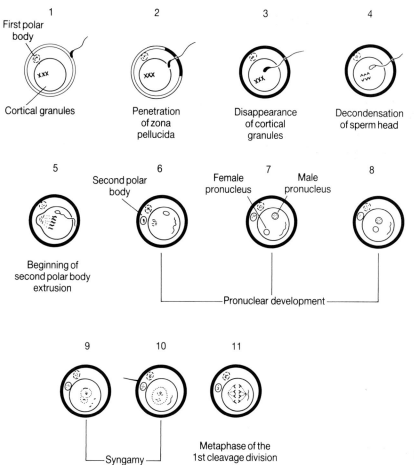

Figure 3.1 Eleven stages of mouse fertilisation

medium containing the oocyte and covered with silicon oil.[4,5]

In a parallel experiment, *in vitro* insemination of oocytes from the same cohort with either C-spermatozoa or C+AR-spermatozoa in concentrations between 30 000 to 100 000/ml was carried out.

Preparation of oocytes

The oocytes were flushed from the oviducts of superovulated mice of the CB6/F1 strain. A cumulus oophorus was removed after digestion with 10 IU/ml of hyaluronidase solution for five minutes. After cumulus separation the oocytes were

washed and put in the droplets of Ham's F-10 medium with 1.5 per cent BSA adjacent to droplets of spermatozoa on the slide.

Micromanipulation

The injection pipettes were prepared by pulling glass capillaries with a Leitz (Hamburg, Germany) pipette puller and were honed with a Bachhofer (Reutlingen, Germany) sharpener. The inner diameter of the injection pipettes was about 10 μm. The oocyte holding pipette was prepared by pulling glass capillary tubes in a small flame. All micromanipulations were performed under the inverted microscope (Olympus, Tokyo, Japan). We used the micromanipulators of Leitz (Hamburg, Germany) with an air injection and vacuum system, connected to an automatic micro-injector (Eppendorf, Hamburg, Germany). Only vital motile spermatozoa were aspirated and injected individually into the perivitelline space (Figures 3.2a–3.2d). If the injected spermatozoa became immotile further actively motile spermatozoa were injected. The injection was done carefully using our S-system (Figure 3.2) (slight pressure and 'S' wise movement while perforating into the perivitelline space).

Observations

Mouse oocytes and sperm

The vitality of the injected oocytes was judged immediately after micromanipulation, as the loss of the membrane integrity of a damaged oocyte can be seen immediately. The criterion for fertilisation was only those oocytes that had two pronuclei and a second polar body. These oocytes were put into colchicine for chromosome analysis, and they were prepared using the air dried method of Tarkowski.[6]

The results were compared to successful fertilisation after routine insemination. Statistical analysis was done using the Chi-square test.

Bovine oocytes and sperm

Bovine ovaries were collected from the slaughterhouse. The ovaries were put into isotonic NaCl solution together with 600 IU/ml of penicillin and washed three times at room temperature. All primary follicles, 2–6 mm in size, were punctured. Isolated oocytes were put into medium 199 with the addition of 20 per cent fetal calf serum, at 39°C, under ambient conditions of 5 per cent CO_2 and 8 per cent 0_2 and washed three times.

For an *in vitro* maturation the oocytes were incubated for 24 hours. The cumulus was digested with 800 IU/ml of hyaluronidase for ten minutes and remaining adhering cells were removed mechanically by using pipettes. Each oocyte was carefully checked for the presence of a polar body. If they were not present, they were cultured for a further two to three hours in 199 medium enriched with 100 μm dibutyryl adenosine cyclic monophosphate (dbc-AMP).

Frozen bovine spermatozoa were thawed by shock thawing at 39°C for 30 seconds and put into Ham's F-10 medium containing 0.75 per cent BSA. The swim up technique was applied for selection of spermatozoa. The spermatozoa were left two hours for capacitation, then 30 minutes for the acrosome reaction in 12 mm dbc-GMP + 10 mm imidazole in Ham's F-10. Micro-injection was performed as described above, followed by three washing steps and transfer into multiwell tissue culture chambers. After 16–18 hours the pronucleus stage was observed, and 48 hours later the two- to four-cell stage embryo.

Results

Mouse oocytes

Acrosome reaction of spermatozoa

Acrosome intact but not acrosome-reacted spermatozoa showed a reaction with Bismarck-brown stain and were rose coloured in the acrosomal area with Bengal-rose. Dead spermatozoa were coloured with Tripane blue. Eleven per cent of the C-spermatozoa, and 91 per cent of the C+AR-spermatozoa acrosomes had reacted.

In vitro fertilisation

The *in vitro* fertilisation rate with oocytes and cumulus cells using C-spermatozoa resulted in a

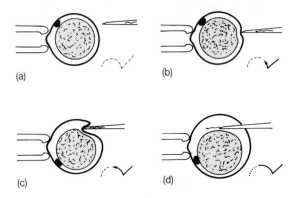

Figure 3.2 Penetration of zona pellucida and injection of a spermatozoon into the perivitelline space

Table 3.1   IVF with capacitated (C)- and capacitated/acrosome-reacted (C+AR)-spermatozoa (mouse)

	Experiments	Oocytes	Fertilised*		
	n	*n*	*n*	%	*Mean fertilisation rates ± SEM %*
C-spermatozoa	16	883	680	77.0	80.27 ± 4.52
C+AR-spermatozoa	10	368	9	2.4	2.47 ± 0.88

Note: *oocyte with a second polar body and two pronuclei.

fertilisation rate of 77 per cent. While C+AR-spermatozoa revealed only 2.4 per cent of fertilisation (Table 3.1), 77 per cent of fertilised oocytes developed to morulae and expanded blastocysts.

Micro-injection of C-spermatozoa and C+AR-spermatozoa into the perivitelline space

The average survival rate of the micromanipulated oocytes was 85 per cent. Fertilisation was achieved only with the injection of motile spermatozoa. The number of the injected oocytes which had developed a second polar body and two pronuclei are specified in Table 3.2. A significantly higher (18.8 per cent) rate of fertilisation occurred using the C+AR-spermatozoa after micro-insemination, compared with C-spermatozoa (5.6 per cent). Figure 3.3 shows a fertilised oocyte with two pronuclei and a second polar body after micro-insemination.

All fertilised oocytes cleaved and in 73.3 per cent four-cell embryos were observed (Figure 3.4). Some of the embryos were prepared by the application of colchicine for chromosome analysis, the remaining embryos developed in 69.2 per cent to the morula stage (Figure 3.5). Both male and female chromosome sets were detected. Into each perivitelline space only one sperm was injected.

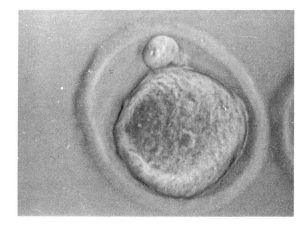

Figure 3.3   Fertilised mouse oocyte after micro-injection × 600

Table 3.2   Micro-insemination of capacitated (C)- and capacitated/acrosome-reacted (C+AR)-spermatozoa into the perivitelline space (mouse)

	Experiments	Oocytes	Fertilised*		
	n	*n*	*n*	%	*Mean fertilisation rates ± SEM %*
C-spermatozoa	8	160	9	5.63	5.65 ± 1.59
C+AR-spermatozoa	38	490	92	18.78	18.34 ± 3.48

Note: *oocyte with a second polar body and two pronuclei.

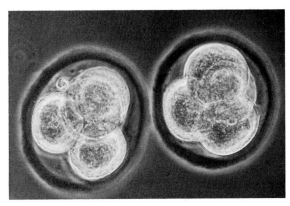

Figure 3.4 Mouse 4-cell stage after micro-injection × 600

Bovine oocytes

Table 3.3 demonstrates the result of the 92 micro-inseminated bovine oocytes which had a diploid fertilisation rate of around 1.5 per cent, although 80.4 per cent of oocytes were successfully injected. None cleaved. The bovine species has a very thick zona pellucida and penetration is considerably more difficult.

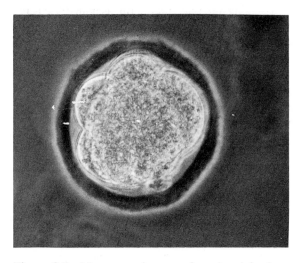

Figure 3.5 Mouse morula stage after micro-injection × 600

Table 3.3 Micro-insemination of capacitated (C)- and capacitated/acrosome-reacted (C+AR)-spermatozoa into the perivitelline space (bovine)

	Injected oocytes	Oocytes	1 PN	2 PN	3 PN	Division
n	92	74	4	1	1	–
%		80.4	5.4	1.4	1.4	0

Discussion

The problems associated with micro-injection of spermatozoa into oocytes have been discussed by numerous authors, and comprehensive discussions can be found in this volume.

Our 'S' shaped insertion of the injecting pipette has enabled us to penetrate the zona pellucida safely without damaging the ooplasma.

Regulating the suction and injection pressures in the injection pipettes can be difficult. To overcome these problems, hydraulic based systems, with oil or with mercury for example, have been tried. All of these systems have potentially detrimental effects upon oocytes when in contact with, or injected into, the living cells. The pneumatic system seemed to present the least difficulty. With our methods the survival rate has reached over 80 per cent and is often as high as 95 per cent.

Mouse oocytes are known to be very susceptible to mechanical stimuli; Thadani[7] used rat oocytes for the micro-injection of mouse spermatozoa.

The relatively low fertilisation rates are probably due to several factors.

Sperm capacitation

The specific molecular events involved in sperm capacitation have not been fully elucidated. It is possible that incubation in an appropriate culture medium and atmosphere for one to two hours causes spermatozoa to be acrosome reacted. This incubation may, however, not capacitate all spermatozoa. In IVF this is sufficient, but may not be enough for micro-insemination (see Chapters 4, 7 and 8).

In the course of the procedure of micro-

Table 3.4 Micro-injection of mouse spermatozoa into the perivitelline space of mouse oocytes

Conditions	Number of oocytes	Number of oocytes that survived	Number of oocytes with pronuclei	
			1 PN	2 PN
Spermatozoa Injection	582	474 (81.4%)	52 (11.0%)	23 (4.8%)
Medium Injection	287	283 (98.6%)	7/232* (3.0%)	0/232* (0.0%)

Note: * number of the observed oocytes.

insemination, it is not possible to assess whether or not the spermatozoon is capacitated or not.

Activation of oocytes

Some researchers report that an injection of sperm heads, procured by homogenization or sonication, directly into the ooplasm activates the oocytes. Cortical granules are released and female pronuclei are developed. This activation of oocytes is not caused only by the injection of sperm heads; oocytes can be activated by pricking in the presence of calcium, i.e. parthenogenesis.

In this study 11 per cent of the sperm micro-injected into the perivitelline space and 3 per cent of the control oocytes showed a single pronucleus in each ooplasm, and on the following day showed apparent cell division (Table 3.4). Perhaps the discrepancies of our results between the sperm injected and control oocytes can be explained by mechanical stimuli, which are produced by the penetration of the zona pellucida, or the injection of medium may cause parthenogenesis.

Selection of the appropriate spermatozoa for successful micro-insemination is a major problem. In routine IVF the oocyte is surrounded by thousands of spermatozoa, after preparation of the latter by centrifugation and swim up. *In vivo*, the oocyte to sperm ratio is thought to be no more than 200. However, in the mouse and hamster the number of spermatozoa does not exceed the number of eggs. Therefore the problem of selecting spermatozoa is not the selection of only one sperm but how to select a fraction that contains 'fertile spermatozoa'. Markert[8] has observed that the phenotype of the sperm does not reflect the genotype in terms of fertilising ability after micro-injection, and immotile and grossly defective sperm produce the same results that are produced by fertilisation with healthy robust sperm. Therefore our attempt in *in vitro* fertilisation to inseminate with the most motile and most vigorous sperm might be necessary only for the initiation of the fertilisation process, but not once the spermatozoa are in direct contact with the ooplasm. Thus the micro-injection of spermatozoa into oocytes may become a more important method for assessing and selecting sperm, as it enables us to facilitate fertilisation even if the penetrating ability of the spermatozoa is weak.

In summary, with this method of micro-insemination, we do not only expect a profound effect in the treatment of human sterility due to andrologic, immunologic, and idiopathic causes, but we also intend to develop potent strategies for studying basic physiologic mechanisms of ovum–sperm interaction.

References

1. Barg PE, Wahrmann MZ, Talansky BE, Gordon HW. Capacitated acrosome reacted but immotile sperm, when microinjected under the mouse zona pellucida, will not fertilize the oocyte. *Journal of Experimental Zoology*. 1986; **237**: 365–74.

2. Santos-Sacchi J, Gordon M. Induction of the

S UNIVERSITY LIBRARY

acrosome reaction in guinea pig spermatozoa by cGMP analogues. *Journal of Cell Biology.* 1980; **85**: 798–803.

3. Talbot P, Chacon RS. A triple stain technique for evaluating normal acrosome reaction of human sperm. *Journal of Experimental Zoology.* 1981; **215**: 201–18.

4. Mettler L, Yamada K, Kuranty A, Michelmann HW, Semm K. Microinjection of spermatozoa into oocytes – reality and wishes. In: *Proceedings of the 5th World Congress on In Vitro Fertilization and Embryo Transfer.* New York, Academy of Science, 1987, pp. 591–600.

5. Yamada K, Stevenson AFG, Mettler L. Fertilization through spermatozoal microinjection: significance of acrosome reaction. *Human Reproduction.* 1988; **3**: 657–61.

6. Tarkowski AK. An air drying method for chromosome preparations from mouse eggs. *Cytogenetics.* 1966; **5**: 394–400.

7. Thadani VM. A study of hetero-specific sperm-egg interactions in the rat, mouse and deer mouse using in vitro fertilization and sperm injection. *Journal of Experimental Zoology.* 1980; **212**: 435–53.

8. Markert CL. Fertilization of mammalian eggs by sperm injection. *Journal of Experimental Zoology.* 1983; **228**: 195–201.

Chapter 4

Techniques for the preparation of spermatozoa and the need for capacitation and the acrosome reaction

David Mortimer

Introduction

Although there is considerable current debate as to the precise location of the acrosome reaction in the fertilising spermatozoon, it is universally accepted that spermatozoa must complete the acrosome reaction in order to penetrate the zona pellucida.[1] Consequently, all spermatozoa that reach the oolemma under physiological conditions have completed the acrosome reaction. Perivitelline spermatozoa therefore lack the anterior cap region of the acrosome but retain an intact equatorial segment. Of particular relevance is the finding that an acrosome reaction is essential for human spermatozoa to penetrate the zona pellucida-free hamster oocyte.[1,2]

Interaction with the oolemma occurs in two stages. First, acrosome reacted spermatozoa attach and bind to the oolemma by a more or less species-specific receptor-mediated process, probably involving the postacrosomal region of the sperm head. Secondly, fusion between the sperm plasma membrane and the oolemma is initiated in the equatorial segment leading ultimately to incorporation of the spermatozoon into the oocyte.[1,3,4] Spermatozoa lacking these structures, e.g. the round head defect or 'globozoospermia', are incapable of oocyte fusion.[5] As the sperm nucleus is taken into the ooplasm its nuclear envelope is lost and, as the chromatin decondenses to form the male pronucleus, with the concomitant replacement of protamines by histones derived from the oocyte, a new nuclear envelope is formed from oocyte components.[1]

Therefore, spermatozoa for micro-injection into the perivitelline space must have completed a physiological acrosome reaction and retain an intact equatorial segment to be capable of inter-action with the oolemma. If spermatozoa are to be injected directly into the ooplasm then we may assume that naked (condensed) chromatin should be injected with appropriate activation of the oocyte to stimulate male pronucleus formation. Spermatozoa for use in zona opening procedures (e.g. partial zona dissection or zona drilling, cracking, tearing, etc.) should also probably be already acrosome reacted, since those that bind to the zona pellucida (where initiation of the acrosome reaction is now believed to occur) will probably not reach the perivitelline space – this being the primary reason for using micro-assisted fertilisation (MAF) in the first place. Whether their reduced or absent fertilising ability is due to their impaired ability to undergo acrosome reactions or hyperactivation is not clear. However, of relevance here is the finding that spermatozoa from men with Kartagener ('immotile cilia') syndrome, which are immotile but capable of undergoing an acrosome reaction, can penetrate zona-free hamster eggs[6] in the hamster egg penetration test (HEPT) and even fuse with human oocytes after subzonal insemination.[7]

This presentation will consider the dynamics of human sperm capacitation and the acrosome reaction *in vitro* and attempt to define minimum requirements for spermatozoa to be used for MAF. Possible methods for optimising the proportion of spermatozoa in a prepared population ready and competent to fuse with the oolemma will be considered, including some discussion of appropriate methods for preparing motile sperm populations from semen for use not only in MAF but also in any assisted reproductive technology (ART), including *in vitro* fertilisation (IVF) and gamete intra-Fallopian transfer (GIFT), avoiding iatrogenic damage.

Capacitation

As for all eutheria, human ejaculate spermatozoa are not capable of undergoing an acrosome reaction and fertilising eggs until they have completed an obligatory final maturation stage, known as capacitation, by which they acquire the capacity to fertilise.[1] This process is obligatory for fertilisation of homologous oocytes both *in vivo* and *in vitro*, as well as for penetration of zona pellucida-free oocytes in both the homologous situation and in the HEPT. By definition, capacitation leaves spermatozoa in a state ready to undergo the acrosome reaction, but does not actually include the acrosome reaction itself. The time required for capacitation seems to be more or less species specific, and to vary between the *in vivo* and *in vitro* situations.[1,8] However, while

the actual time required for human sperm capacitation under either set of conditions is unclear, the entire IVF process of capacitation, penetration of the egg vestments and male pronucleus formation has been described in as little as 2.25 hours.[9] Furthermore, substantial inter-individual variability in capacitation dynamics has been reported[10], and there are many indications that human sperm populations comprise asynchronous subpopulations of spermatozoa with respect to their capacitation in vitro.[11,12,13]

As much as it would be invaluable to be able to monitor capacitation in human sperm populations *in vitro*, no simple, practical technique for this currently exists. Possible techniques have considered changes in lectin labelling of the sperm surface[14], changes in chlortetracycline fluorescence[15] and the expression of hyperactivated motility.[16] However, none of these methods is yet in routine use.

The only commonly used method for assessing acquisition of the capacitated state is the occurrence of spontaneous acrosome reactions determined by the indirect method of hamster egg penetration. Clearly this is a useful bioassay for testing treatments that affect capacitation and the acrosome reaction in combination, but it is of little value for assessing capacitation in isolation.

Even hyperactivation, which is associated with acquisition of the capacitated state in several species, notably laboratory rodents[1], may be of less use for human spermatozoa since substantial levels of hyperactivated motility can be seen very soon after separation of motile spermatozoa from the inhibitory environment of the seminal plasma.[16,17]

Synchronisation of capacitation

Although protocols exist for the synchronisation of capacitation in several experimental models,[18–20,21], there has been little success in similar attempts with human spermatozoa. Calcium deprivation was attempted but, without substitution of another cation for the calcium, was found to cause irreversible loss of motility.[22] Substitution of calcium by the divalent strontium cation during the capacitation pre-incubation was reported to induce significant improvements in human sperm fertilising ability when assessed using the HEPT after washing into calcium-containing medium[23], an effect that was magnified when EGTA was also added during the capacitation pre-incubation to chelate any residual free calcium ions.[24] This approach has been used by several groups to prepare human sperm populations for subzonal microinjection.[25,26] However, although it was originally proposed that this stimulatory effect might be mediated via a synchronisation of capacitation so that a larger cohort of spermatozoa underwent the acrosome reaction together upon exposure to extracellular calcium, studies on the acrosomal status of sperm populations incubated in calcium- and strontium/EGTA-based media revealed this to be incorrect.[27] Consequently, stimulation of human sperm fertilising ability using this technique must be based on a more subtle, as yet unidentified, effect.

Even though the possible benefit of manipulating cyclic AMP levels using analogues and phosphodiesterase inhibitors during capacitation has often been suggested, only limited data are available to support such an approach, and the observed improved HEPT penetration rates may equally be mediated through inducing elevated levels of acrosome reactions.[26–31] However, whilst this may well preclude their usefulness in IVF, since capacitated but acrosome-intact spermatozoa are required for insemination of intact oocyte-cumulus complexes *in vitro*, it would be ideal for MAF procedures.[32,33]

The acrosome reaction

Studies on the human sperm acrosome reaction are confounded by three major difficulties: the inability to visualise the human sperm acrosome directly using phase contrast optics, asynchronous capacitation, and the variable (usually low) level of spontaneously occurring acrosome reactions.

The inability to visualise the human sperm acrosome directly using phase contrast optics has necessitated the use of various indirect techniques to reveal its presence or absence. One of the first techniques described and validated was the triple-stain method[34] which, in spite of its being highly capricious and often rather difficult to assess, is still used in some laboratories. Immunofluorescent techniques have also been used and, although several highly specific monoclonal antibody-based methods have been described[35,36] the most useful techniques of all have been those employing fluorescein-conjugated lectins such as peanut agglutinin (PNA)[37,38], pea agglutinin (PSA)[39] and, most recently, concanavalin A (ConA).[40]

Using such methods to determine acrosome status, numerous workers have reported that, unlike those of many other eutherians, human spermatozoa do not undergo high levels of acrosome reactions spontaneously during culture *in vitro*,[41,42,43], although the proportion of acrosome reacted spermatozoa does seem to be greater if more physiological culture media, and higher albumin concentrations, are used.[44] Even though the levels of spontaneous acrosome reactions after 36 hours of incubation can then reach comparable levels to those inducible by calcium ionophore treatment, the maximal response achievable using ionophore regimens is still substantially below 100 per cent in the majority of men.[44]

Several groups have reported that exposure of capacitated human spermatozoa to follicular fluid will induce high levels of acrosome reactions[45–47], although this has been refuted by others.[48,49] Follicular fluid contains high levels of glycosaminoglycans (GAGs) some of which have been shown to induce the acrosome reaction in other eutheria[50–52], although no such effect has been unequivocally demonstrated for human spermatozoa. In addition, it has recently been shown that progesterone at concentrations of the order of 1 μg/ml induces a calcium flux[53,54], leading to induction of the acrosome reaction.[55] Induction of the human sperm acrosome reaction by the cumulus mass[45,56,57] may also be mediated through progesterone, although a role for GAGs should not be ignored.

While the relatively high progesterone and/or GAG concentrations in ovulatory follicular fluid might well induce acrosome reactions *in vitro*, it is difficult to see a physiological role for such mechanisms if the fertilising spermatozoon actually undergoes its acrosome reaction on the surface of the zona pellucida in response to binding to the sperm receptor molecule known as ZP3.[1,31] Nevertheless, progesterone-triggered or GAG-induced acrosome loss could occur in significant numbers of capacitated, and hence highly labile, spermatozoa although such spermatozoa are unlikely to be involved in the fertilisation of zona-intact eggs.

Artificial induction of the acrosome reaction

Being a calcium-dependent process, the acrosome reaction can be induced artificially by creating elevated intracellular calcium ion concentrations. The most commonly used procedure is treatment with a calcium ionophore, usually the antibiotic A23187 (calcimycin), although ionomycin can also be used. While such treatment can induce high levels of acrosomal changes indistinguishable morphologically from a normal, physiological acrosome reaction, many protocols use excessive amounts of ionophore and cause deleterious side effects, primarily loss of vitality. However, moderate and mild ionophore treatment protocols have been used to induce acrosome reactions in human sperm populations both experimentally and as part of sperm function testing using the HEPT.[44,48,58–60]

Ionophore treatment has been used in experimental studies on human sperm micro-injection into the perivitelline space of hamster oocytes[61], and, although it produced more penetrations than untreated sperm preparations, it was not significantly different to using cryopreserved spermatozoa, which are known to have reduced acrosomal stability.[62] Unfortunately, from the MAF standpoint ionophore treatment of spermatozoa is unacceptable to many workers due to the risk of ionophore carry over and its deleterious effect upon the oocyte.

Manipulation of cyclic AMP levels, primarily using analogues such as cyclic GMP and its dibutyryl derivative, also induces increased levels of acrosome reactions in human spermatozoa, and has made subzonal insemination more successful for some groups.[32,33]

Several authors have described protocols for inducing acrosome reactions in populations of human spermatozoa, or at least improving their performance in the HEPT, using follicular fluid.[63–65] No-one has yet tried using progesterone treatment to augment sperm fertilising ability, but we have shown recently that heparin can induce acrosome reactions in capacitated human spermatozoa above the background level of spontaneous acrosome reactions.[66] Furthermore, this effect seems to be synergistic with that of shifting the pH out of the 'usual' range of 7.4 to 7.6. Treatment with 100 μg heparin/ml for two hours at pH 8.4 after a five hour pre-incubation at pH 7.5 induced comparable levels of acrosome reactions to parallel positive control ionophore treatments. Again, these effects await evaluation of any possible clinical application either to optimise the HEPT or in MAF.

Problems of sperm penetration for direct ooplasmic injection

Success in terms of male pronucleus formation and continued embryonic development has been reported for the injection of isolated sperm nuclei directly into the ooplasm[67–69], and attempts to use this approach with human spermatozoa have also met with some success.[7] However, concern has been raised over the elevated incidence of chromosomal damage induced by the commonly used sperm preparative techniques for producing isolated nuclei, or even isolated sperm heads.[71] In view of such findings direct ooplasmic sperm injection by such methods cannot be considered a valid procedure for clinical application at this time.

Impact of preparative technique on sperm function

The need to separate human spermatozoa from seminal plasma to allow capacitation and expression of their intrinsic fertilising ability is a fundamental requirement of IVF, GIFT, intra-uterine insemination (IUI) and *in vitro* tests of sperm fertilising ability such as the HEPT, sperm-(hemi-)zona binding test and assessment of the acrosome reaction.[1,72] Suitable sperm preparations are usually characterised by extremely high proportions of motile spermatozoa, a preferential selection for morphologically normal spermatozoa, and an absence of the other cell types, anucleate cytoplasmic masses and particulate debris commonly seen in human ejaculates. The 'washed pellet swim up' method has been highly successful in producing sperm preparations for IVF in cases with no male factor. However, as the indications for IVF treatment have expanded beyond simple tubal factor cases to couples with idiopathic infertility and, ultimately, to male factor cases, a problem of fertilisation failure has appeared.[73–75]

Some problem of sperm dysfunction has generally been considered a major contributory factor to IVF fertilisation failures – a concept certainly borne out by in vitro studies on human sperm function.[76,77] However, a landmark paper two years ago by Aitken and Clarkson[78] provided clear evidence for an additional component, that of iatrogenic sperm damage. These authors demonstrated that centrifugal pelleting of unselected ejaculate human sperm populations caused the production of reactive oxygen species, superoxide and hydroxyl radicals, within the pellet which induced irreversible damage to the spermatozoa due to peroxidation of their membrane phospholipids. This damage led to impairment of their fertilising ability in the HEPT.

Within such pellets there are not only 'good' spermatozoa but also senescent and dead spermatozoa, numerous types of leukocytes, germinal line cells (some epithelial cells, anucleate cytoplasmic bodies, presumably residual cytoplasmic masses or 'RCMs' from round spermatids released from the seminiferous epithelium at spermiation), and particulate debris. The reactive oxygen species generated in these pellets come from not only the spermatozoa themselves, but also neutrophils and macrophages present in the original semen sample.[79,80] Separation of spermatozoa on Percoll gradients revealed that it is a population of low density spermatozoa that produce superoxide radicals[78], i.e. spermatozoa with a relatively high cytoplasmic volume. This defective subpopulation therefore includes immature spermatozoa, which typically have cytoplasmic droplets, and also some morphologically abnormal spermatozoa with excess residual cytoplasm.

Even though there have been very many IVF successes using this technique, from a cell biological standpoint we are therefore left with the inescapable conclusion that the plasma membranes of spermatozoa prepared using the 'washed pellet' sperm technique have been rendered less fluid, perhaps to the extent that sperm function may have been compromised. The inter-individual susceptibility to this damage arises from the multifactorial association between the levels of reactive oxygen species produced and semen quality. Normal semen samples from fertile men contain higher proportions of morphologically normal spermatozoa and fewer leukocytes and RCMs. As a consequence, the levels of reactive oxygen species produced in pellets prepared from such samples will be much lower than in pellets from samples containing more abnormal spermatozoa, RCMs and perhaps leukocytes (i.e. typical male factor samples). This has been confirmed in a more recent paper from Aitken's group.[81]

In couples with tubal factor infertility the vast majority of male partners show normal semen characteristics and hence there is only a minimal effect of iatrogenic peroxidation on sperm function, insufficient to noticeably influence IVF fertilisation rates. As the likelihood of a male factor increases, for example in couples with idiopathic infertility, the level of sperm damage in some patients, perhaps those with 'borderline' sperm quality, may be sufficient to impair, and even block, fertilisation. In cases of established male factor, the already poor quality spermatozoa may more frequently be rendered totally incapable of fertilisation. These cases of iatrogenic fertilisation failure would be in addition to any specific lesion of sperm function that might otherwise impair or prevent fertilisation. Such associations are supported by numerous publications from IVF programmes where reduced fertilisation rates are reported for male factor IVF.[75,82]

The evidence of iatrogenic failures of sperm fertilising ability must now be considered incontrovertible[82] and since MAF techniques are primarily indicated in patients with severe male factor infertility, the potential extent of iatrogenic sperm dysfunction must be great, and may account, at least in part, for the low success rates seen to date.

Where do we go from here?

Clearly, in order to minimise the incidence of iatrogenic fertilisation failure, use of the so-called 'classical' sperm preparation procedure of swim-up from a washed sperm pellet must be discontinued forthwith.

Alternative sperm preparation methods such as direct swim up from liquefied semen, with a subsequent washing step, or discontinuous Percoll[78,83,84] or Nycodenz[84,85] gradients should be used to prepare spermatozoa for MAF procedures, and indeed any clinical or experimental procedure that will assess or require sperm fertilising ability. Other techniques based upon the direct migration of spermatozoa from liquefied semen such as the Tea-Jondet tubes[86] and Sperm Select[87] will also provide uncompromised populations of motile spermatozoa.

Greater research effort must be expended upon possible chemical and pharmacological treatment protocols that might synchronise capacitation and/or induction of the acrosome reaction. Particular attention should be paid to the stimulation of asthenozoospermic spermatozoa, probably using pentoxifylline[88], and to the exploitation of non-ionophore pharmacological methods to trigger the acrosome reaction in capacitated sperm populations.[32,33] Also of particular interest here are the reported effects of alkaline pH and heparin in combination[66] and the acrosome reaction-inducing effect of progesterone.[55] Further work

on the practical applications of electrofusion or permeabilisation[89,90] to induce acrosome loss should also receive high priority.

Assessment of improved sperm preparative and pretreatment protocols for human spermatozoa should proceed in three stages before attempting clinical MAF trials:

1. Acrosome reaction studies
2. Studies using the zona-free HEPT[91]
3. Perivitelline micro-injection using zona-intact hamster eggs.[61,92,93]

If higher efficiency sperm preparative and pretreatment protocols can be established, the goal of acceptable levels of fertilisation following the perivitelline micro-injection of single spermatozoa might be attainable. If so, this would become the technique of choice for MAF, since it would preclude not only polyspermic fertilisation but also artifactual egg activation associated with zona drilling and possible impaired embryonic development inside compromised zonae pellucidae.[94]

Acknowledgements

Unpublished studies on the human sperm acrosome reaction were supported by grant MA-9817 from the Medical Research Council of Canada to the author. Additional financial support was provided by the Nat Christie Foundation.

References

1. Yanagimachi R. Mammalian fertilization. In: Knobil E, Neill JD, Ewing LL, Markert CL, Greenwald GS, Pfaff DW (eds.) *The Physiology of Reproduction*. New York: Raven Press, 1988: vol. 1, pp. 135–85.
2. Yanagimachi R. Zona-free hamster eggs: their use in assessing fertilizing capacity and examining chromosomes of human spermatozoa. *Gamete Research*. 1984; **10**: 187–232.
3. Sathananthan AH, Ng SC, Edirisinghe R, Ratnam SS, Wong PC. Human sperm–egg interaction in vitro. *Gamete Research*. 1986; **15**: 317–26.
4. Talbot P, Chacon RS. Ultrastructural observations on binding and membrane fusion between human sperm and zona pellucida-free hamster oocytes. *Fertility and Sterility*. 1982; **37**: 240–8.
5. Aitken RJ, Kerr L, Bolton V, Hargreave T. Analysis of sperm function in globozoospermia: implications for the mechanism of sperm–zona interaction. *Fertility and Sterility*. 1990; **54**: 701–7.
6. Aitken RJ, Ross A, Lees MM. Analysis of sperm function in Kartagener's syndrome. *Fertility and Sterility*. 1983; **40**: 696–8.
7. Bongso TA, Sathananthan AH, Wong PC, Ratnam SS, Ng SC, Anandakumar C, Ganatra S. Human fertilization by micro-injection of immotile spermatozoa. *Human Reproduction.* 1989; **4**: 175–9.
8. Rogers BJ. Mammalian sperm capacitation and fertilization in vitro: a critique of methodology. *Gamete Research*. 1978; **1**: 165–223.
9. McMaster R, Yanagimachi R, Lopata A. Penetra-

tion of human eggs by human spermatozoa in vitro. *Biology of Reproduction.* 1978; **19**: 212–6.

10. Perreault SD, Rogers BJ. Capacitation pattern of human spermatozoa. *Fertility and Sterility.* 1982; **38**: 258–60.

11. Burkman LJ, Coddington CC, Franken DA, Kurger TF, Rosenwaks Z, Hodgen GD. The hemizona assay (HZA): development of a diagnostic test for the binding of human spermatozoa to the human hemizona pellucida to predict fertilization potential. *Fertility and Sterility.* 1988; **49**: 688–97.

12. Bedford JM. Significance of the need for sperm capacitation before fertilization in eutherian mammals. *Biology of Reproduction.* 1983; **28**: 108–20.

13. Franken DR, Burkman LJ, Oehninger SC, Coddington CC, Veeck LL, Kruger TF, Rosenwaks Z, Hodgen GD. Hemizona assay using salt stored human oocytes: Evaluation of zona pellucida capacity for binding human spermatozoa. *Gamete Research.* 1989; **22**: 15–26.

14. Singer SL, Lambert H, Cross NL, Overstreet JW. Alteration of the human sperm surface during in vitro capacitation as assessed by lectin-induced agglutination. *Gamete Research.* 1985; **12**: 291–9.

15. Lee MA, Trucco GS, Bechtol KB, Wummer N, Kopf GS, Blasco L, Storey BT. Capacitation and acrosome reactions in human spermatozoa monitored by a chlortetracycline fluorescence assay. *Fertility and Sterility.* 1987; **48**: 649–58..

16. Burkman LJ. Hyperactivated motility of human spermatozoa during in vitro capacitation and implications for fertility. In: Gagnon C ed. *Controls of Sperm Motility: Biological and Clinical Aspects.* Boca Raton: CRC Press, 1990, pp. 303–29.

17. Mortimer D, Mortimer ST, Anderson SJ, Robertson L. Hyperactivated motility of human spermatozoa. In: Baccetti B ed. *Comparative Spermatology 20 Years After.* New York: Raven Press, 1991, pp. 211–5.

18. Fleming AD, Yanagimachi R. Effects of various lipids on the acrosome reaction and fertilizing capacity of guinea pig spermatozoa with special reference to the possible involvement of lysophospholipids in the acrosome reaction. *Gamete Research.* 1981; **4**: 253–73.

19. Wheeler MB, Seidel Jr GE. Capacitation of bovine spermatozoa by lysophospholipids and trypsin. *Gamete Research.* 1989; **22**: 193204.

20. Yanagimachi R, Suzuke F. A further study of lysolecithin-mediated acrosome reaction of guinea pig spermatozoa. *Gamete Research.* 1985; **11**: 29–40.

21. Parrish JJ, Susko-Parrish J, Winer MA, First NL. Capacitation of bovine sperm by heparin. *Biology of Reproduction.* 1988; **38**: 1171–80.

22. Wolf DP, Sokoloski JE. Synchronization of human sperm capacitation by low extracellular calcium exposure. *Fertility and Sterility.* 1984; **41**: 16S–17S (abstract).

23. Mortimer D. Comparison of the fertilizing ability of human spermatozoa preincubated in calcium- and strontium-containing media. *Journal of Experimental Zoology.* 1986; **237**: 21–4.

24. Mortimer D, Curtis EF, Dravland JE. The use of strontium-substituted media for capacitating human spermatozoa: an improved sperm preparation method for the zona-free hamster egg penetration test. *Fertility and Sterility.* 1986; **46**: 97–103.

25. Laws-King A, Trounson A, Sathananthan H, Kola I. Fertilization of human oocytes by microinjection of a single spermatozoon under the zona pellucida. *Fertility and Sterility.* 1987; **48**: 637–42.

26. Fishel S, Jackson P, Antinori S, Johnson J, Grossi S, Versaci C. Subzonal insemination for the alleviation of infertility. *Fertility and Sterility.* 1990; **54**: 828–35.

27. Mortimer D, Chorney MJ, Curtis EF, Trounson AO. Calcium dependence of human sperm fertilizing ability. *Journal of Experimental Zoology.* 1988; **246**: 194–201.

28. Fraser LR. Mechanisms controlling mammalian fertilisation. In: Clarke JR Jr ed. *Oxford Reviews of Reproductive Biology.* Oxford: Oxford University Press, 1984, vol. 6, pp. 174–225.

29. Perreault SD, Rogers BJ. Relationship between fertilizing ability and cAMP in human spermatozoa. *Journal of Andrology.* 1982; **3**: 396–401.

30. Boatman DE, Bavister BD. Stimulation of rhesus monkey sperm capacitation by cyclic nucleotide mediators. *Journal of Reproduction and Fertility.* 1984; **71**: 357–66.

31. Fraser LR, Ahuja KK. Metabolic and surface events in fertilization. *Gamete Research.* 1988; **20**: 491–519.

32. Yamada K, Stevenson AFG, Mettler L. Fertilization through spermatozoal microinjection: significance of acrosome reaction. *Human Reproduction.* 1988; **3**: 657–661.

33. Lacham O, Trounson A, Holden C, Mann J, Sathananthan H. Fertilization and development of mouse eggs injected under the zona pellucida with single spermatozoa treated to induce the acrosome reaction. *Gamete Research.* 1989; **23**: 233–43.

34. Talbot P, Chacon RS. A triple-stain technique for evaluating normal acrosome reactions of human sperm. *Journal of Experimental Zoology.* 1981; **215**: 201–8.

35. Moore HDM, Smith CA, Hartman TD, Bye AP. Visualization and characterization of the acrosome reaction of human spermatozoa by immunolocalization with monoclonal antibody. *Gamete Research.* 1987; **17**: 245–59.

36. Wolf DP, Boldt J, Byrd W, Bechtol KB. Acrosomal status in human ejaculated sperm with monoclonal antibodies. *Biology of Reproduction.* 1985; **32**: 1157–62.

37. Mortimer D, Curtis EF, Miller RG. Specific label-

ling by peanut agglutinin of the outer acrosome membrane of the human spermatozoon. *Journal of Reproduction and Fertility*. 1987; **81**: 127–35.

38. Mortimer D, Curtis EF, Camenzind AR. Combined use of fluorescent peanut agglutinin lectin and Hoechst 33258 to monitor the acrosomal status and vitality of human spermatozoa. *Human Reproduction*. 1990; **5**: 99–103.

39. Cross NL, Morales P, Overstreet JW, Hanson FW. Two simple methods for detecting acrosome-reacted human sperm. *Gamete Research*. 1986; **15**: 213–26.

40. Holden CA, Hyne RV, Sathananthan AH, Trounson AO. Assessment of the human sperm acrosome reaction using concanavalin A lectin. *Molecular Reproduction and Development*. 1990; **25**: 247–57.

41. Talbot P, Chacon RS. Observations on the acrosome reaction of human sperm in vitro. *American Journal of Primatology*. 1981; **1**: 211–9.

42. Plachot M, Mandelbaum J, Junca A-M. Acrosome reaction of human sperm used for in vitro fertilization. *Fertility and Sterility*. 1984; **42**: 418–23.

43. Stock CE, Fraser LR. The acrosome reaction in human sperm from men of proven fertility. *Human Reproduction*. 1987; **2**: 109–19.

44. Mortimer D, Curtis EF, Camenzind AR, Tanaka S. The spontaneous acrosome reaction of human spermatozoa incubated in vitro. *Human Reproduction*. 1989; **4**: 57–62.

45. Tesařík J. Comparison of acrosome reaction-inducing activities of human cumulus oophorus, follicular fluid and ionophore A23187 in human sperm populations of proven fertilizing ability in vitro. *Journal of Reproduction and Fertility*. 1985; **74**: 383–8.

46. Suarez SS, Wolf DP, Meizel S. Induction of the acrosome reaction in human spermatozoa by a fraction of human follicular fluid. *Gamete Research*. 1986; **14**: 107–21.

47. Siiteri JE, Gottlieb W, Meizel S. Partial characterization of a fraction from human follicular fluid that initiates the human sperm acrosome reaction in vitro. *Gamete Research*. 1988; **20**: 25–42.

48. Mortimer D, Camenzid AR. The role of follicular fluid in inducing the acrosome reaction of human spermatozoa incubated in vitro. *Human Reproduction*. 1989; **4**: 169–74.

49. Stock CE, Bates R, Lindsay KS, Edmonds DK, Fraser LR. Extended exposure to follicular fluid is required for significant stimulation of the acrosome reaction in human spermatozoa. *Journal of Reproduction and Fertility*. 1989; **86**: 401–11.

50. Meizel S, Turner KO. Glycosaminoglycans stimulate the acrosome reaction of previously capacitated hamster sperm. *Journal of Experimental Zoology*. 1986; **237**: 137–9.

51. Handrow RR, Lenz RW, Ax RL. Structural comparisons among glycosaminoglycans to promote an acrosome reaction in bovine spermatozoa. *Biochemical and Biophysics Research Communications*. 1982; **107**: 1326–32.

52. Lenz RW, Bellin ME, Ax RL. Rabbit spermatozoa undergo an acrosome reaction in the presence of glycosaminoglycans. *Gamete Research*. 1983; **8**: 11–9.

53. McLaughlin EA, Ford WCL, Hull MGR. Effect of progesterone on the intracellular calcium concentration of human spermatozoa. *Journal of Reproduction and Fertility Abstract Series*. 1990; **5**: 23 (abstract).

54. Blackmore PF, Beebe SJ, Danforth DR, Alexander N. Progesterone and 17α-hydroxyprogesterone. Novel stimulators of calcium influx in human sperm. *Journal of Biological Chemistry*. 1990; **265**: 1376–80.

55. Osman RA, Andria ML, Jones AD, Meizel S. Steroid induced exocytosis: the human sperm acrosome reaction. *Biochemical and Biophysics Research Communications*. 1989; **160**: 828–33.

56. Siiteri JE, Dandekar P, Meizel S. Human sperm acrosome reaction-initiating activity associated with the human cumulus oophorus and mural granulosa cells. *Journal of Experimental Zoology*. 1988; **246**: 71–80.

57. Stock CE, Bates R, Lindsay KS, Edmonds DK, Fraser LR. Human oocyte-cumulus complexes stimulate the human acrosome reaction. *Journal of Reproduction and Fertility*. 1989; **86**: 723–30.

58. Aitken RJ, Ross A, Hargreave T, Richardson D, Best F. Analysis of human sperm function following exposure to the ionophore A23817. Comparison of normospermic and oligozoospermic men. *Journal of Andrology*. 1984; **5**: 321–9.

59. Aitken RJ, Thatcher S, Glasier AF, Clarkson JS, Wu FCW, Baird DT. Relative ability of modified versions of the hamster oocyte penetration test, incorporating hyperosmotic medium or the ionophore A23187, to predict outcome. *Human Reproduction*. 1987; **2**: 227–31.

60. De Jonge CJ, Mack SR, Zaneveld LJD. Synchronous assay for human sperm capacitation and the acrosome reaction. *Journal of Andrology*. 1989; **10**: 232–9.

61. Lassalle B, Testart J. Human sperm injection into the perivitelline space (SI-PVS) of hamster oocytes: Effect of sperm pretreatment by calcium-ionophore A23187 and freezing-thawing on the penetration rate and polyspermy. *Gamete Research*. 1988; **20**: 301–11

62. Woolley DM, Richardson DW. Ultrastructural injury to human spermatozoa after freezing and thawing. *Journal of Reproduction and Fertility*. 1978; **53**: 389–94.

63. Blumenfeld Z, Nahhas F. Pretreatment of sperm with human follicular fluid for borderline male infertility. *Fertility and Sterility*. 1989; **51**: 863–8.

64. Fukuda M, Cross NL, Cummings-Paulson L, Yee B. Correlation of acrosomal status and sperm per-

formance in the sperm penetration assay. *Fertility and Sterility.* 1989; **52**: 836–41.

65. McClure RD, Tom RA, Dandekar PV. Optimising the sperm penetration assay with human follicular fluid. *Fertility and Sterility.* 1990; **53**: 546–50.

66. Mortimer D, Camenzind AR. Influence of extracellular pH upon the human sperm acrosome reaction. *Journal of Andrology.* 1990; **11**: (suppl. 1), 27 (abstract).

67. Markert CL. Fertilization of mammalian eggs by sperm injection. *Journal of Experimental Zoology.* 1983; **228**: 195–201.

68. Keefer CL. Fertilization by sperm injection in the rabbit. *Gamete Research.* 1989; **22**: 59–69.

69. Lanzendorf S, Maloney M, Ackerman S, Acosta A, Hodgen G. Fertilizing potential of acrosome-defective sperm following microsurgical injection into eggs. *Gamete Research.* 1988; **19**: 329–37.

70. Lanzendorf SE, Maloney MK, Veeck LL, Slusser J, Hodgen GD, Rosenwaks Z. A preclinical evaluation of pronuclear formation by microinjection of human spermatozoa into human oocytes. *Fertility and Sterility.* 1988; **49**: 835–42.

71. Martin RH, Ko E, Rademaker A. Human sperm chromosome complements after microinjection of hamster eggs. *Journal of Reproduction and Fertility.* 1988; **84**: 179–86.

72. Mortimer D. Semen analysis and sperm washing techniques. In: Gagnon C (ed.) *Controls of Sperm Motility: Biological and Clinical Aspects.* Boca Raton: CRC Press, 1990: 263–84.

73. Trounson AO, Leeton JF, Wood C, Webb J, Kovacs G. The investigation of idiopathic infertility by in vitro fertilization. *Fertility and Sterility.* 1980; **34**: 431–8.

74. Mahadevan MM, Trounson AO, Leeton JF. The relationship of tubal blockage, infertility of unknown cause, suspected male infertility, and endometriosis to success of in vitro fertilization and embryo transfer. *Fertility and Sterility.* 1983; **40**: 755–62.

75. Yates CA, de Kretser DM. Male factor infertility and in vitro fertilization. *Journal of In Vitro Fertilization and Embryo Transfer.* 1987; **4**: 141–7.

76. Overstreet JW, Yanagimachi R, Katz DF, Hayashi K, Hanson FW. Penetration of human spermatozoa into the human zona pellucida and the zona-free hamster egg: a study of fertile donors and infertile patients. *Fertility and Sterility.* 1980; **33**: 534–42.

77. Aitken RJ, Best FSM, Templeton AA, Richardson DW, Schats R, Djahanbakhch O, Lees MM. Fertilizing capacity of human spermatozoa: a study of oligozoospermia and unexplained infertility. In: D'Agata R, Lipsett MB, Polosa P, van der Molen JH (eds) *Recent Advances in Male Reproduction: Molecular Basis and Clinical Implications.* New York: Raven Press, 1983, pp. 13–25.

78. Aitken RJ, Clarkson JS. Significance of reactive oxygen species and antioxidants in defining the efficacy of sperm preparation techniques. *Journal of Andrology.* 1988; **9**: 367–76.

79. Aitken RJ, Clarkson JS. Cellular basis of defective sperm function and its association with the genesis of reactive oxygen species by human spermatozoa. *Journal of Reproduction and Fertility.* 1987; **81**: 459–69.

80. Alvarez JG, Touchstone JC, Blasco L, Storey BT. Spontaneous lipid peroxidation and production of hydrogen eproxide and superoxide in human spermatozoa. Superoxide dismutase as major enzyme protectant against oxygen toxicity. *Journal of Andrology.* 1987; **8**: 338–48.

81. Aitken RJ, Clarkson JS, Hargreave TB, Irvine DS, Wu FCW. Analysis of the relationship between defective sperm function and the generation of reactive oxygen species in cases of oligozoospermia. *Journal of Andrology.* 1989; **10**: 214–20.

82. Mortimer D. Sperm preparation techniques and iatrogenic failures of in-vitro fertilization. *Human Reproduction.* 1991; **6**: 173–6.

83. Dravland JE, Mortimer D. A simple discontinuous Percoll gradient procedure for washing human spermatozoa. *International Research Communication Service Medical Science.* 1985; **13**: 16–7.

84. Serafini P, Blank W, Tran C, Mansourian M, Tan T, Batzofin J. Enhanced penetration of zona-free hamster ova by sperm prepared by Nycodenz and Percoll gradient centrifugation. *Fertility and Sterility.* 1990; **53**: 551–5.

85. Gellert-Mortimer ST, Clarke GN, Baker HWG, Hyne RV, Johnston WIH. Evaluation of Nycodenz and Percoll density gradients for the selection of motile human spermatozoa. *Fertility and Sterility.* 198; **49**: 335–41.

86. Lucena E, Lucena C, Gomez M, Ortiz JA, Ruiz J, Arango A, Diaz C, Beuerman C. Recovery of motile sperm using the migration-sedimentation technique in an in vitro fertilization embryo transfer programme. *Human Reproduction.* 1989; **4**: 163–5.

87. Wikland M, Wik O, Steen Y, Qvist K, Söderlund B, Janson PO. A self-migration method for preparation of sperm for in vitro fertilization. *Human Reproduction.* 1987; **2**: 191–5.

88. Yovich JM, Edirisinghe WR, Cummins JM, Yovich JL. Influence of pentoxifylline in severe male factor infertility. *Fertility and Sterility.* 1990; **53**: 715–22.

89. Tomkins PT, Houghton JA. The rapid induction of the acrosome reaction of human spermatozoa by electropermeabilisation. *Fertility and Sterility.* 1988; **50**: 329–36.

90. Rickords LF, White KL, Wiltbank JN. Effect of microinjection and two types of electrical stimuli on bovine sperm-hamster egg penetration. *Molecular Reproduction and Development.* 1990; **27**: 163–7.

91. Vazquez-Levin M, Kaplan P, Sandler B, Garrisi GJ, Gordon J, Navot D. The predictive values of

zona-free hamster egg sperm penetration assay for failure of human in vitro fertilization and subsequent successful zona drilling. *Fertility and Sterility*. 1990; **53**: 1055–9.

92. Lassalle B, Courtot AM, Testart J. In vitro fertilization of hamster and human oocytes by microinjection of human sperm. *Gamete Research*. 1987; **16**: 69–78.

93. Levron J, Manor D, Brandes JM, Itskovitz J.

Human sperm and hamster oocyte interaction: a model system to assess sperm entry into the oocyte after partial zona dissection. *Fertility and Sterility*. 1990; **54**: 342–5.

94. Garrisi GJ, Talansky BE, Grunfeld L, Sapira V, Navot D, Gordon JW. Clinical evaluation of three approaches to micromanipulation-assisted fertilization. *Fertility and Sterility*. 1990; **54**: 671–7.

Section III
Subzonal insemination

Chapter 5

The need for micro-assisted fertilisation in human reproduction

O. Lacham-Kaplan and A. Trounson

Introduction

Men with reduced semen quality may have a very poor prognosis for conception *in vivo*[1], and *in vitro* fertilisation (IVF) has been used to provide a therapy for couples in whom the male partner is infertile.[2] The possibility now exists to isolate the relatively few spermatozoa in an ejaculate using IVF preparation procedures, and inseminate their partner's eggs with around 50 000 motile sperm. In many couples the incidence of fertilisation can approach that for men with normal semen quality. In a major long-term prospective clinical trial[3] we have examined the fertilisation rates and outcome for men with reduced semen quality, using conventional IVF insemination. For this trial, men with male factor infertility were classified according to the criteria described in Table 5.1. The results obtained in this trial are summarised in Table 5.2. Fertilisation rates are significantly reduced for men with single or multiple defects in semen quality, but in most groups at least one embryo is transferred as multiple eggs are recovered. After embryo transfer pregnancy and delivery is similar to that for patients with normal semen quality (Table 5.2); but due to the reduced incidence of fertilisation, the overall expectation for pregnancy or delivery will be progressively reduced as the severity of the male factor problem is increased.

If fertilisation fails on a single occasion, this is not considered significant as fertilisation might occur in a subsequent cycle. The prognosis is then similar to those patients who achieved fertilisation in the first cycle. However, the probability for fertilisation after two consecutive failures is dramatically reduced and this situation usually results in a rec-

Table 5.1 Classification of male factor patients in prospective clinical trial at Monash

Male factor groups	Motility %	Count	Abnormal morphology %
Single defect	< 40	normal	normal
	normal	$5–20 \times 10^6$/ml	normal
	normal	$< 5 \times 10^6$/ml	normal
	normal	normal	> 50
Double defect	< 40	$< 20 \times 10^6$/ml	normal
	< 40	normal	> 50
	normal	$< 20 \times 10^6$/ml	> 50
Triple defect	< 40	$< 20 \times 10^6$/ml	> 50

ommendation that the patients use donor sperm for artificial insemination or IVF.

There also exists a second group of patients who have such severe defects in semen quality and sperm function that standard IVF technology is inappropriate. For both these groups of patients micro-assisted fertilisation has the potential to provide a mode of therapy for their infertility.

In vitro, the major barrier to penetration of the egg by the sperm is the extracellular glycoprotein coat (zona pellucida) which surrounds the egg cell. It is possible to dissolve the zona in acid medium or by protease enzymes, or to tear a hole in the zona with a micromanipulation needle (see Chapters 1, 7 and 8). These are relatively gross procedures which enable spermatozoa to have direct access to the egg cell. Several major problems arise with zona disruption techniques; the incidence of lethal polyspermia is dramatically increased[4] and the viability of eggs is dramatically reduced.[4,5]

We have approached this problem differently. We considered the possibility of micro-injecting a single spermatozoon into the perivitelline space and thereby bypassing the necessity for sperm to penetrate through the zona pellucida. We showed for the first time that human eggs could be fertilised by this approach.[6] Using a mouse model, it was also shown that murine eggs fertilised by micro-injection of a sperm under the zona will develop normally to term.[7] This demonstrated for the first time that eggs fertilised by this procedure were viable.

We elevated the fertilisation rates achieved with subzonal micro-injection of a single sperm in the mouse from around 25 per cent[7] to approximately 40 per cent by technical adjustments of

the procedure[8]; and indeed we observed both acrosome reacted and non-reacted sperm in the perivitelline space of eggs which failed to fertilise.[8] Further increases in fertilisation rates to about 70 per cent have been achieved when mouse sperm were exposed to electric fields to induce electropermeabilisation.[9] It is also possible to elevate fertilisation rates in the mouse by exposure of sperm to chemical inducers of capacitation. We also confirmed the high viability of eggs both *in vitro*[8] and *in vivo*[9] after fertilisation by sperm micro-injection.[8]

In the human, we have also shown that eggs fertilised after micro-injection of sperm under the zona have a similar rate of chromosomal abnormality as eggs fertilised by conventional IVF techniques.[10] In this study we used sperm from men with severe male factor infertility, characterised by the production of very few sperm, or from patients who had failed to fertilise their wives' eggs on repeated occasions. These limited data (Table 5.3) provide some reassurance of the safety of the subzonal micro-insemination technique and the chromosomal normality of the fertilising sperm from these patients.

Clinical trial in subzonal micro-injection

Only patients who had failed on at least two consecutive occasions to fertilise their wives' eggs, or those with too few motile sperm for conventional IVF, were included in the trial of sperm micro-injection.

Table 5.2 Results of IVF for male factor patients in prospective trial at Monash

Group	Patient n	Oocytes collected n	Oocytes fertilised %	Embryos transferred %	Pregnancies transfer %	Deliveries transfer %
Normal semen	1093	2514	71.5	90.6	15.5	10.5
Single defect	120	229	61.6*	83.0*	17.9	13.2
Double defect	124	202	49.9*	72.2*	20.4	13.2
Triple defect	52	103	38.9*	61.2**	11.1	9.5

Notes: * P < 0.5.
   ** P < 0.005.

Table 5.3 Chromosomal abnormality rates in eggs fertilised by sperm micro-insemination and conventional IVF techniques

	Micro-inseminated eggs	*Conventional IVF eggs*
Number of eggs with scorable karyotypes (n patients)	18 (12)	30 (6)
Number of fertilised eggs that were chromosomally abnormal	4 (22%)	9 (30%)
Number of monosomic eggs	2	5
Number of trisomic eggs	2	4
Number of structural abnormalities	0	0

Note: *All male factor patients.
Source: Kola et al., 1990.[10]

The cumulus cells of mature oocyte-cumulus complexes were removed with hyaluronidase and one to ten motile sperm were micro-injected into the perivitelline space as described previously.[6] Sperm were prepared by conventional IVF techniques. The results are summarised in Table 5.4. Only 11 per cent of the eggs fertilised, with increasing polyspermy when the number of sperm micro-injected was increased. Increasing polyspermy has also been observed with injection of multiple sperm in other studies (Table 5.5).

In a study comparing fertilisation rates for normal and infertile sperm we showed that fertilisation rates were approximately three to four times higher with sperm from the normal group (Table 5.6). Hence sperm from the severe male factor patients had a reduced capability to fertilise eggs even after micro-insemination.

We have also compared fertilisation rates with eggs which have been micro-inseminated and either incubated overnight with a dilute solution of the husbands' sperm (5–10 × 10^6 sperm/ml) or cultured without sperm. There was a signifi-

cant (p<0.02) increase in fertilisation rates (Table 5.7) from 11 per cent in the eggs cultured without sperm in the solution to 25 per cent when eggs were cultured with the dilute solution of the husbands' sperm. In a study where a small number (n=6) of patients had their eggs divided into three groups: micro-inseminated with sperm and incubated in dilute sperm overnight, micro-inseminated with sperm but not cultured with sperm and micro-injected with medium (no sperm) and incubated in diluted sperm solution overnight, the fertilisation rates were 18 per cent, 5 per cent and 13 per cent respectively.

There appeared to be an increased incidence of blockage to cleavage at the pronucleate stage in eggs fertilised by sperm from severe male factor patients following subzonal micro-insemination (Table 5.8). The blockage appeared to be related to semen quality rather than micromanipulation, because pronucleate eggs from men with normal semen showed no signs of blockage at the pronucleate stage (Table 5.8). Retarded or blocked cleavage has also been reported for eggs fertilised

Table 5.4 Fertilisation of eggs micro-inseminated with spermatozoa from severe male factor patients

Number of sperm injected	Number of eggs injected	Number of normally fertilised eggs	Number of polyspermic eggs
1	109	9 (8%)	0
2–3	39	4 (10%)	0
4	172	17 (10%)	3 (2%)
5–10	49	3 (6%)	6 (2%)
Total	369	33 (9%)	6 (2%)

Table 5.5 Fertilisation and polyspermy in hamster and human eggs micro-inseminated with multiple human sperm under the zona pellucida

Species of egg	Number of human sperm	Number of eggs injected	Number of eggs fertilised	Number of polyspermic eggs	Reference
Hamster	1–4	66	4 (6%)	0 (0%)	
	5–12	68	18 (26%)	10 (55%)	
	12	36	2 (6%)	2 (100%)	(13)
Human	3–5	7	3 (43%)	0 (0%)	(13)
	10–20	3	2 (67%)	2 (100%)	
Human (male factor)	1–20	585	95 (16%)	35 (39%)	(14)

Table 5.6 Fertilisation with micro-injection using sperm with normal (N) and male factor (MF) parameters

Number of eggs injected	Sperm parameters (number of sperm)	Number of normally fertilised eggs	Number of polyspermic eggs
474	MF (1–10)	43 (9%)*	8 (2%)
43	N (1–10)	12 (28%)*	1 (2%)

Note: *$X^2 = 12.7$; $P < 0.001$.

Table 5.7 Fertilisation results of micro-injected eggs cultured with or without sperm solution for 18–24 hours

Technique	Number of sperm injected	Number of eggs injected	Number of normally fertilised eggs	Number of polyspermic eggs
–	1–3	16	1 (6%)	0
with sperm	1–3	38	4 (11%)	1 (3%)
–	4	61	7 (12%)	0
with sperm	4	84	20 (24%)	4 (5%)
–	5–10	28	2 (7%)	2 (7%)
with sperm	5–10	20	5 (25%)	2 (10%)
Total				
–	1–10	105	10 (10%)*	2 (2%)
with sperm	1–10	142	29 (20%)*	7 (5%)

Note: *$P < 0.02$.

Table 5.8 Development in culture of micro-injected eggs with sperm with normal (N) and male factor (MF) parameters

Treatment	Number of normally fertilised eggs	Number of eggs blocked at 2-pronuclei stage
Eggs micro-inseminated with MF sperm	43	9 (20%)
Eggs micro-inseminated with MF sperm and incubated with sperm overnight	29	7 (24%)
Total	72	16 (22%)
Eggs injected with N sperm	12	0 (0%)

Table 5.9 Comparison of the results from the micro-injection technique in the mouse model with the results from the clinical trial

	Mouse model *%*	*Human clinical trial* *%*
Fertilisation:		
single sperm	25–45	10
multiple > 5	49–53	12–14
polyspermic	5	30–50
Addition of sperm to injected eggs	–	20–25
Development in culture	90–100	70–75
	(0% block at 2PN stage)	(25% block at 2PN stage)
Implantation	82	5
Fetuses	54	0

after zona disruption[4] and zona drilling.[11] We have also observed that mouse eggs fertilised by immature sperm have an increased incidence of retarded cleavage, and cessation of cleavage when compared to eggs fertilised by mature sperm.[12]

Summary

In the initial clinical trial at Monash, 32 of 112 couples undergoing subzonal sperm micro-insemination had embryos transferred and three pregnancies were initiated. Most of the transfers (29) were single embryos at two- to eight-cell stage. In a second clinical trial there are two ongoing pregnancies, one of whom has twins.

When compared with the results for mouse sperm micro-insemination (Table 5.9), it is apparent that substantial improvements are possible for subzonal human sperm micro-insemination. Eventually it should be possible to elevate fertilisation rates with micro-insemination of single sperm to 50 per cent or higher. It is necessary to achieve this level of fertilisation to provide an effective therapy for patients with severe male factor infertility.

References

1. Yates CA, de Kretser MD. Male factor infertility and IVF. *Journal of In Vitro Fertilisation and Embryo Transfer*. 1987; **4**: 141–7.
2. Baker HWG, Burger HG, de Kretser DM, Hudson B. Diagnosis and management of hypogonadism, infertility and impotence. In: Santen RG, Swerd RS (eds) *Male Reproductive Dysfunction*. 1986.
3. Yates CA, de Kretser DK, Trounson A. Unpublished data.
4. Bourne H, Hale L, Vassiiliadis A, Lue DY, Lopata A, Baker G. Viability of embryos resulting from fertilisation of zona opened oocytes. Presented at 9th Annual Meeting, Perth, 26–29 September 1990. Published by the Infertility Society of Australia.
5. Trounson AO, Moore NW. The survival and development of sheep eggs following complete or partial removal of the zona pellucida. *Journal of Reproduction Fertility*. 1974; **41**: 97–105.
6. Laws-King A, Trounson A, Sathananthan H, Kola I. Fertilisation of human oocytes by micro-injection of a single spermatozoon under the zona pellucida. *Fertility and Sterility*. 1987; **48**: 637–42.
7. Mann J. Full term development of mouse eggs fertilised by a spermatozoon micro-injected under the zona pellucida. *Biology of Reproduction*. 1988; **38**: 1077–83.
8. Lacham O, Trounson A, Holden C, Mann J, Sathananthan H. Fertilisation and development of mouse eggs injected under the zona pellucida with single spermatozoa treated to induce the acrosome reaction. *Gamete Research*. 1989; **23**: 233–43.
9. Barnaby E, Trounson A. Unpublished data.
10. Kola I, Lacham O, Jansen PSR, Turner M, Trounson A. Chromosomal analysis of human oocytes fertilised by micro-injection of spermatozoa into the perivitelline space. *Human Reproduction*. 1990; **5**: 575–7.
11. Garrisi GJ, Talansky BE, Grundfeld L, Sapira V,

Navot D, Gordon JW. Clinical evaluation of three approaches to micromanipulation assisted fertilisation. *Fertility and Sterility*. 1990; **54**: 671–7.

12. Lacham O, Trounson A. Fertilizing capacity of epididymal and testicular spermatozoa microinjected under the zona pellucida of the mouse oocyte. *Molecular Reproduction and Development*. 1991; **29**: 85–93.

13. Lassalle B, Courtot AM, Testar J. In vitro fertilisation of hamster and human oocytes by micro-injection of human sperm. *Gamete Research*. 1987; **16**: 89–95.

14. Lippi J, Turner M, Jansen PSR. Pregnancies after in vitro fertilisation by sperm micro-injection into the perivitelline space. Presented at 9th Annual Meeting, Perth, 26–29 September 1990. Published by the Infertility Society of Australia.

Chapter 6

Sperm micro-injection and microfertilisation

A. H. Sathananthan, S-C. Ng, A. Bongso and S. S. Ratnam

Introduction

Micro-insemination sperm transfer (MIST)[1,2], also referred to as subzonal sperm injection (SUZI)[3], is now being used in clinical practice as a technique for the treatment of severe male infertility, since the first baby was conceived by this technique in 1988.[1] The development and use of the technique have been described elsewhere in this volume. Despite the numerous pregnancies and live births, the actual success rates (1 to 5 per cent) to date has been rather disappointing considering the research, expertise, technology and cost that have gone into the development of this technique.[2–9] Evidently the treatment of severe male infertility seems to be the challenge as there is presently limited hope for men with the triple sperm defects of reduced sperm number, motility and morphology, by conventional *in vitro* fertilisation (IVF) or spontaneous conception[10]. Since SUZI is also used for cases of repeated failed fertilisation during IVF, an inherent egg factor may also exist and affect the success rates of this technique. We present here the clinical results of sperm micro-injection (MI) obtained at the National University Hospital, Singapore, and some of the scientific work preceding the development of this technology in the human.

Indications for SUZI

Since SUZI is expensive and time consuming it needs to be justified to the patient. It is very much a research procedure at present and mainly confined to the larger IVF centres. Four indications for SUZI have been considered in our clinical trials:

1. Severe oligozoospermia where the sperm count was less than 5 million/ml
2. Oligoasthenoteratozoospermia – severe male factor infertility involving sperm number, motility and morphology (triple sperm defects)
3. Complete asthenozoospermia – totally immotile sperm
4. Repeated failed fertilisation during conventional IVF, although sperm and oocytes seemed normal (our transmission electron microscopy [TEM] analysis of unfertilised oocytes over the years has shown many instances where sperm have failed to bind or penetrate the zona pellucida (ZP)). Rare sperm abnormalities such as round headed acrosomeless sperm, globozoospermia, may also require sperm injection.

Technique of SUZI

The technique of SUZI is now well established, since it was first shown that human oocytes could be fertilised by sperm MI.[4] In a subsequent study we showed conclusively by transmission electron microscopy (TEM) that normal fertilisation of human oocytes could be achieved by injection of either single or multiple sperm into the perivitelline space (PVS).[8,9] The specific details of our sperm injection procedure have been reviewed by Ng et al.[2] and will be dealt with only briefly.

Sperm preparation

Since poor sperm quality was a major factor justifying SUZI, the entire semen sample was used and sperm were prepared by the Ficoll entrapment procedure.[11] This procedure improves sperm quality from the World Health Organisation (WHO) grade I to grade II motility with concomitant improvement in fertilisation.[12] The semen after liquefaction was centrifuged ($450\times$gravity (g)) to pellet the sperm which was then mixed with 0.5 ml of 5 per cent Ficoll in phosphate buffered saline (PBS). This mixture (0.1 ml) was then introduced gently under Whittingham's T_6 medium (0.5 ml) and incubated in 5 per cent CO_2, 5 per cent O_2 and 90 per cent N_2 (5:5:90) at 37°C for one to two hours. The motile sperm from the supernatant were then subjected to high speed centrifugation in a microcentrifuge at $3352\times$g for 10 minutes. Recently a further one to two hours incubation of sperm was done prior to microcentrifugation to enhance the acrosome reaction (AR) which is a prerequisite to gamete fusion.[13–15] The final sperm suspension was

made in T_6 medium with 20 mM Hepes and 10 per cent heat-activated human serum (HS) instead of 5 per cent Ficoll in PBS.

Immotile sperm for SUZI were treated differently. Semen was washed twice in T_6 medium, pelleted, resuspended and incubated for six to eight hours in the same medium before micro-injection.[16] Sperm parameters used for SUZI are shown in Table 6.1.[17]

Oocyte collection

The women were stimulated with either: (1) clomiphene and human menopausal gonadotrophin (HMG), (2) purified follicle-stimulating hormone (FSH) and HMG, or (3) buserelin 'down regulation' and FSH. Serum oestradiol (E_2) was monitored and follicle size was estimated by ultrasound scanning. Human chorionic gonadotrophin (HCG) was administered when at least two follicles reached an average of 16 mm and E_2 reached > 300 pg/ml/follicle $\geq$ 14 mm. The oocytes were collected by transvaginal ultrasound 34 hours after HCG and incubated at 37°C in T_6 medium with heat-activated HS for four to six hours. The cumulus was removed by gentle micropipetting after exposure to 0.1 per cent bovine hyaluronidase in T_6 medium, and only metaphase II oocytes were micro-injected within an hour after this procedure. Each oocyte was manipulated in T_6 medium with 20 mM Hepes and 10 per cent HS.

Micro-injection

Prepared sperm were introduced into a micro-pipette (Drummond, Pennsylvania) from the rear end and this was attached to a micro-injector 5242 (Eppendorf, Hamburg). The micropipette was made with a micropuller and microgrinder (Narishige, Tokyo) (see Chapter 2). The external diameter of its tip was 10–15 μm, while the internal diameter was 8–12 μm. The tip was bevelled at an angle 25°–35°. The holding pipette for the oocyte was drawn out from a Pasteur pipette over an ethanol flame. Both pipettes were bent to allow horizontal manipulation over the microscope stage. Seven to 10 motile sperm were injected into

Table 6.1 SUZI with initial sperm density of less than 10.0×10^6/ml

Previous total density (10^6/ml)	0.1 − 5.0	5.1 − 10.0
Number of cases	46	32
Previous density	2.40 ± 1.30	7.30 ± 1.4
Fresh density	1.10 ± 1.27	2.66 ± 4.4
Postwash density	0.13 ± 0.19	0.22 ± 0.2
Postcentrifugation density	1.20 ± 1.09	1.52 ± 1.2

Source: Ng et al., 1990.[17]

the PVS using a micromanipulator fitted to an inverted microscope with a warm stage set at 37°C (Carl Zeiss, Germany). After manipulation oocytes were washed three times in T_6 medium before incubation overnight. Pronuclei were checked 14–22 hours after SUZI and normal 2PN zygotes were transferred into the Fallopian tube.[2] The outcome of SUZI is shown in Table 6.2.[17]

Sperm assessment for SUZI

In our evaluation of sperm for SUZI we have endeavoured to assess sperm quality objectively by TEM[18], in addition to routine assessment by light microscopy (LM) or computerised semen analysis. TEM examination of sperm in pellets left over after preparation of SUZI, assessment of sperm in the PVS and of those in the ooplasm after incorporation have enabled us to assess sperm quality. Both morphological features and the AR were studied in these situations especially when the sperm had triple defects or were completely immotile. The effect of ultracentrifugation was also studied since it has been reported that centrifugation at speeds in excess of 800 ×g can be detrimental.[19] Sperm head morphology has now come into focus as a salient factor determining the outcome of IVF.[21,22] Abnormalities of the head not only include bizarre shapes and forms but could also affect the acrosome, nucleus and the postacrosomal region.[22] Poor quality sperm invariably have midpiece and tail defects in addition to head defects. Acrosome, midpiece

and tail aberrations could affect zona penetration and motility, but these are not of major importance in SUZI, where the sperm are introduced into the PVS. Nuclear or chromatin defects that are so prevalent even in normal sperm samples[23] may result in genetic defects or abnormal development, though this has yet to be established in ART.[2] Sperm with nuclear defects have been shown to penetrate the cumulus, ZP and even the oocyte.[24,25] We have shown a variety of head defects of sperm injected into the PVS and in a few after incorporation into the oocyte (Figure 6.1). Abnormal sperm were also seen to fuse with the oocyte after SUZI (Figure 6.2). So it is evident that abnormal sperm have an even chance of fertilising the oocyte after MI, and sperm selection for SUZI is a dilemma since it is not possible to visualise head defects with the injecting microscope. This raises ethical concerns as to the selection of sperm for MI, especially if a single sperm is used. Our earlier studies concentrated on the injection of single sperm[8] and since it was shown that some mammalian oocytes

Table 6.2 Outcome of SUZI: initial sperm density of less than 10.0×10^6/ml

Previous total density (10^6/ml)	0.1 − 5.0	5.1 − 10.0
Metaphase II oocytes	284	175
Sperm (n) transferred	5.9 ± 3.5	6.4 ± 2.8
2PN ova	36 (12.7%)	20 (11.4%)
3PN ova	9 (3.2%)	1 (0.06%)
Patient transfers	23	14
Pregnancies	3 (13.0%)*	1 (7.1%)†
Delivered	1	−

Note: *One ectopic, one missed abortion;
†biochemical.

Source: Ng et al. 1990.[17]

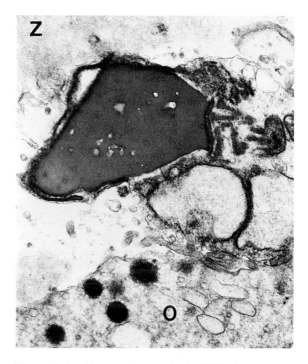

Figure 6.1 Abnormal sperm in the PVS of an unfertilised oocyte after SUZI

have vitelline blocks to polyspermy to varying degrees[26,27] we decided to attempt the multiple sperm injection technique in Singapore so that there might be some degree of natural selection of sperm at the level of the oolemma.[9] Our TEM studies have shown that 33 per cent of sperm located in the PVS after SUZI were highly abnormal in structure[9] and further studies of unfertilised oocytes have revealed that there is even a higher incidence (50–60 per cent) of abnormal sperm in the PVS, since men with multiple sperm defects are usually chosen for this procedure. Chromosome analyses of a limited number of oocytes after micro-injection of sperm from male factor patients have shown no significant differences in chromosomal abnormality, when compared to oocytes fertilised by conventional IVF.[28] This was done mainly to test the safety of the technique of MI since there is arbitrary selection of sperm. The incidence of chromosomal

anomalies in sperm and oocytes has been reviewed by Ng et al.[2] in relation to SUZI. The overall incidence of chromosomal anomalies in human sperm (8–12 per cent) is lower than that for oocytes (20–21 per cent). Haploid karyotypes of sperm with three or more defects need to be investigated to determine whether such sperm could contribute significantly to chromosomal aberrations in the embryo. The best stage to detect such anomolies is at syngamy[28], especially if there is a delay in pronuclear breakdown or the first cleavage division.

Acrosome reaction in microfertilisation

It is now well established that sperm capacitation and the AR are important prerequisites for gamete membrane fusion both during IVF and microfertilisation.[9,25,29] The AR is the morphological expression of sperm capacitation, a physiological process which begins in the sperm preparation medium and is completed either in the cumulus or at the surface of the ZP during conventional IVF.[15,24] We have shown that the AR could occur in the PVS of oocytes (Figures 6.3 and 6.4) after SUZI.[9] Earlier studies showed that acrosome reacting sperm could fuse with the oocyte if they are brought into close proximity of the oolemma.[25] Hence the selection of an acrosome-reacted sperm is not as critical as selecting a normal sperm for SUZI, neither of which is possible with the light microscope (LM). However, it is desirable to have a population of capacitated or acrosome-reacted sperm for micro-injection to ensure better chances of fertilisation. This is particularly relevant if the sperm sample is of poor quality with few motile sperm or if a single sperm is injected into the PVS.[8] Hence methods to synchronise sperm capacitation[8,30,31] may be desirable to increase the number of acrosome-reacted sperm for micro-injection. Routine sperm preparation methods have been used for successful microfertilisation[16,32]; we have used the Ficoll method of sperm separation for poor quality semen.[12] The human sperm AR is rather difficult to assess by LM unless fluorescent staining methods are used.[33,34] The most reliable

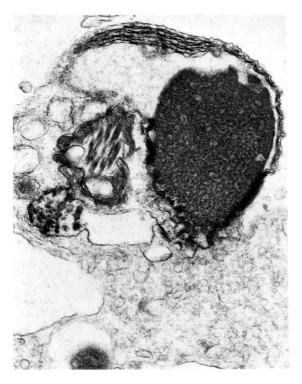

Figure 6.2 Abnormal sperm in the PVS fusing with the oocyte after SUZI. Evidently the postacrosomal region had fused with the egg as observed in serial sections × 27 300

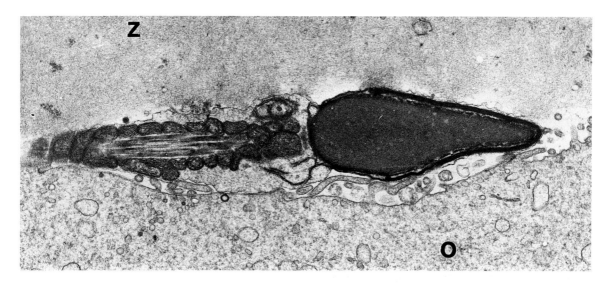

Figure 6.3 Acrosome intact sperm in the PVS of an oocyte after SUZI. (Reproduced from Ng et al[55])

method of assessment is by TEM, though laborious and time consuming. Further, the early stages of the AR can only be visualised by TEM[14] and this is quite important to objectively assess sperm function *in vitro*. Our preliminary TEM studies on poor quality and immotile sperm used for micro-

injection show that the incidence of the AR is quite low (10–15 per cent) even after four to six hours incubation in T_6 medium. The presence of dead sperm among immotile sperm makes it difficult to assess the AR accurately since many of the dead sperm are nude and resemble acrosome-reacted

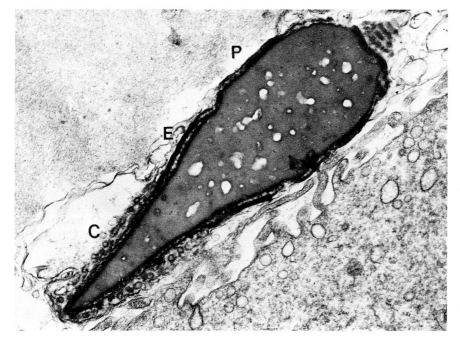

Figure 6.4 Acrosome-reacting sperm in the PVS of a fertilised ovum four hours after SUZI. The acrosome cap has vesiculated. (Reproduced from Ng et al[55])

sperm. Human sperm, unlike mouse sperm, are slow to capacitate *in vitro*.[31] In the first one to six hours incubation only about 10 per cent of sperm show evidence of the AR in pellets.[35] There is also no significant difference in the incidence of the AR in different IVF media. Further the rates of capacitation assessed by the morphology of the acrosome seem to vary considerably in different sperm samples incubated in the same medium. In our assessment of over 120 unfertilised micro-injected oocytes by TEM we found sperm showing various stages of the AR. In a previous study[9] of 100 sperm assessed in the PVS three to 48 hours after SUZI, only 24 per cent were acrosome reacting or reacted, while the others were intact (unreacted). Even sperm with nuclear and head defects were seen to undergo the AR in the PVS. Thus the AR could occur or be completed at the surface of the oocyte.

Microfertilisation

The process of microfertilisation after SUZI is no different to fertilisation *in vitro*.[9,14,15] All criteria of fertilisation, namely sperm incorporation, cortical granule (CG) exocytosis, abstriction of second polar body and pronuclear formation were documented (Figures 6.5–6.10), in addition to evidence of sperm midpieces and tails in the ooplasm.[8,9,30] Sperm/oocyte membrane fusion was observed in two oocytes but the sperm were grossly abnormal (Figure 6.2). Evidently the postacrosomal region had fused with the oolemma. Sperm/oocyte fusion has also been confirmed in the mouse.[37] Incorporated sperm showed decondensation of chromatin and were still associated with remnants of the

midpiece (Figure 6.5). A sperm with nuclear defects was also incorporated and was expanding chromatin.[9] Hence it is more than likely that abnormal sperm can fertilise the oocyte. The majority (85 per cent) of the oocytes were unfertilised and parthenogenetic activation was a rare occurrence. Karyotypes of unfertilised oocytes show that most of them are haploid (Table 6.3). Ng et al.[36] have reviewed the genetic aspects of

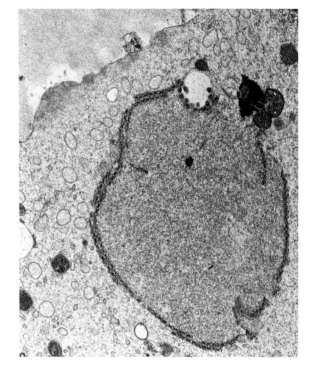

Figure 6.5 Sperm head soon after incorporation into the ooplasm after SUZI. Its chromatin has decondensed and a remnant of the centriolar complex is associated with the basal region of the sperm head × 17 500. (Reproduced from Sathananthan et al[9])

Table 6.3 Karyotypes of human oocytes that failed to fertilise after micro-injection[36]

	Haploid n = 23	Diploid n = 26	Hyperploid n = 25/26	Hypoploid n = 11	Parthenogenetic	Degenerated	Total
Fresh oocytes:							
SUZI	19	1	1	0	1	14	36
MI into egg	6	1	0	0	0	7	14
Aged oocytes:							
SUZI	17	5	3	0	2	29	56
MI into egg	2	0	0	1	1	3	7

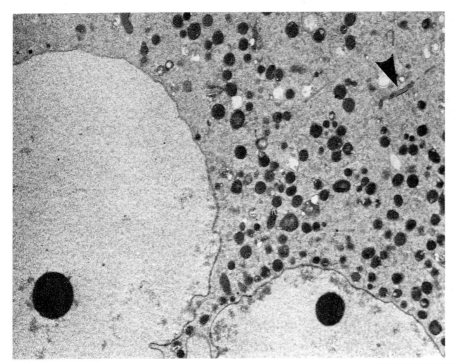

Figure 6.6 Normally fertilised ovum 12 hours after single sperm injection into the PVS. Two pronuclei are associated with a sperm tail (arrow) × 11 900. (Reproduced from Laws-King et al[8])

micro-injection. Spontaneous release of CG was not observed, unless the oocytes were perforated by micro-injection. Most of the fertilised ova (85 per cent) showed evidence of two pronuclei assessed by Normarski microscopy and only 2 to 3 per cent had multiple pronuclei. Normal fertilisation has been confirmed by TEM both after single (Figures 6.6–6.8) and multiple sperm injection.[7,9] A tripronuclear oocyte revealed two sperm tails associated with two pronuclei proving that two sperm had penetrated the oocyte, possibly simultaneously (Figure 6.11).

Block to polyspermy/sperm receptors

It is evident from the results of microfertilisation (Table 6.2) that monospermic penetration is the usual outcome, even though seven to 10 sperm were used for SUZI. We thus postulated that a vitelline block to polyspermy may exist in the human.[9] Results of assisted fertilisation from other groups[3,4] (Chapter 5) seem to support this theory and the

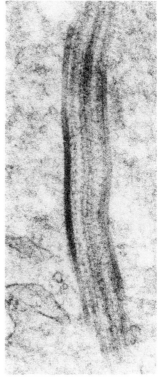

Figure 6.7 Sperm tail axoneme at high magnification in Figure 6.6 × 70 000. (Reproduced from Laws-King et al[8])

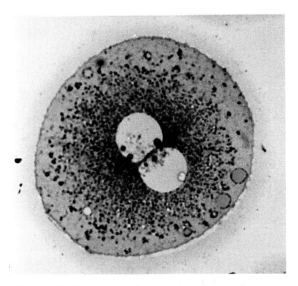

Figure 6.8 Two-pronuclear ovum 14 hours after single sperm injection into the PVS. The male and female pronuclei are closely associated in central ooplasm × 600. (Reproduced from Sathananthan et al[9])

technique of micro-injecting multiple sperm is now an accepted procedure. Research at Monash University on MI of mouse oocytes[37] also confirms a block to polyspermy at the oolemma, though this was suspected for some time.[26,27] The technique of MI has enabled us to explore this phenomenon further and there is little doubt now that there is a secondary block to polyspermy at the oolemma in both the human and mouse, in addition to the primary block at the ZP. Hence multiple sperm injection should be the preferred method of insemination. However, the Sydney IVF group (Table 6.4) has encountered high rates of polyspermy (49.8 per cent) after injecting an average of six sperm/oocyte within a range of one to 20 or 30 sperm/oocyte. The reason for this is unclear but if over 10 sperm/oocyte are injected the chances of polyspermy may be greater.[52] It appears that the optimum number of sperm for SUZI is in the range of three to 10 sperm/oocyte[2,3,4] to ensure high rates of monospermic fertilisation, the number of sperm

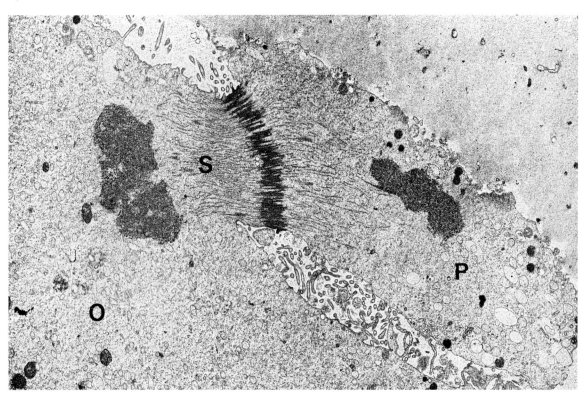

Figure 6.9 Abstriction of the second polar body at fertilisation four hours after SUZI. (Reproduced from Ng et al[55])

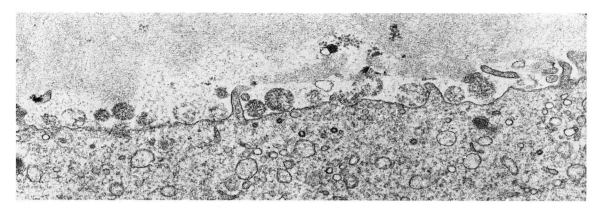

Figure 6.10   Cortical granule release at fertilisation four hours after SUZI. Note contents in PVS × 19 600

injected depending on the severity of male factor infertility.

Ng et al.[2,17] have advanced an hypothesis on the nature of the sperm block based on animal and human studies. They postulate that there are sperm receptors resident on the oolemma of zona-intact oocytes which bind to complementary sites on the postacrosomal fusogenic region of the sperm plasma membrane.[15,25] These receptors are probably modified by exocytosis of CG, when their

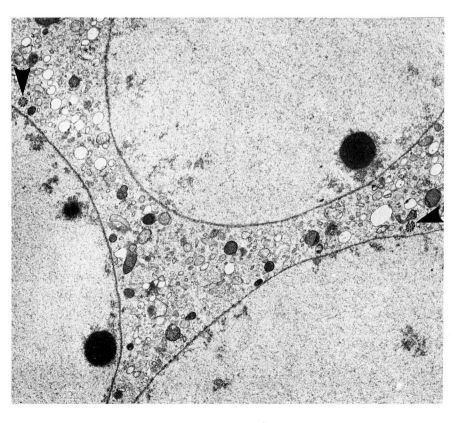

Figure 6.11
Tripronuclear ovum 24 hours after SUZI. Two sperm tails are seen in two different locations (arrows) indicating dispermy × 15 400. (Reproduced from Sathananthan et al[9])

membranes are incorporated with the oolemma. The first direct evidence of oolemmal receptors in mouse oocytes came from a study of SUZI after alcohol activation.[2] Dispermy is sometimes encountered after SUZI in the few instances of polyspermy recorded and confirmed by TEM (Figure 6.11).[9] This may be explained by the simultaneous binding and fusion of two sperm prior to CG release. Future research needs to be directed to the characterisation of the specific molecules involved in fertilisation, using immunological techniques.

Table 6.5 Development of embryos after zona opening

Patients*	15	
Oocytes inseminated	151	
Fertilised	32	(21%)
Cleavage	16	(50%)
Late fertilisation	3	(2%)
1PN oocytes	3	(2%)
Spontaneous cleavage	22	(15%)
Blastocysts	0	
ET patients	0	

Note: *Severe male factor patients.

Embryonic cleavage after SUZI/sperm centrioles

Our results show that pregnancy rates are low (seven to 13 per cent per transfer) and only one healthy baby has been born to date, although 78 women and 459 oocytes were subjected to SUZI (Table 6.2). Monospermic fertilisation was about 12 per cent in the two categories of patients. Since the embryos were transferred at the 2PN stage their potential for further development *in vitro* could not be ascertained. Monash studies on micro-injection of sperm from severe male factor patients have shown that about 20–25 per cent of the oocytes normally fertilised were blocked at the 2PN stage, whereas in the mouse such a block was not evident (Chapter 5). This block was attributed to semen quality rather than the micromanipulation technique. Blocked or retarded cleavage has also been

reported for oocytes fertilised after zona opening (Table 6.5)[38] and zona drilling.[39]

This raises an important question as to whether embryonic development is compromised when sperm quality is very poor. Recent studies on 2PN and 3PN ova in syngamy have shown that the sperm centriole is inherited by the human zygote and seems to organise at least one pole of the first mitotic spindle.[40] This exciting discovery led us to postulate in 1990 a new hypothesis on the role of sperm centrioles in the assessment of male infertility. Centrioles with centrosomes organise or nucleate microtubules in cilia, flagella and sperm tails.[41] The mature human sperm has only one functional centriole, the proximal next to the basal plate, while the distal gives rise to the sperm tail axoneme during spermiogenesis. The functional centriole shows the typical $9 + 0$ organisation of microtubule (MT) triplets resembling a pinwheel and is associated with osmiophilic centrosomal material. Since centrioles with centrosomes nucleate the sperm tail axoneme consisting of MT showing the $9 + 2$ organisation they must play a functional role in sperm motility mediated by interaction of MT. An abnormal tail axoneme should reflect abnormal sperm centriolar function, which in turn may cause anomalies in the organisation of the first mitotic spindle after fertilisation, arresting development or causing aberrant development. Our preliminary studies show centriolar anomalies in poor quality and immotile sperm from patients with immotile cilia syndrome.[42] The failure of a considerable number of embryos to cleave nor-

Table 6.4 Sydney IVF sperm micro-injection results[5]

Patients	118*	
Oocytes micro-injected	996	
Fertilised	223	(22.4%)
Polyspermy	111	(49.8%)
Embryo transfers	65	(55.1%)
Pregnancies	4	(6.2%)†
		(3.4%)=
	2 delivered (singletons)	
	1 miscarried	
	1 ongoing	

Notes: * includes 3 cases using epididymal sperm and one Kartagener's syndrome.
† per embryo transfer.
= per patient.

mally after micro-insemination with sperm having predominantly motility problems may partly be attributed to aberrant centriolar or centrosomal function inherited from the father. Further research needs to be done to determine the precise roles of both paternal and maternal centrioles/centrosomes in human development and their implications in the treatment of male infertility.

Sperm exit and entry after SUZI

In our earlier studies on SUZI[9], we showed that some of the sperm injected into the PVS may swim outwards through the perforation made by the injecting needle. This narrow perforation slit remains open even three days after sperm injection although the edges on either side of the slit have come closer together (Figure 6.12). This is large enough to allow sperm exit since they swim vigorously in the PVS long after MI. Occasionally

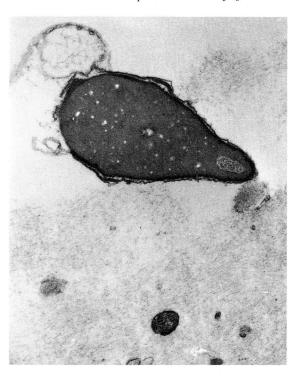

Figure 6.13 Acrosome-reacted sperm penetrating the outer ZP, 24 hours after SUZI. This sperm had probably escaped from the PVS × 27 300

sperm, both acrosome intact and reacted, were located in the slit and others that had swum out were seen re-entering the ZP in the usual manner after vesiculation of surface membranes (Figure 6.13). Since great care had been taken to inject single or multiple sperm into the PVS there was no question of sperm contamination from the injecting needle in the medium. Sperm exit through the perforation has also been demonstrated in the mouse after MI.[37]

As sperm could exit through the perforation slit in the ZP, it seemed logical to us that sperm could penetrate the oocyte through this slit, since it does not close after MI.[9] The Monash group has recently adopted the method of leaving the MI oocytes overnight (18–24 hours) in the medium containing five to 10×10^6 sperm/ml (Chapter 5). This has significantly enhanced the fertilisation rate twofold, although there was a slight increase in polyspermy. The technique seems to be a compromise between

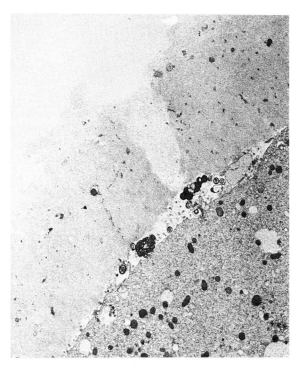

Figure 6.12 Penetration slit in ZP 48 hours after SUZI, which still remains open × 9 100

the SUZI and partial zona dissection methods[43] discussed elsewhere in this book (Chapter 5). It seems to be a better method of controlling unrestricted sperm penetration into the PVS that might cause high rates of polyspermy. Indeed, if the ZP is partially denuded by mechanical means and the oocyte exposed, sperm/egg fusion and early sperm incorporation may occur unabated and asynchronously after insemination *in vitro* and result in polyspermic penetration.[25] The early stages of sperm penetration cannot be visualised by LM and if such stages are found in ova with two pronuclei then in effect we have polyspermy. Preservation of the integrity of the ZP is also important to protect the embryo in the first week of development. Another advantage of postinsemination after MI is that the sperm AR could be enhanced at the surface of the ZP or in the vicinity of cumulus cells that remain attached to the ZP. It is now becoming increasingly apparent that the ZP[44] and cumulus[45] induce the AR. Consequently hyperactivation of capacitated motile sperm present in the defective sperm sample surrounding the oocyte could ultimately result in a better quality of sperm entering the PVS for microfertilisation. Further, cumulus and corona cells at the surface of MI oocytes may occasionally show phagocytic incorporation of sperm, a phenomenon prevalent during conventional IVF where large numbers of sperm are used for insemination.[24] This might well be a method of weeding out the weaker and functionally abnormal sperm before they reach the oocyte. The site of induction of the sperm AR during IVF seems to be the surface of the ZP, where specific glycoprotein inducers have been identified in the mouse.[44] Whether the inner zona is as good a site of AR induction for sperm in the PVS[9] needs to be investigated both in the mouse and human. Considering these reasons it might well be a better technique to postincubate the MI oocytes with remaining sperm to ensure higher fertilisation rates[4] and viable pregnancies which is the ultimate goal in ART.

Sperm injection into the oocyte

Direct sperm injection into the oocyte cytoplasm has been attempted by Lazendorf and co-workers.[46]

This technique results in a higher mortality rate of oocytes (Table 6.6)[2], since the oolemma is punctured causing localised or extensive disorganisation of the ooplasm.[9] Most of our recent studies have been on oocytes after accidental injection of sperm into the ooplasm during SUZI. We have demonstrated that the injected sperm are often located in membrane-bound vacuoles (Figure 6.14) and that possible sperm/oocyte membrane fusion can occur in these vacuoles.[9,17] Pronuclear development has also been demonstrated in a few oocytes.[9,17] However, a few sperm heads within the ooplasm remain unexpanded 24 hours after multiple sperm injection and these show various stages of the AR

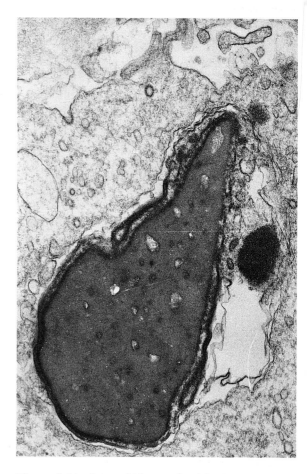

Figure 6.14 Sperm 24 hours after injection directly into the ooplasm. Its acrosome is reacting by vesiculation and a membrane-bound vacuole surrounds the sperm head × 35 700. (Reproduced from Sathananthan et al[9])

(Figures 6.14 and 6.15). Parts of the ZP and pockets of the oolemma with released products of CG may be evident in the ooplasm. Some sperm also show aberrant nuclear decondensation.[9] Abnormal sperm were also encountered within the ooplasm and if a single sperm is injected, which is usually the case, the chance of selecting an abnormal sperm is quite high, considering the quality of sperm used for MI. The wisdom of separating sperm heads from tails by sonication[2] is now open to question, since we have shown that the sperm centriole/centrosome is inherited by the fertilised ovum and could play a role in embryonic cleavage. There seems little advantage in direct sperm injection over SUZI, since the egg plays an active role in sperm incorporation by phagocytosis,[25,29] even if the sperm are immotile.[16] No pregnancies have yet been reported after direct sperm injection.

Micro-injection of immotile sperm

Immotile sperm from patients with Kartagener's syndrome, a rare clinical condition,[47] will fertilise human oocytes after SUZI resulting in embryonic cleavage.[16] Earlier, Laws-King et al.[8] and Ng et al.[48] showed that fertilisation could be achieved with immotile sperm. Our original findings on sperm incorporation *in vitro*[15,29,49] demonstrated that sperm motility was not essential for sperm/oocyte membrane fusion and consequent sperm incorporation, since some sperm were phagocytosed by the oocyte tail first. We have examined washed immotile sperm from five donors in pellets,[18] which reveal a population of sperm with

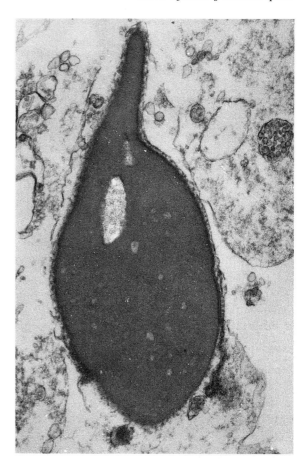

Figure 6.15 Acrosome-reacted sperm head in a degenerating oocyte 24 hours after direct sperm injection × 35 700. (Reproduced from Ng et al[55])

Table 6.6 Results of direct sperm injection into oocytes in 3 patients[7]

Pretreatment motile sperm density	1.10 ± 1.67 M/ml
Posttreatment motile sperm density	0.23 ± 0.01 M/ml
Sperm transferred	1
Metaphase II oocytes	38
Damaged after MIMIC	12
2 pronuclear zygotes	4
3 or more pronuclei	0
1 pronucleus	3
Tubal embryo transfer (patients)	2

normal heads undergoing stages of the AR. Sperm located in the PVS after MI also showed intact or reacting acrosomes (Figure 6.16). Immotile sperm have a variety of head, tail and midpiece defects.[18] The axonemal MT are often disorganised and lack dynein arms.[47,48] Hence the sperm are immotile, though a few may exhibit wriggling movements with no forward progression.[18] A larger percentage of sperm were also dead in some samples assessed by LM and these could well have been used for MI. Dead sperm have no acrosomes (nude) or may have disorganised surface membranes or have degenerating midpieces and tails.[18] There are also ethical concerns regarding treatment of

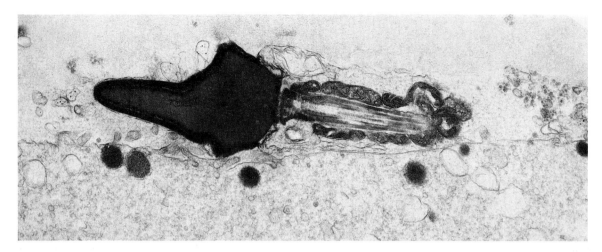

Figure 6.16 Immotile sperm in the PVS of an unfertilised oocyte. Note normal head structure and intact acrosome × 19 600

patients with Kartagener's syndrome, since it is an autosomal recessive genetic condition.

Micro-injection of round headed sperm

Since round headed sperm have no acrosomes and postacrosomal sheaths[18,50] they are unable to penetrate the ZP and fertilise the oocyte. This syndrome is also very rare. We attempted SUZI with round headed sperm after demembranation of the sperm heads by plunging into liquid N_2. The sperm were found in the PVS (Figure 6.17) and had not fused with the oocyte. Those injected directly into the ooplasm remained unexpanded but the oocytes showed evidence of degeneration (Figure 6.18). It has been shown that round headed

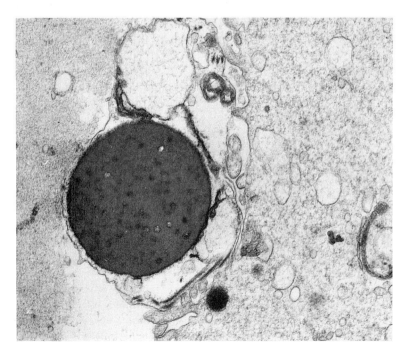

Figure 6.17 Round headed sperm in the PVS of an unfertilised oocyte 48 hours after SUZI × 27 300

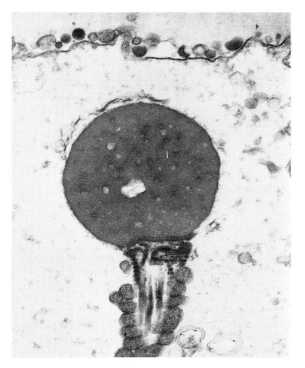

Figure 6.18 Round headed sperm injected directly into the ooplasm. The ooplasm has degenerated × 27 300

sperm fail to bind or penetrate the oocyte in the egg penetration test.[50] Examination of sperm pellets of one patient revealed that 98 per cent of sperm were round headed, while 2 per cent had the usual head structure.[18] Whether round headed sperm could fertilise the egg after cytoplasmic injection remains to be explored.

Micro-injection of epididymal sperm

Epididymal sperm from patients with obstructive azoospermia can fertilise oocytes but success rates are low (10 per cent),[51] as is the case with sperm having multiple defects.[7,10] There are evidently few progressively motile sperm in the caput, and these are unable to bind or penetrate the ZP[52] and SUZI seems warranted. However, epididymal sperm from other regions of the epididymis can penetrate the ZP.[24] Sperm aspirated from the caput epididymis have recently been micro-injected into the PVS resulting in fertilisation and embryo development.[53] Capacitation and acrosomal activity of caput sperm need to be assessed by TEM to improve the chance of microfertilisation in obstructive azoospermia.

SUZI into embryos

In a recent study we micro-injected sperm into the PVS of human embryos to determine whether there is sperm fusion and incorporation after fertilisation.[54] This study was necessary since supernumerary sperm are usually present in the PVS after microfertilisation.[9] Sperm (10–30) were injected into one- to 10-cell embryos and cultured further for 6–24 hours *in vitro* for TEM.[54] Acrosome intact and reacted sperm were seen in the PVS and between blastomeres. Sperm/blastomere membrane fusion was not observed even as early as the pronuclear stage but sperm heads were incorporated into embryonic cells and were often located in membrane bound vacuoles. Both acrosome intact and reacted sperm were seen in vacuoles and sperm chromatin decondensation was not evident (Figure 6.19). Sperm heads with swollen and complex surface membranes and those undergoing chromatin degeneration were seen in eight- to 16-cell stage embryos developed *in vitro*. Evidently, the phagocytic capability of the oocyte at fertilisation seems to have been retained by early embryonic cells, while its fusigenic potential has declined or has been lost after pronuclear development.

Conclusion

Multiple sperm transfer seems to be the preferred method of treatment for male factor patients having three or more sperm defects, since conventional IVF yields low fertilisation rates, and even lower pregnancy rates. Sperm MI combined with incubation of oocytes in culture medium could be the rational way of improving both the sperm AR and microfertilisation. Since there is apparently a block

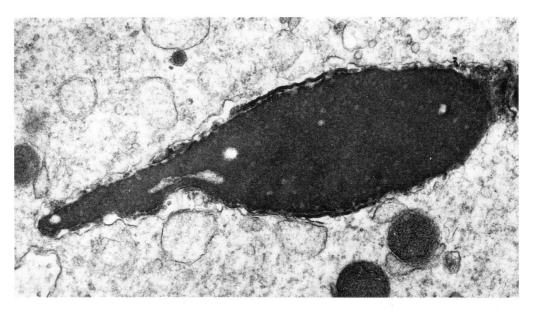

Figure 6.19 Partially reacted sperm head 24 hours after SUZI into a 3PN ovum. A membrane-bound vacuole surrounds the sperm and its chromatin has not decondensed × 35 700

at the one-cell stage of development after MI of poor quality sperm, it is advisable to develop embryos to the two- or four-cell stage before transfer. The wisdom of transferring pronuclear stage ova in conventional IVF seems to be now debatable. Methods to optimise and synchronise the AR during the sperm preparation phase for MI need to be researched. The importance of sperm morphology, prevalent in poor quality sperm, should not be underestimated in the assessment of sperm function in the treatment of male infertility.

References

1. Ng SC, Bongso A, Sathananthan AH, Chan CLK, Wong PC, Hagglund L, Anandakumar C, Wong YC, Goh VHH. Pregnancy after transfer of multiple sperm under the zona. *Lancet.* 1988; **2**; 790.
2. Ng SC, Bongso A, Sathananthan AH, Ratnam SS. Micro-insemination sperm transfer (MIST) into human oocytes and embryos. In: Dale B ed. *Mechanism of Fertilisation: Plants to Humans.* Berlin, Springer Verlag, 1990, pp. 351–76.
3. Fishel S, Antinori S, Jackson P, Johnson J, Lisi F, Chiariello F, Versaci C. Twin birth after subzonal insemination. *Lancet.* 1990; **335**: 772.
4. Metka M, Harmony T, Huber J, Schurz B. Artificial insemination using a micromanipulator. *Fertilitat.* 1985; **1**: 41–4.
5. Fishel S, Antinori S, Jackson P, Johnson J, Rinaldi L. Presentation of six pregnancies established by subzonal insemination (SUZI). *Human Reproduction.* 1991; **6**: 124–30.
6. Cohen J, Alikani M, Malter HE, Adler A, Talansky BE, Rosenwaks Z. Partial zona dissection or subzonal sperm insertion: microsurgical fertilization alternatives based on evaluation of sperm and embryo morphology. *Fertility and Sterility.* 1991; 696–706.
7. Ng S-C, Bongso A, Ratnam SS. Microinjection of human oocytes: a technique for severe oligoasthenoteratozoospermia. *Fertility and Sterility.* 1991; **56**: 1117–23.
8. Laws-King A, Trounson A, Sathananthan AH, Kola I. Fertilisation of human oocytes by micro-injection of a single spermatozoon under the zona pellucida. *Fertility and Sterility.* 1987; **48**: 637–42.
9. Sathananthan AH, Ng SC, Trounson AO, Bongso

A, Laws-King A, Ratnam SS. Human micro-insemination by injection of single or multiple sperm: ultrastructure. *Human Reproduction*. 1989; **4**: 574–83.

10. Yates CA, Thomas CJ, Kovacs GT, de Kretser DM. Andrology, male factor infertility and IVF. In: Wood C, Trounson A (eds) *Clinical In Vitro Fertilisation*. Berlin: Springer-Verlag, 1989.

11. Cummings JM, Breen TM. Separation of progressive motile sperm from human semen by 'sperm-rise' through a density gradient. *Australian Journal of Laboratory Science*. 1984; **2**: 15–20.

12. Bongso TA, Ng SC, Mok H, Lim MN, Teo HL, Wong PC, Ratnam SS. Improved sperm density, motility and fertilization rates following Ficoll treatment of sperm in a human in vitro fertilisation programme. *Fertility and Sterility*. 1989; **51**: 850–54.

13. Sathananthan AH, Trounson A. The micro-injection technique and the role of the acrosome reaction in microfertilization. In: Mashiach S, Ben-Rafael Z, Laufer N, Schenker JG (eds.) *Advances in Assisted Reproductive Techniques*. New York: Plenum, 1990, pp. 825–39.

14. Sathananthan AH, Ng SC, Trounson A, Ratnam SS. Transmission electron microscopy in the assessment of infertility for assisted reproductive technology. In: Ratnam SS, Ng SC, Sen DK, Arulkumaran S (eds) *Contributions to Obstetrics and Gynaecology*. London: Churchill Livingstone 1991, pp. 61–87.

15. Sathananthan AH, Ng SC, Trounson AO, Ratnam SS, Bongso TA. Human sperm-oocyte fusion. In: Dale B (ed.) *Mechanism of Fertilisation*. Berlin: Springer-Verlag, 1990, pp. 329–50.

16. Bongso TA, Sathananthan AH, Wong PC, Ratnam SS, Ng SC, Anandakumar C, Ganatra S. Human fertilization by micro-injection of immotile spermatozoa. *Human Reproduction*. 1989; **4**: 175–9.

17. Ng SC, Bongso A, Sathananthan AH, Ratnam SS. Micro-insemination of human oocytes. In: Mashiach S, Ben-Rafael Z, Laufer N, Schenker JG (eds.) *Advances in Assisted Reproductive Techniques*. New York: Plenum, 1990, pp. 841–9.

18. Sathananthan AH, Ng SC, Ho J, Tok V, Ratnam SS. Ultrastructural assessment of human sperm for techniques in assisted reproductive technology. (In preparation, 1992.)

19. Jeulin C, Serres C, Jouannet P. The effects of centrifugation, various synthetic media and temperature on the motility and vitality of human spermatozoa. *Reproduction Nutrition and Development*. 1982; **22**: 81–91.

20. Kruger TF, Acosta AA, Simmons KF, Swanson RJ, Matta JF, Oehninger S. Predictive values of abnormal sperm morphology in in vitro fertilization. *Fertility and Sterility*. 1988; **49**: 112–17.

21. Jinno M, Kabayashi T, Sugimura K, Nozawa S, Katayama E, Iida E. IVF/sperm morphology. *Molecular Andrology*. 1990; **2**: 161–8.

22. Zamboni L. The ultrastructural pathology of the spermatozoon as a cause of infertility: the role of electron microscopy in the evaluation of semen quality. *Fertility and Sterility*. 1987; **48**: 711–34.

23. Carlon N, Navarro A, Giorgetti C, Roulier R. Ultrastructure study of sperm in unexplained failure of in vitro fertilization. (In press.)

24. Sathananthan AH, Trounson AO, Wood C. *Atlas of Fine Structure of Human Sperm Penetration, Eggs and Embryos Cultured In Vitro*. Philadelphia: Praeger, 1986.

25. Sathananthan AH, Ng SC, Edirisinghe R, Ratnam SS, Wong PC. Sperm–oocyte interaction in the human during polyspermic fertilisation in vitro. *Gamete Research*. 1986; **15**: 317–26.

26. Wolf DP. The block to sperm penetration in zona-free mouse eggs. *Developmental Biology*. 1978; **64**: 1–10.

27. Yanagimachi R. Mammalian fertilization. In: Knobil E, Neill J (eds.) *The Physiology of Reproduction*. New York: Raven Press, 1988.

28. Kola I, Lacham O, Jansen PRS, Turner M, Trounson A. Chromosomal analysis of human oocytes fertilised by micro-injection of spermatozoa into the perivitelline space. *Human Reproduction*. 1990; **5**: 575–7.

29. Sathananthan H, Chen C. Sperm–oocyte membrane fusion in the human during monospermic fertilisation. *Gamete Research*. 1986; **16**: 177–86.

30. Mortimer D, Curtis EF, Dravland JE. The use of strontium substituted media for capacitating human spermatozoa: an improved sperm preparation method for the zona-free hamster egg penetration test. *Fertility and Sterility*. 1986; **46**: 97–103.

31. Mortimer D, Chorney MJ, Curtis EF, Trounson AO. Calcium dependence of human sperm fertilising ability. *Journal of Experimental Zoology*. 1988; **246**: 194–201.

32. Lassalle B, Courtot AM, Testart J. In vitro fertilisation of hamsters and human oocytes by micro-injection of human sperm. *Gamete Research*. 1987; **16**: 69–78.

33. Holden CA, Hyne RV, Sathananthan AH, Trounson AO. Assessment of the human sperm acrosome reaction using concanavalin A lectin. *Molecular Reproduction and Development*. 1990; **25**: 247–57.

34. Moore HDM, Smith CA, Hartman TD, Bye AP. Visualisation and characterisation of the acrosome reaction of human spermatozoa by immunolocalisation with monoclonal antibody. *Gamete Research*. 1987; **17**: 245–59.

35. Stock CE, Fraser LR. The acrosome reaction in human sperm from men of proven fertility. *Human Reproduction*. 1987; **2**: 109–19.

36. Ng SC, Bongso TA, Ratnam SS. Micro-insemi-

nation: genetic aspects. *Archives of Andrology.* 1990; **25**: 261–70.

37. Sathananthan AH, Trounson A, Peura A, Lacham O. Mouse fertilisation by single or multiple sperm injection: ultrastructure. *Assisted Reproductive Technology/Andrology.* 1992, suppl. III, 1–14.

38. Bourne H, Baker G, Lopata A. Unpublished work.

39. Garrisi GJ, Talansky BE, Grundfeld L, Sapira V, Navot D, Gordon JW. Clinical evaluation of three approaches to micromanipulation assisted fertilization. *Fertility and Sterility.* 1990; **54**: 671–7.

40. Sathananthan AH, Kola I, Osborne J, Trounson A, Ng SC, Bongso A, Ratnam SS. Centrioles in the beginning of human development. *Proceedings of the National Academy of Sciences, USA.* 1991; **88**: 4806–10.

41. Fawcett DW. *A Text Book of Histology,* 11th ed. Philadelphia: Saunders, 1986.

42. Sathananthan AH. Inheritance of paternal centrioles and male fertility. XIII World Congress, Gynaecology and Obstetrics (FIGO), Singapore, 1991, Abstract No. 1629 (p. 209).

43. Malter HE, Cohen J. Partial zona dissection of the human oocytes: a nontraumatic method using micromanipulation to assist zona pellucida penetration. *Fertility and Sterility.* 1989; **51**: 139–48.

44. Wassarman P. Cellular and molecular elements of mammalian fertilization. In: Dale B (ed.) *Plants to Humans.* New York: Plenum, 1990.

45. Stock CE, Bates R, Lindsay KS, Edmonds DK, Fraser LR. Human oocyte–cumulus complexes stimulate the human acrosome reaction. *Journal of Reproduction and Fertility.* 1989; **86**: 723–30.

46. Lazendorf SE, Slusser MS, Maloney MK, Hodgen GD, Veeck LL, Rosenwaks Z. A preclinical evaluation of pronuclear formation by micro-injection of human spermatozoa into human oocytes. *Fertility and Sterility.* 1988; **49**: 835–42.

47. Palmblad J, Mossberg B, Afzelius BA. Ultrastructural cellular and clinical features of the immotile cilia syndrome. *Annals of Reviews in Medicine.* 1984; **35**: 481–5.

48. Ng SC, Sathananthan AH, Edirisinghe WR, Chue JHK, Wong PC, Ratnam SS, Sarla G. Fertilisation of a human egg with sperm from a patients with immotile cilia syndrome: case report. In: Ratnam SS, Teoh ES, Anandakumar C (eds.) *Advances in Fertility and Sterility.* Lancaster: Parthenon, 1987: **4**: 71–6.

49. Sathananthan AH, Trounson A, Freeman L. Morphology and fertilisability of frozen oocytes. *Gamete Research.* 1987; **16**: 343–54.

50. La Londe L, Langlais J, Antaki P, Chapdelaine A, Roberts KD, Bleau G. Male infertility associated with round headed acrosomeless spermatozoa. *Fertility and Sterility.* 1988; **49**: 316–21.

51. Temple-Smith PD, Southwick GJ, Yates CA, Trounson AO, de Kretser DM. Human pregnancy by in vitro fertilisation (IVF) using sperm aspirated from the epididymis. *Journal of In Vitro Fertilisation and Embryo Transfer.* 1985; **2**: 119–22.

52. Trounson A, Peura A, Lacham O. Fertilisation of mouse and human eggs by micro-injection of single sperm under the zona pellucida. *Journal of Reproduction and Fertility.* 1989; **38**: 145–52.

53. Olar TT, La Nasa J, Dickey RP, Taylor SN, Curole DN. Fertilisation of human oocytes by micro-injection of human sperm aspirated from the caput epididymis of an individual with obstructive azoospermia. *Journal of In Vitro Fertilisation and Embryo Transfer.* 1990; **7**: 160–4.

54. Ng SC, Sathananthan AH, Bongso TA, Ratnam SS, Tok VCN, Ho JKC. Subzonal transfer of multiple sperm (MIST) into early human embryos. *Molecular Reproduction and Development.* 1990; **26**: 253–60.

55. Ng SC, Bongso TA, Sathananthan AH, Ratnam SS. Micromanipulation: its relevance to human IVF. *Fertil. Steril.* 1990; **53**: 203–19.

Chapter 7

Subzonal insemination and zona breaching techniques for assisted fertilisation

S. Fishel, J. Timson, S. Antinori, F. Lisi and L. Rinaldi

Introduction

Previous chapters in this volume have described the development of micro-insemination procedures (Chapters 1, 2). Similar to other workers, our approach was to try to procure fertilisation for those couples who had previously failed to achieve fertilisation *in vitro*, and those who were unacceptable for *in vitro* fertilisation (IVF) due to severe male infertility.

Our main techniques were subzonal insemination (SUZI) and partial zona dissection (PZD). In an early series, the technique of zona drilling (ZD) was used. In total, 472 patients presented for micro-assisted fertilisation (MAF) and the data is presented.

Patients, materials and methods

Patients

Male factor infertility or previous failure of fertilisation were the criteria for inclusion in this study. Each couple was given an extensive consultation to explain the practicalities of the procedure involved and was informed about the lack of information concerning this technique in the human. Women were between 22 and 45 years of age. No female factors were obvious which may have affected outcome. Couples in this series were referred for male infertility. Ethical deliberations for this work have been commented on previously.[1]

Follicular stimulation

Each patient was administered a GnRH agonist (Suprefact: Hoechst, Hounslow, UK) as a nasal spray to desensitise the pituitary gonadotrophs. The dosage was two sprays per nostril every eight hours, commencing on day 21 of the cycle before treatment. The start of menses was designated day one of the treatment cycle. Patients who were not synchronised with the proposed starting date of treatment were maintained on Suprefact.

Follicular stimulation was initiated with 150 IU of follicle stimulating hormone (FSH: Metrodin; Serono, Rome, Italy), administered either on days one and two or days one, two and three, i.e. a dose of four or six ampoules of Metrodin in total. On day three of follicular stimulation, patients were administered either two, three or four ampoules of human menopausal gonadotrophin (HMG: Pergonal; Serono), according to their age, weight and previous response, until the administration of 10 000 IU human chorionic gonadotrophin (HCG: Profasi; Serono) to induce ovulation. Throughout follicular stimulation, patients continued with daily doses of Suprefact to maintain pituitary desensitization. Evaluation of data according to variations in stimulation regimes showed no statistical differences.

Oocyte recovery and embryology

Oocytes were recovered by the sonographic transvaginal technique. The procedures for culturing oocytes, embryology and replacement of embryos have been described previously.[2] In a number of patients all their oocyte–cumulus complexes were subject to digestion by hyaluronidase (Chapter 3), either in previous treatments or as control studies for comparing SUZI, PZD and IVF in sibling oocytes. For the latter it was important to evaluate the maturity of the oocytes, and to compare only those at metaphase II. Patients had their oocyte–cumulus complexes subject to hyaluronidase as an additional step in the IVF procedure, generally because of a very low sperm count, to isolate the individual oocytes for insemination in a single microdrop containing the spermatozoa concentrated from the whole ejaculate. This is referred to in the text as microdrop IVF.

Preparation of spermatozoa

During the early work, spermatozoa were prepared using the standard procedures of double centrifugation and resuspension. Approximately 30 minutes before subzonal insemination, up to eight hours after preparation, the suspension of spermatozoa was centrifuged a third time and the pellet was overlaid with a small amount of medium. The tube was placed at 37°C to encourage motile spermatozoa to swim free of immotile cells and debris. The overlay medium was aspirated from the sediment and used for SUZI. In some cases, as a trial, spermatozoa were initially resuspended for

the eight hour period in medium containing strontium chloride as a substitute for calcium.[3,4] This had no significant effect on fertilisation, and the results of these studies are published elsewhere.[5]

However, the majority of seminal plasma samples were prepared utilising Percoll (Sigma, Poole, UK) with two discontinuous gradients of 45 per cent and 90 per cent. For SUZI no statistical differences were calculated between the use of Percoll or the centrifugation methods.

Evaluation of the morphology of spermatozoa

All semen samples were delivered after a split ejaculate. Both portions were assessed independently, and combined for the total morphology for the purposes of this analysis. Slides were thoroughly washed with 70 per cent ethyl alcohol before use. Staining was by the Diff Quik Staining Kit methodology (Baxter Dade Diagnostics AG, Dubinger, Switzerland). After the fixing and staining protocol, slides were air dried and cover slips were applied using Xam neutral medium (Searle, Hopkin & Williams, UK). The morphology of spermatozoa was assessed according to the parameters in Table 7.1. For each assessment 200 spermatozoa were counted.

Preparation of the oocyte and the micro-insemination procedures

Details of the procedures used for SUZI have been given elsewhere[1,5] (Chapter 2). The procedures for partial zona dissection were performed as described elsewhere in this volume (Chapter 8), and for zona drilling, as detailed by Gordon and Talansky.[6]

Control studies

The great difficulty that practitioners face in this work is to strike a balance between offering what is perceived to be the 'best' treatment for the patient to establish a pregnancy, against the necessity to validate the data with matched controls. Where possible in a group of patients, sibling oocytes from the same cohort were divided into a group undergoing *in vitro* insemination and micro-assisted fertilisation (MAF). All oocytes were subject to hyaluronidase to ensure that the oocytes used for both IVF and MAF were at metaphase II. Conditions which prevented the use of control studies in some patients included: too few spermatozoa or inhibited progressive motility to reasonably attempt IVF, too few oocytes, and those patients who had previous failures of IVF who expressly wished their oocytes to be used for SUZI only.

Statistics

Statistical evaluation between groups was assessed using the X^2 test. The Student's t-test was used where appropriate.

Results

Overall data for SUZI patients and oocytes

Of the 307 patients undergoing oocyte recovery, 47.9 per cent of them achieved fertilisation with

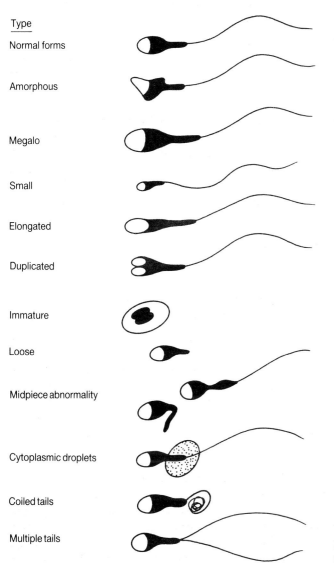

Type

Normal forms

Amorphous

Megalo

Small

Elongated

Duplicated

Immature

Loose

Midpiece abnormality

Cytoplasmic droplets

Coiled tails

Multiple tails

Figure 7.1 Category of abnormal forms of human spermatozoa

43.6 per cent having embryo transfer. Thirty-one pregnancies were established representing an over-all incidence of pregnancy of 23.1 per cent per transfer and 10.1 per cent of all oocyte recoveries. Approximately 54 per cent of patients had one embryo transferred compared with 28 per cent and 17 per cent having two and three embryos transferred, respectively (Table 7.1). There was no difference in the mean age of patients who became pregnant ($\bar{x}$ 34.6 ± 5.01 SD), whose embryos did not cleave ($\bar{x}$ 34.8 ± 4.78 SD), and in those patients where fertilisation failed to occur ($\bar{x}$ 32.9 ± 4.17 SD). Overall, the mean age of patients was 34.9 ± 5.87 SD. The status of oocytes recovered before SUZI is shown in Table 7.2. Of all the oocytes that appeared to have a mature oocyte-cumulus complex before digestion with hyaluronidase (2476), 82 per cent were observed in metaphase II compared with 14.6 per cent in metaphase I. Three per cent still had a germinal vesicle and 8 (0.32 per cent) appeared to have been parthenogenetically activated *in vivo* as a single pronucleus was pres-ent after the removal of the cumulus cells. The number of oocytes available for SUZI was 1384. Of all the oocytes undergoing SUZI, 21 per cent were fertilised, 92.4 per cent cleaved and 77.3 per cent of the fertilised oocytes were replaced, or 16.3 per cent of the total number of oocytes undergoing SUZI. The highest order of multiple pronucleate eggs observed was five pronuclei which arose in 1 per cent of oocytes. Overall, 9 per cent of fertilised

Table 7.2 Status of oocytes recovered before SUZI

Total number of oocytes recovered	2476	
Number in metaphase II	2030	(82%)
Number in metaphase I	362	(14.6%)
Number with germinal vesicle	76	(3.1%)
Number parthenogenetic	8	(0.32%)
Number for SUZI	1384	(68.2%)†
		(55.9%)*
Other=	646	(31.8%)
		(26.1%)*

Notes: † % of metaphase II oocytes.
* % of all oocytes.
= includes oocytes inseminated in vitro with husband or donor sperm, those used for zona breaching procedures or donation.

oocytes were multi-pronucleate. The incidence of parthenogenetic activation by SUZI was observed at 0.58 per cent (Table 7.3).

The mean number of spermatozoa injected for all oocytes was 5.13 ± 1.06 (SEM). The mean number of spermatozoa injected into oocytes that were not fertilised, or that achieved fertilisation with two or three pronuclei was 4.07 ± 0.14 (SEM), 4.91 ± 0.28 (SEM) and 7.11 ± 0.97 (SEM), respectively. The difference in the mean number of spermatozoa injected in the fertilised oocytes was significantly greater than those injected into the oocytes that were not fertilised (P < 0.001), and similarly for the oocytes that had three pronuclei com-pared to those with two pronuclei (P < 0.002). The assessment of fertilisation compared to the number of spermatozoa injected is shown in Table 7.5. It was not easy to be sure of the number of spermatozoa injected in all oocytes, but data was collated on 1209 oocytes. The majority of oocytes were injected with either three (23.2 per cent) or four (26.4 per cent) sperms, with two, five and six sperms being injected into 10.9 per cent, 13.2 per cent, and 12.2 per cent of oocytes, respectively (Table 7.4).

SUZI v. IVF with sibling oocytes

Table 7.5 shows the outcome of fertilisation in those patients for whom it was possible to compare IVF with SUZI in the same cohort of oocytes. Sig-

Table 7.1 Overall data from those patients having SUZI embryo transfers only

Total number of patients	307	
Number with fertilisation	147	(47.9%)
Number with cleavage	134	(91.2%)
Number with replacement	134	(43.6%)
Number of clinical pregnancies	31	(23.1%)†
		(10.1%)*
Number with one conceptus replaced	73	(54.4%)†
Number pregnant	8	(10.9%)
Number with two conceptus replaced	38	(28.4%)†
Number pregnant	11	(28.9%)
Number with three conceptus replaced	23	(17.2%)†
Number pregnant	12	(52.2%)

Notes: † % of replacements.
* % of all oocyte recoveries.

nificantly more patients (44 per cent) achieved fertilisation with SUZI compared to those who achieved fertilisation with both SUZI and IVF (8.4 per cent). Only 1.6 per cent of patients achieved fertilisation with IVF only.

In this group of patients the incidence of fertilisation per egg with subzonal insemination was significantly higher (26.8 per cent) than with IVF (4.4 per cent).

Assessment and classification of semen parameters

Six parameters were used to assess the semen: volume (ml), total count (TC x 10^6), total motility (TM – percentage), total count x 10^6/ml (TC/ml), total motile count x 10^6 (TMC) and progression (P – on a scale 0–4). The arithmetic mean (x) and the standard error of the mean (SEM) for volume, TC, TM, TC/ml and P were 3.64 ± (0.09), 33.87 ± (3.90), 18.20 ± (1.10), 10.68 ± (1.34), 7.62 ± (1.31), 1.62 ± (0.05), respectively.[5] In earlier studies assessing the semen parameters according to four groups of patients (those patients in whom fertilisation did not occur (non-fertilised), where fertilisation occurred but no cleavage, the occurrence of fertilisation and those patients in whom pregnancy occurred), it was found that only the total motile count and progression showed a significant difference. There was a higher total motile count (TMC) (P < 0.005) in the group of patients which achieved fertilisation compared with those which failed to achieve fertilisation, and similarly for a rating of progression of spermatozoa (P < 0.0001) for the same two groups (see Table 7.6).

The incidence of fertilisation was assessed according to two classifications of seminal parameters. Classification of seminal parameters into the standard World Health Organisation (WHO) characteristics (Classification 1) was difficult as these parameters do not consider the various degrees of severity of asthenozoospermia and oligozoospermia and the various combinations. For example, Table 7.7 shows the classification according to asthenozoospermia and oligozoospermia only, which resulted in 16 groups (A–P) ranging from the 'normal' to the very severe oligozoospermic/very severe asthenozoospermic samples. The division into 16 groups resulted in some

Table 7.3   Outcome of oocytes with SUZI

Number of oocytes with SUZI	1384	
Number fertilised	291	(21.0%)
Number cleaved	269	(92.4%)
Number replaced	225	(77.3%)†
		(16.3%)*
Number 2PN not cleaved	23	(7.9%)†
Number 2PN cleaved but not replaced	109	(3.1%)†
Number 3PN	18	(6.2%)†
Number 4PN	5	(1.7%)†
Number 5PN	3	(1.0%)†
Number 1PN	8	(0.58%)*

Notes: †   % of fertilised oocytes.
　　　　 *   % of all oocytes with SUZI.

Table 7.4   Assessment of fertilisation v. number of sperms injected

Number of sperms injected	Total number of oocytes	Number 2PN	Number >2PN		Total number fertilised	
1	11	0	0		0	
2	132	9	0		9	(6.8%)
3	280	38	0		38	(13.6%)
4	319	66	2	(0.6%)	68	(21.3%)
5	160	27	2	(1.3%)	29	(18.1%)
6	147	53	1	(0.7%)	54	(36.7%)
7	53	8	2	(3.8%)	10	(18.9%)
8	34	11	4	(11.8%)	15	(44.1%)
9	30	3	3	(10.0%)	6	(20.0%)
10	15	4	2	(13.3%)	6	(40.0%)
>10	28	14	8	(28.6%)	22	(78.6%)

Table 7.5 Comparison between SUZI and IVF in sibling oocytes

Total number of patients with both SUZI and IVF	191	
Number with fertilisation with SUZI and IVF	16	(8.4%)†
Number of patients with fertilisation with SUZI only	84	(44%)†
Number of patients with fertilisation with IVF only	3	(1.6%)
Total number of eggs with SUZI	821	
Number fertilised	220	(26.8%)*
Total number of eggs with IVF	571	
Number fertilised	25	(4.4%)*

Notes: † P < 0.0001.
  * P < 0.0001.

groups having very few patients, thus presenting a difficulty for valid analysis. Table 7.8 demonstrates the incidence of fertilisation per patient and per egg for each of the 16 groups according to Classification 1. Given the numbers available for analysis there was no clear statistical trend for assessing the value of SUZI for each particular classification.[5]

The incidence of fertilisation for the 'normal' group (28 per cent) was not significantly different from a patient with very severe oligozoospermia/very severe asthenozoospermia (34 per cent – Classification P). The majority of patients (Groups G, H and I) fell into the categories of very severe oligozoospermia, oligoasthenozoospermia

Table 7.6 Mean semen parameters for each group

Parameter		Non-fertilised	Fertilised no cleavage	Fertilised	Pregnant
Volume	n	133	4	74	11
(ml)	x	3.68	4.63	3.64	2.80
	SD	1.36	1.31	1.33	0.88
	SEM	0.12	0.65	0.15	0.27
Total	n	133	4	74	11
count	x	30.00	29.25	43.01	21.41
($\times 10^6$)	SD	56.23	17.19	65.61	22.93
	SEM	4.88	8.59	7.63	6.91
Total	n	133	4	74	11
motility	x	16.73	29.25	19.39	21.36
(%)	SD	22.21	23.99	15.99	12.2
	SEM	1.93	11.99	1.86	3.68
Total	n	133	4	74	11
count/ml	x	10.08	6.88	12.06	10.02
($\times 10^6$)	SD	22.21	4.05	16.99	13.90
	SEM	1.93	2.02	1.98	4.19
Total	n	133	4	74	11
motile	x	5.79*	5.63	11.53*	4.17
count	SD	14.65	2.98	27.17	4.90
($\times 10^6$)	SEM	1.27	1.49	3.16	1.48
Progression	n	133	4	74	11
	x	1.46†	1.75	1.84†	1.91
	SD	0.75	0.50	0.71	0.77
	SEM	0.07	0.25	0.08	0.23

Notes: * P < 0.05.
  † P < 0.0001.

Table 7.7 Classification of seminal parameters 1

Code	Definition	$\times 10^6ml$	Parameters % Motile	Group
NML	Normal	> 20	> 40	A
AS	Asthenozoospermia	> 20	15–40	B
SA	Severe asthenozoospermia	> 20	5–14	C
VSA	Very severe asthenozoospermia	> 20	< 5	D
OS	Oligozoospermia	10–20	> 40	E
SOS	Severe oligozoospermia	5–9	> 40	F
VSOS	Very severe oligozoospermia	< 5	> 40	G
OAS	Oligoasthenozoospermia	10–20	15–40	H
OSSAS	Oligozoospermia/severe asthenozoospermia	10–20	5–14	I
OSVSAS	Oligozoospermia/very severe asthenozoospermia	10–20	< 5	J
SOAS	Severe oligozoospermia/asthenozoospermia	5–9	15–40	K
SOSAS	Severe oligozoospermia/severe asthenozoospermia	5–9	5–14	L
SOVSAS	Severe oligozoospermia/very severe asthenozoospermia	5–9	< 5	M
VSOAS	Very severe oligozoospermia/asthenozoospermia	< 5	15–40	N
VSOSAS	Very severe oligozoospermia/severe asthenozoospermia	< 5	5–14	O
VSOVSAS	Very severe oligozoospermia/very severe asthenozoospermia	< 5	< 5	P

and oligozoospermia/severe asthenozoospermia, which represented a total of 47.1 per cent (Table 7.8).

According to the fertilisation data (Table 7.6), the incidence of fertilisation was significantly affected when the total motile count (TMC) was taken into consideration. The calculation of TMC takes into account the volume of semen and the density and motility of spermatozoa, providing information on the total number of motile spermatozoa available. A second classification (Classification 2) was therefore devised expressing five groups of patients according to the TMC, Groups 1–5 (Table 7.9). The incidence of fertilisation with SUZI according to the new classification is shown in Tables 7.11 and 7.12. The majority of patients were in Groups

Table 7.8 Fertilisation according to seminal parameters (Classification 1)

Group	Code	Incidence (%)	Number of patients	Number fertilised	Number of eggs	Number fertilised
A	NML	8.9	18	12 (17%)	72	20 (28%)
B	AS	8.4	17	8 (47%)	74	11 (15%)
C	SA	2.0	4	3 (75%)	15	3 (20%)
D	VSA	7.4	15	8 (53%)	65	17 (26%)
E	OS	4.4	9	4 (44%)	38	4 (11%)
F	SOS	1.5	3	1 (33%)	10	1 (10%)
G	VSOS	15.2	32	10 (31%)	121	27 (22%)
H	OAS	20.0	43	17 (40%)	178	28 (16%)
I	OSSAS	11.9	25	6 (24%)	134	8 (6%)
J	OSVSAS	2.0	4	4 (100%)	40	11 (28%)
K	SOAS	3.0	6	1 (17%)	24	1 (4%)
L	SOSAS	3.4	7	2 (29%)	23	3 (13%)
M	SOVSAS	0	0	–	–	–
N	VSOAS	2.0	4	3 (75%)	12	5 (42%)
O	VSOSAS	7.4	15	5 (33%)	51	10 (20%)
P	VSOVSAS	3.9	8	5 (63%)	38	13 (34%)

1 and 2, i.e. 68 per cent (Table 7.10) The incidence of fertilisation per patient was approximately 40 per cent, or per oocyte approximately 21 per cent (Table 7.11). On a per patient basis, there was a trend to decreasing fertilisation with increasing total motile count (Table 7.10). In Groups 1 and 2, significantly more patients achieved fertilisation with SUZI than with IVF. In Group 1, none of the 72 patients had fertilisation with IVF.

Evaluating the data on a per egg basis, all groups excepting Group 4 had a significant increase in the incidence of fertilisation with SUZI compared with IVF (Table 7.12).

Sperm morphology v. SUZI

Using Classification 2, the incidence of fertilisation, cleavage and fragmentation after SUZI was evaluated (Table 7.12). Patients with the severest morphology (> 95 per cent abnormal forms) tended to

a reduced incidence of fertilisation between groups and within each group, the lowest incidence of fertilisation occurring in patients with a TMC <1 and > 95 abnormal forms. In TMC Group 1, a high incidence of patients had a sperm morphology of > 95 per cent abnormal forms (36 per cent). The incidence of pronuclear stage arrest and, possibly, the level of cytoplasmic fragments appeared to be related more to the degree of abnormal forms than the actual TMC (Table 7.13). Overall, there was a significant reduction in the incidence of fertilisa-

Table 7.9 Seminal parameters: Classification 2

Group	Total motile count (TMC) ($\times 10^6$)
1	< 1
2	1–5
3	6–10
4	11–20
5	> 20

Table 7.10 SUZI v. IVF and sperm: Classification 2: patients

Classification	Total number	Incidence	Fertilisation SUZI only %	Fertilisation SUZI and IVF %
Group 1	72	0.40	28 (38.9%)	0
Group 2	49	0.28	26 (53.1%)	4 (8.2%)
Group 3	16	0.09	57 (43.8%)	2 (12.5%)
Group 4	16	0.09	3 (18.8%)	3 (18.8%)
Group 5	25	0.14	7 (28.0%)	2 (8.0%)

Table 7.11 SUZI v. IVF and sperm: Classification 2: eggs

| Classification | SUZI | | IVF | |
	Total number	Number fertilised %	Total number	Number fertilised %
Group 1	424	89 (21.0%)[a]	252	0[a]
Group 2	281	66 (23.5%)[b]	172	11 (6.4%)[b]
Group 3	79	15 (19.0%)[c]	59	6 (10.2%)[c]
Group 4	67	12 (18.0%)[d]	70	5 (7.1%)[d]
Group 5	129	22 (17.1%)[e]	98	5 (5.1%)[e]

Notes: [a] $x^2 = 59.094$, P < 0.0001.
  [b] $x^2 = 20.898$, P < 0.0001.
  [c] $x^2 = 65.014$, P < 0.0001.
  [d] N.S.
  [e] $x^2 = 6.494$, P < 0.011.

Table 7.12 SUZI in relation to sperm morphology and Classification 2

Classification	Number of abnormal forms %	Number of patients	Number of oocytes	Number fertilised	Number cleaved	Number grade 2 & 3 fragments (0–3)
Group 1	> 95%	9	45	4 (8.9%)	2	2
	70–95%	10	41	9 (21.9%)	7	2
	< 70%	6	28	8 (28.6%)	7	1
Group 2	> 95%	5	23	4 (17.4%)	3	2
	70–95%	18	82	19 (23.2%)	18	2
	< 70%	7	31	8 (25.8%)	8	1
Group 3	> 95%	3	13	2 (15.4%)	1	1
	70–95%	4	17	5 (29.4%)	4	1
	< 70%	3	12	5 (41.7%)	5	2
Group 4	> 95%	2	8	3 (37.5%)	3	1
	70–95%	4	19	4 (21.1%)	4	1
	< 70%	1	4	2 (50.0%)	1	0
Group 5	> 95%	3	13	2 (15.4%)	0	–
	70–95%	6	26	10 (38.5%)	8	0
	< 70%	5	24	8 (33.3%)	7	1

tion, multipronucleate oocytes and cleavage, and a significant increase in cytoplasmic fragments in patients with > 95 per cent abnormal forms (Table 7.13).

SUZI v. zona drilling (ZD) and IVF

For the preliminary evaluation of ZD, the results from 34 patients were compared. During this period, 222 patients also underwent SUZI. The mean TMC for patients undergoing SUZI and ZD was 7.62 ± 1.31 (SEM) and 16.23 ± 6.68 (SEM), respectively ($P < 0.05$). The significantly higher

TMC is a result of a requirement for adequate numbers of progressively motile spermatozoa to achieve fertilisation by ZD.

Each of these patients had sibling oocytes subjected either to SUZI, ZD or IVF. Significantly more patients achieved fertilisation with SUZI only, compared with IVF only (Table 7.14). The incidence of patients with fertilisation with SUZI only (29.4 per cent) was similar to those achieving fertilisation with ZD only (20.6 per cent), and 14.7 per cent of patients had fertilisation with both techniques. Assessing fertilisation per egg revealed a similar incidence between SUZI (17.6 per cent) and ZD (21.3 per cent), both significantly higher than

Table 7.13 Summary of SUZI and sperm morphology v. fertilisation, pronuclei, cleavage and cytoplasmic fragments

Sperm morphology (% abnormal forms)	Number of oocytes	Fertilisation	Multipronuclei	Cleavage	Fragments (grade 2 & 3)
> 95	102	15 (14.7%)*	0	9 (60.0%)†	6 (66.7%)=
70–95	185	47 (25.4%)*	3 (6.4%)	41 (87.2%)†	6 (14.6%)=
< 70	99	31 (31.3%)	4 (12.9%)	28 (90.3%)	5 (16.1%)

Notes:
* $x^2 = 3.835$, P = 0.05.   † $x^2 = 11.377$, P < 0.0001.   = $x^2 = 8.287$, P = 0.004.

Table 7.14 Comparison between SUZI and zona drilling (ZD) and IVF in sibling oocytes: patients

Number of patients with SUZI and ZD and IVF	34
Number with fertilisation	25 (73.5%)
Number with SUZI fertilisation only	10 (29.4%)*
Number with SUZI and ZD fertilisation only	5 (14.7%)
Number with SUZI and ZD and IVF fertilisation only	1 (2.9%)
Number with ZD fertilisation only	7 (20.6%)
Number with ZD and IVF fertilisation only	1 (2.9%)
Number with IVF fertilisation only	1 (2.9%)*

Note: * $x^2 = 6.941$, P $= 0.008$.

with IVF (6.8 per cent) (Table 7.15). However, those oocytes that fertilised with ZD had a significantly reduced incidence of cleavage, with 45 per cent arresting at the pronuclear stage, compared to those oocytes fertilised by SUZI (14.9 per cent).

SUZI v. PZD and IVF

One hundred and thirty one patients underwent MAF, each with a proportion of their oocytes subjected to either SUZI, PZD or IVF. In TMC Group 1, a subgroup of patients (Subgroup A) consisted of 30 patients who had not had IVF previously, because of their severely low sperm count. A further subgroup (Subgroup B) consisted of 12 patients who had undergone microdrop IVF, but failed to achieve fertilisation.

Group 2 patients were also subdivided as 19 who had previously failed routine IVF, and 30 who had microdrop IVF, without successful fertilisation. Groups 3, 4 and 5 consisted of 32 patients who had failed IVF on at least one previous attempt. A further group of eight patients were identified as having a titre of antisperm auto-antibodies > 128 in conjunction with failed IVF.

In the TMC Group 1 patients, 45.2 per cent achieved fertilisation with SUZI only compared with 4.8 per cent (P < 0.0001) having PZD (Table 7.17). Four (9.5 per cent) patients achieved fertilisation with both SUZI and PZD. No patient achieved fertilisation with IVF. More patients achieved fertilisation with SUZI and PZD in Subgroup A compared to Subgroup B (TMC Groups 1 and 2). As the concentration of TMC increased, the incidence of fertilisation per patient

with PZD increased, but overall significantly more patients (P $= 0.006$) achieved fertilisation with SUZI only compared to PZD only. Of the patients with antisperm auto-antibodies, five of the eight achieved fertilisation, two with SUZI only, one with PZD only, two with both PZD and SUZI, and none with IVF (Table 7.17).

Assessing the data on a per egg basis (Table 7.18), significantly more oocytes from patients in TMC Groups 1 and 2 fertilised with SUZI, compared with PZD (Table 7.18). In TMC Group 1, the incidence of fertilisation was higher from those in Subgroup A compared with Subgroup B for SUZI, but not PZD. The overall incidence of fertilisation was generally higher for SUZI than PZD in TMC Groups 1–5, and, including the group with antisperm auto-antibodies, significantly more oocytes (P $< .0001$) were fertilised with SUZI than with PZD. The incidence of fertilisation with the group expressing antisperm auto-antibodies was,

Table 7.15 Comparison between SUZI and zona drilling (ZD) and IVF in sibling oocytes: eggs

Number of oocytes for SUZI	153
Number fertilised	27 (17.6%)*
Number cleaved	23 (85.1%)=
Number of oocytes for ZD	94
Number fertilised	20 (21.3%)†
Number cleaved	11 (55.0%)=
Number of oocytes for IVF	44
Number fertilised	3 (6.8%)*†
Number cleaved	3

Notes: * $x^2 = 82.950$, P < 0.0001.
　　　　† $x^2 = 3.530$, P $= 0.6$.
　　　　= $x^2 = 3.832$, P $= 0.05$.

Table 7.16 The incidence of fertilisation and cleavage per patient undergoing SUZI, partial zona dissection (PZD) or IVF in sibling oocytes

Classification of sperm	Number of patients	Total number with fertilisation	Total number with cleavage	SUZI only — Number with cleavage (2 or more PN)	SUZI only — Number with fertilisation & E.T.	PZD only — Number with cleavage (2 or more PN)	PZD only — Number with fertilisation & E.T.	IVF† — Number with cleavage (2 or more PN)	IVF† — Number with fertilisation & E.T.	SUZI & PZD — Number with cleavage (2 or more PN)	SUZI & PZD — Number with cleavage (2 or more PN) & E.T.
Group 1											
Subgroup A	30	19 (63.3)	17 (89.5)	15 (50.0)	13 (86.7)	2 (6.7)	2	0	—	2 (6.7)	2 (100)
Subgroup B	12	6 (50.0)	5 (83.3)	4 (33.3)	3 (75.0)	0	—	0	—	2 (33.2)	2 (100)
Total	42	25 (59.5)	22 (88)	19* (45.2)	16 (84.2)	2* (4.8)	2 (100)	0	—	4 (9.5)	4 (100)
Group 2											
Subgroup A	19	11 (57.9)	10	6 (31.5)	5 (83.3)	3 (15.8)*	3 (100)	0	—	2 (10.5)	2 (100)
Subgroup B	30	14 (46.7)	12 (85.7)	5 (16.7)	4 (80)	4 (13.3)	3 (75)	1 (3.3)	1	5 (16.7)	5 (100)
Total	49	25 (51)	22 (88)	11 (22.4)	9 (81.8)	7 (14.2)	6 (85.7)	1 (2.0)	1	7 (14.2)	7 (100)
Group 3	9	7 (77.8)	6 (85.7)	2 (22.2)	2 (100)	2 (22.2)	1 (50)	0	—	3 (33.3)	3 (33.3)
Group 4	12	7 (58)	9 (100)	2 (16.7)	2 (100)	2 (16.7)	2 (100)	1 (8.3)	1	3 (25)	3 (100)
Group 5	11	6 (54.5)	8 (100)	2 (18.2)	1	3 (27.3)	3 (100)	2 (18.2)	2 (100)	1 (9.1)	1 (100)
Antisperm autoantibodies (failed IVF × 2)	8	5 (62.5)	5 (100)	2 (25)	2 (100)	1 (12.5)*	1	0	—	2 (25)	2
Total	131	75 (57.3)	67 (91.1)	36‡ (27.5)	32 (86.5)	17‡ (13)	15 (11.5)	4 (3.1)	4 (100)	20 (15.3)	20 (100)

†IVF never occurred in isolation of the other treatments so is not an addition to the total number.

Figures in parenthesis are percentages.

*: $\chi^2 = 16.254$, $P < 0.0001$; ‡: $\chi^2 = 7.663$, $P = 0.006$.

Table 7.17 Incidence of fertilisation and cleavage in sibling oocytes undergoing SUZI, partial zona dissection (PZD) or IVF

Classification of sperm	Number of oocytes	Total number with fertilisation	Total number with cleavage	SUZI		PZD		IVF	
				Oocytes	Number with fertilisation (2 or more PN)	Oocytes	Number with fertilisation (2 or more PN)	Oocytes	Number with fertilisation (2 or more PN)
Group 1									
Subgroup A	131	37 (28.2)	31 (83.8)	62	28 (45.1)	38	4 (10.5)	31	0
Subgroup B	76	10 (13.2)	8 (80)	31	6 (19.4)	26	3 (11.5)	19	0
Total	207	47 (22.7)	39 (83)	93	34* (36.6)	64	7* (10.9)	50	0
Group 2									
Subgroup A	133	20 (15)	17 (85)	44	11 (25)	52	6 (11.5)	37	0
Subgroup B	191	36 (18.8)	31 (86.1)	67	20 (29.9)	59	7 (11.9)	65	2 (3.1)
Total	324	56 (17.3)	48 (85.7)	111	31† (27.9)	111	13† (11.7)	103	2 (2)
Group 3	72	23 (31.9)	21 (91.3)	24	9 (37.5)	33	8 (24.2)	15	0
Group 4	81	22 (25.7)	21 (95.4)	27	8 (29.6)	29	5 (17.2)	25	3 (12)
Group 5	105	27 (25.7)	23 (85.1)	39	8 (20.5)	38	7 (18.4)	28	4 (14.3)
Antisperm autoantibodies (failed IVF × 2)	70	28 (40)	27 (96.4)	25	11 (44)	25	17 (68)	20	0
Total	859	203 (23.6)	179 (83.2)	319	101‡ (31.3)	300	57‡ (19)	240	9 (3.8)

Figures in parenthesis are percentages.
*: $\chi^2 = 15.208$, $P < 0.0001$. †: $\chi^2 = 8.192$, $P = 0.004$. ‡: $\chi^2 = 12.380$, $P < 0.0001$.

however, higher with PZD (68 per cent) than with SUZI (44 per cent). There was a general trend indicating a higher incidence of fertilisation with SUZI, but a higher incidence with PZD as the TMC increased.

The data expressed in Table 7.19 suggested that as the TMC increased, the incidence of polyspermia increased with SUZI and PZD, although this was more marked in the latter group (overall, 10.9 per cent v. 24.6 per cent, respectively: $P = 0.042$). Conversely, there appeared to be a higher incidence of moderate to severe cytoplasmic fragments in embryos from SUZI when sperm from TMC Groups 1 and 2 were used. Although there was an overall higher incidence of cytoplasmic fragments in embryos resulting from SUZI (31 per cent) compared to PZD (19.6 per cent), this was not statistically significant. Should this trend prove to be significant, it is likely to be a reflection of the high incidence of abnormal sperm morphology in these TMC Groups 1 and 2 (Tables 7.12 and 7.13). The incidence of cleavage in zygotes resulting from SUZI or PZD was similar, overall 86.1 per cent and 89.2 per cent, respectively; but this is generally lower than that observed after routine IVF. Even in the four oocytes fertilised by IVF in this study, cleavage was 100 per cent (Tables 7.17 and 7.18).

By re-assessing the data according to whether the patients had a single or multiple failure of IVF, a different pattern emerged (Table 7.19). Combining TMC Groups 2–5 resulted in 123 patients, 42 of whom had failed IVF only on one occasion, and 81 of whom had had multiple failures of IVF. In all cases, the incidence of fertilisation was less with both MAF techniques when the patients failed on more than one occasion. This was more marked with oocytes undergoing PZD. Fertilisation after PZD was greatly reduced when the patients had more than one failure after IVF – 29 per cent versus 3 per cent after multiple failure. Of the four patients whose oocytes were fertilised with IVF, three were in the group having had only a single IVF failure (Table 7.19).

Discussion

In this series of 472 patients, 307 underwent oocyte recovery for SUZI only. From these 2476 oocytes were recovered, 1384 underwent SUZI, and 291 from 147 patients were fertilised. That SUZI can achieve fertilisation even with the most severe seminal defects associated with spermatozoa density, motility and morphology has been recently confirmed by a number of reports.[1,7–12] The procedure per se has not resulted in a significant increase in abnormal embryos,[8] nor in the birth of abnormal babies.[1,9,13] However, the efficiency of the technique and which type of patient may benefit has yet to be established. The efficacy of any micro-assisted fertilisation procedure can only be assessed, where possible, by (i) the use of *in vitro* insemination using sibling oocytes for comparison; and (ii) a clear classification of the sperm used.

This study demonstrated that SUZI significantly increased the number of oocytes fertilised and the number of patients with fertilisation compared with standard *in vitro* insemination. Studies using sibling oocytes to assess SUZI versus IVF for the same population of spermatozoa resulted in only 6 per cent of eggs fertilised with IVF compared with 20.8 per cent with SUZI (Table 7.11).

In a trial of 131 patients in which SUZI, PZD and IVF were compared using sibling oocytes, more patients, and oocytes overall, achieved fertilisation with SUZI. This limited series of data indicated that with PZD there was a greater risk of polyspermia overall. However, significantly more embryos with moderate to severe cytoplasmic fragments resulted from SUZI with sperm from TMC Groups 1 and 2. This suggests that although fertilisation can be achieved by SUZI in the severest cases, perhaps a higher number of embryos produced are abnormal, and this is reflected in the incidence of cytoplasmic fragmentations. Of particular relevance to therapy was the observation that the efficacy of PZD significantly decreased if patients had had more than one failure of IVF (Table 7.19).

In both the classifications used in this study to assess the spermatozoa, SUZI also appeared to increase the number of oocytes and patients achieving fertilisation in each individual grouping

Table 7.18 Incidence of polyspermy, cleavage and cytoplasmic fragments in sibling oocytes undergoing SUZI, partial zona dissection (PZD) or IVF

Classification of sperm	SUZI				PZD				IVF			
	Number of fertilised oocytes	Number with >2PN	Number with cleavage	Number with fragments (grade 2 & 3)	Number of fertilised oocytes	Number with >2PN	Number with cleavage	Number with fragments (grade 2 & 3)	Number of fertilised oocytes	Number with >2PN	Number with cleavage	Number with fragments (grade 2 & 3)
Group 1	34	2* (5.9)	28 (82.4)	12 (42.9)	7	1* (14.3)	6 (85.7)	2 (28.6)	0	–	–	–
Group 2	31	2* (6.5)	26 (83.9)	8 (30.8)	13	2* (15.4)	11 (84.6)	2 (18.2)	2	0	2	0
Group 3	9	2 (22.2)	8 (88.9)	2 (25)	8	2 (25)	7 (87.5)	2 (28.6)	0	–	–	–
Group 4	8	1 (12.5)	7 (87.5)	2 (28.6)	5	2 (40)	5 (100)	1 (20)	3	0	3	1 (33.3)
Group 5	8	2 (25)	7 (87.5)	1 (14.3)	7	3 (42.9)	6 (85.7)	2 (33.3)	4	0	4	0
Antisperm autoantibodies (failed IVF × 2)	11	2 (18.2)	11 (100)	2 (18.2)	17	4 (23.5)	16 (94.1)	1 6.25	0	–	–	–
Total	101	11† (10.9)	87 (86.1)	27‡ (31)	57	14† (24.6)	51 (89.5)	10‡ (19.6)	9	–	9	1 (11.1)

Numbers in parenthesis are percentages.
*: P < 0.0001. †: P = 0.942. ‡: NS.

Table 7.19 Incidence of fertilisation in patients with single or multiple failure of IVF after micro-assisted fertilisation with SUZI and PZD on sibling oocytes (sperm Classification Groups 2–5 combined: n = 123)

Type of successful insemination per patient	Single failure of IVF		> 2 failures of IVF		Total	
	Number of patients	*Number with fertilisation*	*Number of patients*	*Number with fertilisation*	*Number of patients*	*Number with fertilisation*
	42		81		123	
Total with fertilisation		33 (79%)		12 (15%)		45 (37%)
Total with SUZI*		21 (50%)		10 (12%)		31 (25%)
Total with PZD*		25 (60%)		3 (4%)		28 (23%)
SUZI and PZD		13 (31%)		1 (1%)		14 (11%)
IVF		3 (7%)		1 (1%)		4 (3%)
SUZI only		8 (19%)		9 (11%)		17 (14%)
PZD only		12 (29%)		2 (3%)		14 (11%)

* Includes patients who had fertilisation with PZD and SUZI simultaneously (n = 14) and PZD only (n = 14) or SUZI only (n = 17).

(i.e. Groups A–P, Classification 1 or Groups 1–5, Classification 2). An attempt to delineate between different categories of male infertility in order to assign a fertilisation rate for each level of severity proved non-viable on a basis of Classification 1. Despite a demarcation in the incidence of fertilisation using the TMC Classification in a previous study,[4] by increasing the numbers of sperm used for SUZI in TMC Group 1, i.e. the numbers injected into the perivitelline space, the incidence of fertilisation was increased. In this data, there was no clear distinction in the incidence of fertilisation between the Groups (Table 7.17), although in Group 1, oocytes from Subgroup A had a higher incidence (45.1 per cent) of fertilisation than Subgroup B (19.4 per cent). This may reflect an inherent defect in the spermatozoa that is different, as the sperm in Subgroup B had been assessed as adequate for microdrop IVF previously. These two groups need to be evaluated more strictly.

The relevance of sperm morphology to micro-assisted fertilisation procedures, especially to SUZI, needs to be clarified. A mechanistic relationship (i.e. sperm function) to particular morphological abnormalities remains unclear. Sperm morphology has consistently been shown to be of value as a prognosticator of spermatozoa function, with the zona free hamster egg assay[14,15] and human oocyte fertilising ability.[16–18] However, the particular relevance of sperm morphology in relation to SUZI is unclear. One third of spermatozoa located in the perivitelline space after SUZI for men with severe oligospermia were found abnormal;[12] and defects of the nucleus, acrosome, midpiece and axoneme have been observed in spermatozoa penetrating the ooplasm after SUZI.[19] A discussion of the relevance of spermatozoa attachment, binding to, and penetration of the zona pellucida in relation to SUZI has been considered elsewhere.[1,13]

In this study, a critical assessment of sperm morphology (Figure 7.1) revealed 26 per cent of patients with > 95 per cent abnormal forms (Table 7.13). The incidence of fertilisation was clearly affected by the severity of both the TMC and the morphology of spermatozoa (Table 7.12). By distinguishing the groups of patients before SUZI, it is necessary to evaluate the need to modulate the numbers of sperm used for SUZI in each particular

group. For example, with TMC Group 1 and a morphology of > 95 per cent abnormal forms – the group with the lowest incidence of fertilisation – would it be advantageous to use more sperm for SUZI? The incidence of polyspermia was lowest in this group, but the incidence of cleavage arrest was highest (Table 7.18). Previous studies[5,20] (Chapter 7) have suggested that there is possibly a high viability of embryos produced by SUZI, and not significantly different from embryos produced after IVF. The data in the present series does not confirm this.

The main inefficiency in MAF is at the level of achieving sperm/egg fusion and subsequent fertilisation. Factors associated with this are the numbers and quality of the spermatozoa actually injected into the perivitelline space with SUZI. These particular problems can be circumvented with a motile population of spermatozoa by techniques which create a breach in the zona pellucida before the egg is inseminated[21–23] (see Chapters 8, 11) Increasing the number of spermatozoa inserted into the perivitelline space during SUZI significantly increased, overall, the incidence of fertilisation in this study (approximately 10 per cent). However, the incidence of polyspermia was also a function of TMC. Whether there is a maximum number of sperm that should be deposited in the perivitelline space, above which there is a negative correlation with fertilisation, or an unacceptably high incidence of multipronucleate oocytes is as yet undetermined. Individual cases, i.e. those with particular anomalies, may reflect a different outcome. Spermatozoa are often seen swimming around the perivitelline space 14–20 hours after SUZI in oocytes with and without the pronuclei of fertilisation and in embryos up to 96 hours. It is unknown whether the presence of many active or degenerating spermatozoa in the perivitelline space would compromise cleavage.

In this study there was a higher incidence and a higher order of polyspermic oocytes than published previously;[5] this is a reflection of increasing the numbers of spermatozoa deposited in the perivitelline space. That there is not a higher incidence of polyspermia is probably a function of some degree of block to polyspermy existing at the level of the oolemma, and/or the reduced chance of sperm/oocyte fusion due to the poor quality of the spermatozoa. Techniques causing a breach in the zona pellucida prior to insemination with motile sperm[22,24] have been reported to result in higher polyspermy rates than SUZI[1,12] (Chapter 8): which is also confirmed in this study (Table 7.18). However, a recent report of Payne et al.[30] using PZD resulted in a polyspermy rate between 4.6 per cent and 6.4 per cent. Lassalle and co-workers[25] demonstrated that SUZI with multiple spermatozoa resulted in monospermic fertilisation of human oocytes. The existence of slow and fast blocks to polyspermy and the respective roles of the oolemma and zona pellucida in human oocytes has been discussed extensively elsewhere.[1,11,12,23,25]

Only acrosome-reacted spermatozoa can fuse with the oolemma[26] (Chapter 4), although this can apparently occur at the surface of the oolemma.[27] In previous studies,[6,7] an attempt was made to increase the numbers of acrosome-reacted spermatozoa selected for SUZI using culture medium depleted of calcium but replaced by $SrCl_2$ for the preparation of spermatozoa. This was based on the theory of 'stalling' those spermatozoa capable of undergoing the acrosome reaction by substituting calcium ions with strontium ions as described by Mortimer.[3] Mortimer's early work[3] suggested that subsequent transfer of the spermatozoa to medium containing calcium may synchronise a high population of the spermatozoa to undergo the acrosome reaction, increasing the chances of selecting acrosome-reacted spermatozoa for SUZI.

Preliminary data using strontium ions suggested that this may be beneficial for increasing the incidence of fertilisation for SUZI.[1] However, the results of a later study,[5] based on a larger number of oocytes and using sibling oocytes, demonstrated that the incidence of fertilisation is not increased by replacing calcium ions with strontium ions prior to SUZI. This confirmed the later work of Mortimer et al.[4] which indicated that, by removing calcium ions from the culture medium, the incidence of acrosome-reacted spermatozoa is similar to that when spermatozoa are cultured with calcium ions.

After hyaluronidase treatment of the oocytes prior to SUZI, 0.32 per cent appeared to contain a single pronucleus with a single polar body and this has been reported previously.[1] This may be indicative of the incidence of parthenogenetically activated oocytes *in vivo*. Single pronucleate oocytes have been observed after IVF with an incidence of 1.6 per cent to 5 per cent,[28] but it is unclear that these can be considered, in a strict sense, parthenogenetic, as they have been in contact with spermatozoa, as discussed elsewhere.[1] However, the incidence of single pronucleate oocytes after the SUZI procedures in this study was 0.58 per cent, which may represent the incidence of parthenogenetic activation due to the subzonal insemination technique *per se*. The total manipulation of the oocyte which includes removal of the cumulus mass after exposure to hyaluronidase, pipetting the oocyte through a finely drawn Pasteur pipette to remove the corona radiata, exposure to sucrose and the distortion which may occur during the SUZI procedure may all contribute to activate the oocyte.

Summary

In the studies using zona drilling, it was apparent that although fertilisation could be achieved, and at a similar rate to SUZI, subsequent cleavage was inhibited in a high percentage of zygotes. In a recent clinical trial published by Gordon and co-workers[29] 21.3 per cent of oocytes fertilised, of which 50 per cent were polyspermic. Although the majority of the oocytes were subject to acid Tyrode's, some were 'drilled' using chymotrypsin or mechanically perforated after softening with chymotrypsin. To date there have been no reports of a human pregnancy with this technique. Ng et al.[30] demonstrated that ZD may cause arrest of the second meiotic division at anaphase II.[30] This is in contrast to creating a breach mechanically in which there was no evidence of such arrest.

In the comparative study between SUZI, PZD and IVF in 131 patients, it was apparent that if the patients had failed IVF on more than one occasion, PZD would be likely to be less successful than SUZI. It is probable that the morphology is also relevant and, although not assessed in this data, has been discussed elsewhere (Chapter 7).

The current data suggests that PZD should be

the first approach with antisperm auto-antibodies, but care should be given to the insemination concentration as there is a high incidence of polyspermia. However, for patients with a TMC < 1 SUZI would be the preferred approach.

There was no distinction in the incidence of cleavage between PZD and SUZI in all groups assessed.

During this early developmental period for the clinical use of SUZI and PZD it is apparent that these techniques can achieve fertilisation, pregnancy and birth in couples unable to conceive by non-MAF procedures. The underlying concern that the incidence of abnormal embryos may increase after SUZI, or, by bypassing the selection criteria for spermatozoa at the level of the zona pellucida, there may be an increase in the demise of embryos cannot be emphatically dismissed. However, the numbers of normal, ongoing pregnancies and births to date have alleviated much of the initial concerns. Subzonal insemination and PZD are now proving a viable option for certain causes of infertility.

The barrier to improving the success of SUZI is at the level of fertilisation. By adjusting the numbers of spermatozoa used for SUZI, based on the TMC, the morphology of spermatozoa, and possibly certain sperm function tests, and comparing these with the incidence of fertilisation, polyspermia, cytoplasmic fragmentation and cleavage arrest, we may be able to attain a formula for the optimal procurement of viable embryos. An increase in the fundamental research studies relating particularly to human gametes and techniques to aid fusion of the gametes (see Chapter 12), thus limiting the numbers of sperm used for SUZI, will undoubtedly increase the incidence of fertilisation as well as the procurement of fertilisation in specific cases hitherto unamenable to conception *in vitro*.

Acknowledgements

The authors are very grateful to Miss Jenny Hall for the provision of Figure 7.1.

References

1. Fishel S, Jackson P, Antinori S, Johnson J, Lisi F, Chiariello F, Versaci C, Lisi R. Sub-zonal insemination (SUZI) for the alleviation of infertility. *Fertility and Sterility*. 1990; **54**: 828–35.
2. Fishel S, Symonds EM (eds.) *In-Vitro Fertilisation – Past, Present and Future*. Oxford: IRL Press, 1986.
3. Mortimer D. Comparison of the fertilising ability of human spermatozoa pre-incubated in calcium- and strontium-containing media. *Journal of Experimental Zoology*. 1986; **237**: 21–4.
4. Mortimer D, Chorney MJ, Curtis EF, Trounson AO. Calcium dependence of human sperm fertilizing ability. *Journal of Experimental Zoology*. 1988; **246**: 194–201.
5. Fishel S, Timson J, Lisi F, Rinaldi L. Evaluation of 225 patients undergoing subzonal insemination for the procurement of fertilization in vitro. *Fertility and Sterility*. 1992 (in press).
6. Gordon JW, Grunfeld L, Garrisi GJ, Talansky BE, Richards C, Laufer N. Fertilization of human oocytes by sperm from infertile males after zona pellucida drilling. *Fertility and Sterility*. 1988; **50**: 68–73.
7. Ng S-C, Bongso A, Ratnam SS, Sathananthan H, Chan CLK, Wong PC, Hagglund L, Anandakumar C, Wong YC, Goh VHH. Pregnancy after transfer of sperm under zona. *Lancet*. 1988; **2**: 790.
8. Kola I, Lacham O, Jansen RPS, Turner M, Trounson A. Chromosomal analysis of human oocytes fertilized by micro-injection of spermatozoa into the perivitelline space. *Human Reproduction*. 1990; **5**: 575–7.
9. Fishel S, Antinori S, Jackson P, Johnson J, Lisi F, Chiariello F, Versaci C. Twin birth after sub-zonal insemination. *Lancet*. 1990; **335**: 722–3.
10. Bongso TA, Sathananthan AH, Wong PC, Ratnam SS, Ng S-C, Anandakumar C, Ganatra S. Human fertilization by micro-injection of immotile spermatozoa. *Human Reproduction*. 1989; **4**: 175–9.
11. Ng S-C, Bongso TA, Sathananthan H, Ratnam SS. Micromanipulation: its relevance to human in vitro fertilization. *Fertility and Sterility*. 1990; **53**: 203–19.
12. Sathananthan AH, Ng S-C, Trounson A, Bongso A, Laws-King A, Ratnam SS. Human micro-insemination by injection of single or multiple sperm: ultrastructure. *Human Reproduction*. 1989; **4**: 574–83.
13. Fishel S, Antinori S, Jackson P, Johnson J, Rinaldi L. Presentation of six pregnancies established by sub-zonal insemination (SUZI). *Human Reproduction*.

1991; **6**: 124–30.

14. Shalgi R, Dor J, Rudak E, Lusky A, Goldman B, Mashiach S, Nebel L. Penetration of sperm from teratospermic men into zona-free hamster eggs. *International Journal of Andrology*. 1985; **8**: 285–94.

15. Marsh SK, Bolton VN, Braude PR. The effect of morphology on the ability of human spermatozoa to penetrate zona free hamster oocytes. *Human Reproduction*. 1987; **2**: 499–503.

16. Kruger TF, Menkveld R, Stander FSH, Lombard CF, van der Merwe JP, van Zyl JA, Smith K. Sperm morphologic features as a prognostic factor in in-vitro fertilization. *Fertility and Sterility*. 1986; **46**: 1118–23.

17. Kruger TF, Acosta AA, Simmons KF, Swanson RJ, Matta JF, Oehninger S. Predicted value of abnormal sperm morphology in IVF. *Fertility and Sterility*. 1988; **49**: 112–17.

18. Menkveld R, Stander FSH, Kotze TJvW, Kruger FT, van Zyl JA. The evaluation of morphological characteristics of human spermatozoa according to stricter criteria. *Human Reproduction*. 1990; **5**: 586–92.

19. Sathananthan AH, Trounson A, Wood C. *Atlas of Fine Structure of Human Sperm Penetration, Eggs and Embryos Cultured In Vitro*. Philadelphia: Praeger Scientific, 1986.

20. Cohen J, Alikani M, Malter HE, Adler A, Talansky BE, Rosenwaks Z. Partial zona dissection or subzonal sperm insertion: microsurgical fertilization alternatives based on evaluation of sperm morphology. *Fertility and Sterility*. 1991; **56**: 696–706.

21. Cohen J, Malter H, Fehilly C, Wright G, Elsner C, Kort H, Massey J. Implantation of embryos after partial opening of oocyte zona pellucida to facilitate sperm penetration. *Lancet*. 1988; **2**: 162.

22. Malter HE, Cohen J. Partial zona dissection of the human oocyte: a non-traumatic method using micromanipulation to assist zona pellucida penetration. *Fertility and Sterility*. 1989; **51**: 139–48.

23. Payne D, McLaughlin KJ, Depypere HT, Kirby CA, Warnes GM, Matthews CD. Experience with zona drilling and zona cutting to improve fertilization rates of human oocytes in vitro. *Human Reproduction*. 1991; **6**: 423–31.

24. Cohen J, Malter H, Wright G, Kort H, Massey J, Metchell D. Partial zona dissection of human oocytes when failure of zona pellucida penetration is anticipated. *Human Reproduction*. 1989; **4**: 435–42.

25. Malter H, Talansky B, Gordon J, Cohen J. Monospermy and polyspermy after partial zona dissection of reinseminated human oocytes. *Gamete Research*. 1989; **23**: 377–86.

26. Yanagimachi R. Mammalian fertilisation. In: Knobil E, Neill J (eds.) *The Physiology of Reproduction*. New York: Raven Press, 1988, pp. 135.

27. Sathananthan AH, Chen C. Sperm-oocyte membrane fusion in the human during monospermic fertilization. *Gamete Research*. 1986; **15**: 177–8.

28. Plachot M, Gunca AM, Mandelbaum J, de Grouchy J, Salat-Baroux J, Cohen J. Chromosome investigation in early life. II. Human pre-implantation embryos. *Human Reproduction*. 1987; **2**: 29–35.

29. Gordon JW, Grunfeld L, Garrisi GJ, Talansky BE, Richards C, Laufer N. Fertilization of human oocytes by sperm from infertile males after zona pellucida drilling. *Fertility and Sterility*. 1988; **50**: 68–73.

30. Ng S-C, Bongso TA, Chang SI, Sathananthan AH, Ratnam SS. Transfer of human sperm into the perivitelline space of human oocytes after zona-drilling or zona-puncture. *Fertility and Sterility*. 1989; **52**: 73–9.

Section IV
Partial zona pellucida dissection (PZD)

Chapter 8

Microsurgical fertilisation and zona pellucida micro-manipulation

H E Malter, J Cohen, J Alikani, J Grifo, B E Talansky
and Z Rosenwaks

Introduction

The human *in vitro* fertilisation (IVF) laboratory has recently undergone a minor revolution in the treatment of infertility resulting from a deficiency in the male partner. Micromanipulation techniques are being used to obtain fertilisation and pregnancies in cases that would have been considered hopeless only a few years ago. Over 75 pregnancies have been established worldwide following the use of microsurgical fertilisation (MF) techniques. Besides fertilisation failure, micromanipulation has been used to address other problems associated with human embryology.

In this chapter, we will discuss different aspects of our experience with clinical micromanipulation. First, micromanipulation techniques for the promotion of fertilisation will be evaluated. These techniques mainly involve circumventing the zona pellucida (ZP), a major barrier to gamete fusion in instances of male factor related infertility. Secondly, the consequences of ZP manipulation will be addressed. Some of these are detrimental, such as an increase in polyspermy, while others may be beneficial, such as an improvement in embryonic hatching. The creation of an opening in the ZP is a simple procedure with profound consequences.

Fertilisation and assisted fertilisation

Monospermic fertilisation results from the fine coordination of two intricate reproductive systems. The molecular and physical processes that occur in the male and female mammalian tracts are subject to dysfunction at many levels. Additionally, the concurrence of events necessary for normal fertilisation is particularly sensitive to interruption. The development of gamete micromanipulation technology has enabled the reproductive biologist to circumvent any inefficient steps in the fertilisation process that might prevent sperm–egg fusion from reaching completion.

To date, three major categories of assisted fertilisation by gamete micromanipulation have been explored in several mammalian systems. The first involves the creation of an artificial gap in the ZP. Subsequently, the micromanipulated oocyte is inseminated according to standard IVF protocols.

These procedures have been broadly termed 'zona drilling'. A second category of micromanipulation techniques directed at facilitating sperm–egg interaction is the subzonal insertion (SZI) of sperm. More invasive than zona drilling, SZI completely bypasses the ZP and involves direct placement of sperm into the perivitelline space. Finally, the third and most invasive form of microsurgical fertilisation is the micro-injection of sperm into the cytoplasm of the oocyte. This method entails the traversal of all outer barriers of the oocyte: the cumulus-corona complex, the ZP and the oolemma.

Zona drilling

In the original zona drilling procedure, developed in the mouse, a minute volume of acidic solution was gently released from a microneedle on a small portion of the ZP until the point at which it was breached.[1] Routine insemination followed the procedure. In this model, the creation of an artificial gap in the ZP was associated with increased rates of fertilisation at both normal and reduced sperm concentrations. Initial pronuclear formation was observed about 45 minutes earlier in manipulated groups than in controls. In addition, zona drilling resulted in rates of supernumerary sperm penetration which did not differ from the incidence of polyspermy in zona-intact controls. Mouse zygotes that resulted from assisted fertilisation by zona drilling, when transferred to the oviducts of pseudopregnant foster female mice, gave rise to normal live young. The zona drilling procedure exposed sperm to a region of direct access to the oocyte and allowed the ZP to retain its many physiological functions following fertilisation.

In order to develop zona drilling as a potential tool for clinical IVF, additional animal studies were undertaken. It was demonstrated that frequently, after the creation of a relatively large hole in the ZP, the embryo tended to protrude through the gap as development progressed. This sometimes resulted in embryonic development both inside and outside the zona, or in the loss of intact blastomeres. When a portion of the blastocyst protruded through the small gap in the zona, the resulting constriction frequently caused the formation of twin blastocysts.[2,3] Also, hatching routinely occurred one day earlier in micromanipulated than in ZP-intact control embryos.[3]

Removal of a portion of the ZP is effective in exposing sperm directly to the oocyte. Several experiments have shown that the sperm are actually utilising the artificially created gap to gain access to the egg. It is known that in the mouse premature induction of the acrosome reaction (AR) prevents fertilisation of zona-intact oocytes.[4] With this in mind, Gordon and Talansky induced the AR in populations of mouse sperm with dibutryl cyclic guanosine monophosphate (dB cGMP), and demonstrated that these acrosomeless sperm were able to penetrate zona-drilled, but not zona-intact oocytes.[1] Conover and Gwatkin exposed oocytes to an antibody to ZP-3, and showed that these oocytes could not be penetrated without micromanipulation by zona drilling.[5] Recently we showed that a method of zona drilling greatly increased the rate of fertilisation in a strain of random-bred mice, which is normally refractory to sperm penetration *in vitro*.[6] These results all indicate that sperm are indeed traversing the opening in the ZP following micromanipulation.

Since the results of the initial animal studies were encouraging, micromanipulation-assisted fertilisation was applied to clinical IVF.[7,8] While fertilisation was frequently achieved, embryonic cleavage was abnormal, and no pregnancies resulted after uterine replacement. The human ZP differed from the mouse zona in its response to acid Tyrode's solution. While the outer layer of the human ZP was easily dissolved by the acidic solution, the inner, more resistant layer required longer exposure in order to be completely breached. Enzymatic methods for zona opening were also not effective for use with human oocytes.[9]

Various alternative methods for opening the ZP were proposed, for example, zona cutting and cracking.[10,11] A mechanical procedure for introducing a gap in the mammalian ZP was developed, which resulted in the first human pregnancy from microsurgical fertilisation.[12] This method, termed partial zona dissection (PZD), involves the use of a sucrose solution to shrink the oocyte so that a glass microneedle can be introduced into the PVS without damaging the oocyte. The clinical use of PZD appears promising. To date, over 30 live births have resulted from this method of microsurgical fertilisation, and many pregnancies are ongoing.

What types of fertilisation disorders may be alleviated by zona micromanipulation procedures such as zona drilling or PZD? The motility which is acquired and enhanced during sperm development is important for penetration through outer egg investments. It has been shown, however, that motility may not be necessary for traversal through the plasma membrane.[13,14] Thus, sperm with non-progressive, abnormal or limited motility may be relatively inefficient in traversing only the outermost barriers of the oocyte. Micromanipulation may also be useful when the ZP is impenetrable by even 'normal' sperm. Alteration of ZP glycoproteins may cause the ZP to be refractile to sperm binding and penetration. In the human, antibodies to sperm can be present in the follicle and may result in infertility due to prevention of fertilisation.[15] Additionally, properties of the ZP are altered with time in culture and exposure to serum.[16,17] The zona hardening that results from *in vitro* culture can inhibit sperm penetration. In both of these instances, it may be possible to bypass the zona barrier with microsurgical fertilisation.

Subzonal sperm insertion

A second method of assisted fertilisation utilising micromanipulation is SZI. In the procedure, the ZP is not merely opened, but is functionally and physically bypassed. Sperm are aspirated into a hollow microneedle, and are deposited into the PVS. Like zona drilling methods, SZI has been attempted in both animal and human models. Only sperm which have undergone capacitation and the AR will be capable of fusing with the oolemma. Several researchers have argued that since the ZP is no longer involved in the selection process, it may be necessary to use artificial induction of the AR in order to ensure that the 'selected' sperm will be capable of fertilisation. However, spermatozoa of most mammalian species are fragile and easily prone to physical damage.[18,19] Full embryonic development and live birth was achieved in a study during which mouse sperm, capacitated

under 'normal' conditions in a viscous solution of methyl cellulose, were placed subzonally.[20] This treatment served to slow the motility and facilitate capture of the spermatozoa into the microneedle. It is likely that exposure to the methyl cellulose protected vulnerable mouse sperm from the mechanical and physiological damage caused by aspiration into the microneedle that was reported in previous studies.[18] Others have tried to combine the use of methyl cellulose with various methods of AR induction in order to improve the results of SZI by generating more uniform populations of acrosome-reacted sperm.[21]

Recently, some of the developmental work on SZI has come to fruition in the clinical laboratory. Successful application of a method for synchronising capacitation in which sperm are incubated in medium in which strontium chloride is substituted for calcium has been reported.[22,23] This method enabled the investigators, for the first time, to obtain fertilisation after a single, motile spermatozoon was placed under the human ZP. Subsequently, others reported pregnancies[24,25] and the first births[26] after transfer of multiple (3-10) sperm under the ZP. Special methods of sperm preparation were not employed in these studies. Fertilisation in human oocytes injected with immotile sperm from a male with Kartagener's disease has also been reported.[27] Recently, we have applied SZI to severe cases of male factor infertility.[28] The data obtained from these clinical trials has clarified several biological principles and has raised interesting questions pertaining to mammalian fertilisation. For example, although both PZD and SZI may be effective treatments for cases of extreme teratozoospermia, it has become clear that those embryos derived from SZI implant at a significantly higher rate than those resulting from the PZD procedure.[28] A possible explanation for this phenomenon, as well as further results, are offered below.

Physiological aspects of zona pellucida micromanipulation

The evolution of gamete micromanipulation has not only introduced an important and novel approach to treating fertilisation disorders, but has also provided new insight into the biology of fertilisation in different mammalian systems.

Results of several studies have clarified the role served by the ZP in the oocytes' block to polyspermy. While limited levels of polyspermy were reported in the mouse model, using zona drilling and PZD, these rates increase when such techniques are applied to the human oocyte.[27,29] It is known that in the mouse, there is a slow and partial block to polyspermy at the level of the plasma membrane.[30] On the other hand, polyspermy control in the human oocyte seems to be more dependent on the ZP.[7,29] Whether or not the human vitelline membrane maintains a slow and/or transient function has not yet been defined. However, results of clinical trials of SZI, which show that polyspermy increases with increased numbers of sperm placed in the PVS, emphasise the minor role played by the plasma membrane in polyspermy prevention.[31,32]

During the initial phase of clinical PZD application, it was noted that the degree of polyspermic fertilisation was reduced as the interval between exposure to sucrose and insemination was increased.[29] It was postulated that sucrose was somehow affecting sperm receptivity of the plasma membrane. This effect became increasingly apparent with time. The hypothesis was tested further in a trial of PZD performed on one day old re-inseminated oocytes.[33] By varying the periods of exposure to sucrose following micromanipulation, it was demonstrated that polyspermy rates were significantly altered by changing the interval during which oocytes were

exposed to sucrose. The investigators suggested that the changes in the cell membrane resembling activation were triggered by sucrose. Whether such changes involve any of the biological processes associated with physiological 'activation',[24] such as calcium oscillations and/or metabolic alterations, remains unclear. Whatever the mechanism, however, the receptivity and fusogenic characteristics of the oocyte plasma membrane are subject to effects of the micromanipulation protocol (probably related to sucrose exposure). Such technical details appear to have profound consequences for subsequent sperm–egg interaction.

Zona manipulation has also helped to elucidate the biological role of the mammalian egg surface during fertilisation. In a recent investigation, PZD was used in conjunction with IVF to study the function of the heterogeneous surface structure of the mouse and hamster oocyte.[6] Specifically, the function of the microvillus-free area of the vitellus associated with the first polar body was examined by performing PZD both in proximity, and opposite to this area of the egg surface. Inseminations of such oocytes revealed clear differences in sperm–egg interactions which were dependent on the site of zona manipulation (Table 8.1). The experimental design supported the fact that sperm made contact and interacted with the oocyte at the site of micromanipulation. Further, manipulation of the ZP at a region opposite the first polar body and therefore away from the microvillus-free area consistently resulted in higher rates of fertilisation than when PZD was performed near the polar body. This data therefore indicates that in some

Table 8.1 Fertilisation (penetration) following the application of PZD distal or next to the first polar body (PB1) in mouse oocytes (mouse sperm) and hamster eggs (mouse sperm)

Species	Location of PZD on ZP	Proportion of micromanipulated eggs with fertilisation	
Mouse	Next to PB1	26/206	(12.6%)*
(random bred)	Distal to PB1	84/225	(37.3%)*
	No PZD	4/119	(3.4%)
Hamster	Next to PB1	77/224	(34.4%)†
(mouse sperm)	Distal to PB1	117/192	(60.9%)†
	Zona-free	98/101	(97.0%)

Source: Talansky et al.,1991.[6]
Notes: * P < 0.01.
  † P < 0.001.

consistently resulted in higher rates of fertilisation than when PZD was performed near the polar body. This data therefore indicates that in some mammalian species, zona manipulation for assisting fertilisation should be done at a region away from the polar body. Whether these results are applicable to human IVF is not clear. However, clinical data in which the site of PZD in relation to the polar body has been carefully recorded suggests that the human oocyte may not have a functional microvillus-free area (Table 8.2). In fact, the results seem to indicate that in the human oocyte, zona dissection near the polar body favours supernumerary sperm entry. It may be that in the absence of a (functional) microvillus-free region, the enlarged PVS created by the polar body acts as a 'sink' in which sperm may accumulate.

Clinical microsurgical fertilisation

Human IVF can be considered a treatment of limited gamete interaction since sperm and eggs are placed in close proximity under carefully optimised conditions.[35] However, the presence of sperm and possibly oocyte abnormalities as well often results in a complete failure of fertilisation

even by the most carefully optimised application of the standard technique. In addition, a number of infertile men with very few live spermatozoa in their semen are refused access to IVF centres. Various micromanipulation strategies discussed in the previous section have been suggested for the promotion of sperm–egg fusion in these couples. Of these methods, only PZD and SZI have been applied successfully in the human.[12,24,25]

Partial zona dissection

Partial zona dissection has produced over 60 pregnancies in more than 10 different IVF centres. We have applied this procedure to 177 couples with male factor infertility at Reproductive Biology Associates in Atlanta and The Centre for Reproductive Medicine and Infertility of The New York Hospital, Cornell Medical Centre. Basically, three groups of patients were admitted for these studies (Table 8.3). The first group which comprises approximately half of the total number of patients had severely abnormal semen analyses and failed to fertilise all oocytes in a previous IVF cycle.[28,36] Some of these patients failed to fertilise when IVF

Table 8.2 Fertilisation and polyspermy following the application of PZD distal or next to the first polar body (PB1) in 10 patients

Location of PZD on ZP	Proportion of micromanipulated eggs with					
	Monospermy		Polyspermy		Fertilisation	
Next to PB1	8/29	(28%)	7/29	(24%)	15/29	(52%)
Distal to PB1	14/31	(45%)	1/31	(3%)	15/31	(48%)

Table 8.3 Selection criteria for MF and regular IVF in instances of male factor infertility

Group	Selection criterion	< 50 000 motile sperm recovered	Highest semen cut-off criterion			Treatments		
			Count (× 10^6/m)	Motility	Morphology	PZD	SZI	IVF
A	Previous failure of fertilisation	occasionally	10	20%	10%	+	+	optional
B	Semen analysis unacceptable for regular IVF	always	5	10%	2%	optional	+	–
C	Semen analysis acceptable for IVF	not applicable but reduced progression and survival	20	30%	10%	+	+	+
D	Semen analysis acceptable for IVF	not applicable	20	30%	10%	–	–	+

was repeated several times. The second group had not been accepted for regular IVF by any other programmes, including our own. These patients' semen analyses were considered highly abnormal; only a maximum of 50 000 motile spermatozoa could be retrieved from their semen, even if the final sperm pellet was resuspended in a small volume of 20 to 50 μl.[28] Such patients were advised to have microsurgical fertilisation rather than a standard IVF cycle. The third group (approximately 30 per cent of those selected for PZD) had not attempted IVF previously (some were not acceptable to other IVF programmes) and all had male factor infertility of intermediate severity.[28] Since the chances of fertilisation would be somewhat reduced among these patients, micromanipulation was performed on some of their oocytes, while other oocytes were left intact. A fourth group of patients with abnormal semen analyses were not considered suitable for PZD since many motile spermatozoa were recovered from their semen and they had never had a previous IVF attempt. Results of the first three groups are summarised in Table 8.4. Fertilisation rates were significantly higher in PZD oocytes than in zona-intact oocytes.[28,29,36] However, one should not compare fertilisation rates of both groups of oocytes in men who were selected according to different criteria. For example, the fertilisation of PZD oocytes by spermatozoa from men who were not able to fertilise oocytes in a previous regular IVF cycle is significantly higher than that of PZ-intact control oocytes.[28] However, it is approximately the same as that of regular IVF in couples who were selected for PZD, but who never had IVF before. Some of the patients received only PZD embryos, whereas others received ZP-intact controls and PZD embryos. A small number of patients had only ZP-intact control embryos replaced and two of them became pregnant.[28] Overall though, at least 11 pregnancies were produced following replacement of only PZD embryos, and in several other patients twin pregnancies were obtained following replacement of one control embryo combined with one or more PZD embryos (Table 8.4). Twenty-one per cent of all embryos implanted successfully and 22 per cent of the patients had a clinical pregnancy. We have postulated recently that the high incidence of implantation could be explained by the presence of the artificial gap in the ZP, facilitating the blastocysts to shed the ZP during hatching.[37,38] This assumption has led to several investigations attempting to introduce a micromanipulation method, which we have named 'assisted hatching', possibly suitable for all IVF embryos and applied shortly before transfer (see below).

Subzonal sperm insertion and frequency of gamete fusion

The concept that most spermatozoa in the ejaculate are unable to fertilise – even those from fertile men – and represent chiasmatic errors occurring during

Table 8.4 Results of PZD trials with ZP intact (ZI) controls (117 cycles in male factor couples) performed at Reproductive Biology Associates (RBA, Atlanta, Georgia) between March 1988 and September 1990 and 60 similar cycles performed at the Centre for Reproductive Medicine and Infertility (The New York Hospital, Cornell Medical Centre, New York) between October 1989 and December 1990

Parameter	Cohen et al. 1990[37]	Tucker et al. 1991[35]	Cohen et al. 1991[31]*	Total
Fertilisation of ZP intact (ZI) eggs	42/129 (33%)	33/254 (13%)	n.a.	n.a.
Fertilisation (PZD eggs)	75/138 (54%)	73/281 (26%)	101/282 (36%)	149/701 (36%)
Replacements/cycles	37/47 (79%)	30/70 (43%)	41/60 (68%)	108/177 (61%)
Number ZI embryos replaced	24	20	21	65
Number PZD embryos replaced	55	40	82	177
Number fetuses/Number embryos replaced	15/79 (19%)	17/60 (28%)	17/103 (17%)	49/242 (20%)
Clinical pregnancy	10	16	13	39
Ongoing/delivered	8	13	10	31
Pregnancies from PZD embryos only	2	4	5	11
Pregnancies from PZD/ZI mixed	8	12	6	26
Clinical pregnancies/cycle	10/47 (21%)	16/70 (23%)	13/60 (22%)	39/177 (22%)
Clinical pregnancies/transfer	10/37 (27%)	16/30 (53%)	13/41 (32%)	39/108 (36%)

Note: *ZI control oocytes only occasionally used.

spermatogenesis is not well founded. The question related to the fertilising ability of individual human spermatozoa is not only intriguing scientifically; it is also important to know how many spermatozoa from fertile and infertile men can fuse with the oolemma if SZI is to be used rather than IVF, as an alternate mode for obtaining fertilisation.

Recently we performed an SZI study in couples with male factor infertility by inserting between one and 20 motile spermatozoa in the perivitelline space (PVS) of fresh mature oocytes.[31] Sixteen per cent of individual spermatozoa were able to fuse with the oolemma and form a pronucleus. It is therefore not surprising that fertilisation following SZI increased when more spermatozoa were inserted. However, the incidence of polyspermy also increased, especially when more than two motile sperm cells were introduced into the PVS. Insertion of more than eight spermatozoa resulted in 100 per cent polyspermy indicating that sperm cells derived from infertile men are frequently capable of fusion with the oolemma. More than half of motile spermatozoa from men with normal semen analyses are able to fuse with the oolemma when inserted directly into the PVS of morphologically normal mature one day old oocytes. This conclusion was obtained from the use of SZI techniques in oocytes which failed to fertilise following insemination in a group of couples with various types of infertility. Instead of regular re-insemination, SZI was performed.[32]

Subzonal sperm insertion for treatment of infertile men

Subzonal sperm insertion in oocytes from couples in whom the men were considered infertile has led to pregnancies at five different centres.[24,25,28,39,40] In order to evaluate the potential applications of PZD and SZI, we have recently assessed both techniques simultaneously by comparing them in sibling oocytes in couples with male factor infertility in whom regular IVF had failed previously or in whom normal fertilisation was likely to be reduced due to severe semen abnormalities (Table 8.3, groups A and B).[28] In addition, the embryonic morphology and implantation potential of PZD and

SZI embryos from couples with extreme forms of teratozoospermia was compared using retrospective analyses of videotapes of microsurgically fertilised embryos shortly before replacement. The morphology of these micromanipulated embryos was compared to those of ZP-intact embryos cultured under identical conditions and replaced concurrently. Previously, it was demonstrated that the percentage of spermatozoa with normal shape assessed with strict criteria was the only semen parameter correlated with the implanting capacity of PZD embryos.[31,41]

To date 68 couples have been referred to us for microsurgical fertilisation (MF) in whom we applied SZI. The oocytes were subjected to various treatments according to the selection criteria presented in Table 8.3. Recently we demonstrated in the first 48 patients recruited for this treatment that the rate of fertilisation in SZI eggs (37/125, 30 per cent) was significantly higher ($P < 0.01$) than in PZD eggs (11/86, 13 per cent) in cases where ZP-intact control eggs could not be included due to extremely low sperm numbers.[28] This indicates that the PZD technique requires higher motile sperm concentrations than SZI. Surprisingly, fertilisation appeared higher in SZI eggs from patients with a previous failure of fertilisation (48/129, 37 per cent) than in patients who never had an IVF attempt before (17/125, 14 per cent). This possibly demonstrates that the latter group of patients were selected using very low cut-off criteria.

Despite the severity of their sperm profiles, 71 per cent of the patients had an embryo replacement and 13 of them became clinically pregnant (19 per cent (Table 8.5)). Eight of these pregnancies were established in patients in whom only SZI embryos were available. One of these was a twin and another a triplet pregnancy. One quadruplet pregnancy was established in a patient who had two SZI, one PZD and one ZP-intact embryo replaced. One patient became pregnant after replacement of control embryos only, and two other pregnancies were established in patients who had both PZD and SZI embryos replaced. The range and number of possible implantations attributed to microsurgical embryos are indicated for each group in Table 8.5.

Recently we correlated the implanting ability of 74 MF embryos with teratozoospermia.[28]

Subzonally inserted embryos (n = 15) from men with extreme teratozoospermia were able to implant at a significantly higher rate than PZD embryos (n = 18) from a comparable group of men (Table 8.6).[28] Due to the possibility of mixed embryo transfers (SZI and/or PZD and/or ZP-intact control), the range of minimum and maximum implantation rates was compared for each group; both analyses were significant. If it is assumed that a minimum number of embryos from microsurgical fertilisation implanted, then none of the 18 PZD embryos from couples with extreme teratozoospermia implanted. Under these conditions, SZI appeared significantly more successful; at least 6/15 (40 per cent) of the embryos implanted. The same significance was found when

the assumption was made that the maximum number of embryos implanted was derived from MF. Again SZI appeared more effective than PZD in this particular group of patients. Using the same mode of comparison, PZD appeared more successful than SZI in men with moderate teratozoospermia; however the trend was not significant due to the small sample size.

The total number of abnormal embryo characteristics (score between 0 and 11) in PZD embryos was not different from that of SZI embryos (an average of 2.4 and 2.9 respectively). However, the distribution of abnormal embryos in both groups was different when it was correlated with teratozoospermia. For example, PZD embryos from extreme teratozoospermic patients were more fre-

Table 8.5 Results of SZI performed in 68 couples. PZD and ZP-intact oocytes were occasionally included according to the criteria used in Table 8.1

Cycles		68 (a)
Replacements		48 (b) (71% of a)
Positive βHCG		15
Clinically pregnant (fetal heart beat)		13 (19% of a; 27% of b)

Type of embryo(s) replaced	*Proportion of pregnancy per replacement*	*Incidence of embryos implanting*
SZI exclusively	8/25	11/48 (23%)
PZD and SZI	1/4	1/13
PZD exclusively	1/4	1/6
PZD and/or SZI and/or ZP-intact	2/14	5/42
ZP-intact†	1/1	1/2
Total	13/48 (27%)	19/111 (17%)

Notes: a SZI oocytes were not fertilised.
b SZI and PZD oocytes not fertilised.

Table 8.6 Correlation between sperm morphology and ability of SZI and PZD embryos to implant

	Percentage normal sperm in semen			
	0.5% *Incidence of embryonic implantation*		*6–10%* *Incidence of embryonic implantation*	
Mode of micromanipulation	*Minimum*	*Maximum*	*Minimum*	*Maximum*
PZD	0/18 (0%)*	3/18 (20%)†	5/25 (20%)	7/25 (28%)
SZI	6/15 (40%)*,=	7/15 (47%)†,×	1/16 (7%)=	1/16 (7%)×

Notes: *† P < 0.05.
= P < 0.05.
× P < 0.02.

quently abnormal (defined as having at least two abnormalities) than embryos from moderate teratozoospermic patients (94 per cent versus 56 per cent, respectively). On the other hand, most abnormal SZI embryos (87 per cent) were associated with cases of moderate teratozoospermia. Plausible explanations for these observations are given elsewhere.[32]

In conclusion, techniques such as PZD and SZI are advantageous in cases of extreme male factor infertility. They can be used either simultaneously on sibling oocytes or if indicated, individually. Based on the preliminary findings presented above, SZI should be applied to extreme forms of male factor infertility, whereas PZD may be more beneficial in cases of moderately abnormal semen profiles.

Microsurgical fertilisation in patients with normal semen in whom IVF failed

Microsurgical fertilisation was performed in two groups of 158 couples. Couples from Group A (n = 128) had severe forms of male factor infertility based on abnormal semen analysis. Over 75 per cent of these patients failed IVF previously or were rejected due to insufficient sperm numbers. Oocytes of 68 Group A patients were micromanipulated with PZD (Table 8.4). Oocytes from the 60 other patients were micromanipulated with SZI (Table 8.5). Couples in Group B (n = 30) had normal semen analyses, but had failed to fertilise during regular *in vitro* fertilisation (IVF) previously. A few of the female partners in Group B had immunological infertility, some had morphologically abnormal oocytes, but most appeared to have completely normal gametes. Oocytes from 15 patients were

treated with PZD. The oocytes from the other 15 patients were micromanipulated with SZI. The incidences of fertilisation in these (sub)groups of patients were not different and ranged between 15 per cent to 35 per cent, depending on the selection criterion used. The proportion of replacements (at least one monospermic embryo) was 89/128 (70 per cent) for Group A and 26/30 (87 per cent) for Group B (Table 8.7). The proportion of clinical pregnancy per cycle was 26/128 (20 per cent for Group A and 1/30 (3 per cent) for Group B ($0.05 < P < 0.10$)). The proportions of replaced embryos implanting were 36/214 (17 per cent) and 1/47 (2 per cent) for Groups A and B respectively ($P < 0.05$). In Group A, 13 fetuses were derived definitely from SZI-embryos and 10 from PZD-embryos. The other 13 fetuses resulted from replacements of mixtures of PZD/SZI and zona-intact embryos. The single fetus in Group B originated from a PZD embryo. It can be concluded that PZD and SZI are promising techniques for treatment of severe male factor infertility, whereas MF embryos from patients who failed regular IVF with apparently normal gametes rarely implant.

Polyspermy correction by enucleation

Considering the increase in polyspermy observed following microsurgical fertilisation it would be highly desirable to be able to reduce the incidence of polyspermy or correct the abnormal zygotes which result from it. We have reported previously on a technique for the correction of polyspermic zygotes through the microsurgical removal of the extra sperm pronucleus.[42] We report here on improved results using a modification of this technique and

Table 8.7 Reduced implanting ability of microsurgical embryos from couples with normal semen analysis who failed to fertilise following standard IVF

Number of patients	Semen analysis	Proportion of replacements	Proportion of clinical pregnancies	Proportion of embryos implanting
30	normal	26/39 (87%)	1/30 (3%)	1/47 (2%)
128	abnormal	89/128 (70%)	26/128 (20%)	36/214 (17%)
P-value		not significant	0.05–0.10	< 0.05

on the application of enucleation in determining pronuclear 'gender'. Seventy polyspermic human zygotes (with three [n = 58] or four [n = 12] pronuclei) were enucleated by aspiration using a 5–7 μm sharp glass microneedle. Before insertion of the needle, a flow of acidic Tyrode's solution was used to create a slight opening in the zona pellucida. An important factor is that zygotes were not exposed to cytoskeletal relaxants. The survival rate following the procedure was 87 per cent. Cleavage was observed in 73 per cent of the surviving enucleated embryos. However, 12 apparently healthy embryos were fixed for analysis prematurely at the zygote stage. The cleavage rate could therefore be as high as 93 per cent. The current success rates are higher than previously reported and would probably be satisfactory for clinical application. A serious question remaining is that of the identification of sperm pronuclei. Our hypothesis is that the egg pronucleus is situated at the closest proximity to the second polar body and the remaining pronuclei are derived from sperm. Efforts are currently underway using polymerase chain reaction (PCR) analysis to elucidate pronuclear gender. The genetic material from individual pronuclei or zygotes in which the putative sperm pronuclei have been removed is analysed by PCR amplification with X and Y chromosome specific probes. Theoretically, the putative egg pronucleus will always have only an X chromosome while the sperm pronuclei will exhibit signals from either X or Y probes. If this result is consistently obtained, it will confirm the validity of our selection criteria.

The effects of zona micromanipulation on the embryo

The molecular structure of the mammalian embryonic ZP as it undergoes hatching is largely unknown but it appears that the ZP matrix changes with time. Evidence suggests that hatching may occur via any of the following three mechanisms; (i) uterine enzymes digest the ZP from the outside; (ii) embryonic proteases digest the zona from the inside; and (iii) the zona is thinned through increased proliferation and pressure from the expanding blastocyst, sodium being pumped

into the blastocoele. Evidence for these three routes exist in the mouse, whereas embryonic proteases appear to be absent in several other species.[43] Expansion and thinning of the ZP appears to be essential for hatching and are observed in most mammalian species. In the rabbit, hatching only occurs when there are a minimal number of cells and ZP rupture appears to be associated with proliferation and physical expansion. Rhesus monkey blastocysts also require a minimal diameter in order for hatching to occur.[44]

Human embryos are usually transferred at the cleaved embryo stage, due to increased embryonic demise with prolonged culture. Only one in four fully expanded blastocysts derived from *in vitro* fertilised ovarian human oocytes will hatch.[44,45] This provides evidence that human blastocysts are capable of hatching in the absence of uterine lysins, but also demonstrates that zonae are often resistant to dissolution. The incidence of blastocyst formation and hatching can be increased by culturing human embryos on monolayers of reproductive tract cells.[46,47] This finding supports the argument that many *in vitro* fertilised embryos are deficient in the amount of zona lysins needed to initiate and complete hatching.

Although introducing an incision in the zona pellucida is a simple procedure, it may have important consequences for further embryonic development. For instance, micro-organisms, viruses and cytotoxins present in the insemination suspension could invade and infect the embryo via the artificially produced gap in the ZP (see section on microsurgical fertilisation). Immune cell invasion through gaps in the zona may cause embryonic death, prior to the formation of tight junctions.[48] Blastomeres may be lost through large holes, possibly causing embryonic death or vesiculation.[2] In addition embryos may be partly or completely lost through the artificial hole during transfer. Although it is difficult to monitor such events following embryo replacement, a trial which addressed some of these problems has been conducted in PZD patients.[49] Every other patient received corticosteroids and antibiotics for four days in order to counteract the potential effects of immune cell invasion. The rationale for corticosteroid administration was to reduce the number of intra-uterine immune cells. Seven of the eight pregnancies obtained following PZD occurred in the experimental group and although this represented a relatively small group of patients, immunosuppression is now routinely applied to patients whose oocytes or embryos are micromanipulated.

Disruption of the ZP by micromanipulation may not only lead to loss of embryonic tissue, but may also have profound consequences on the hatching process, a prerequisite for implantation. Both the timing and morphology of the hatching process *in vitro* of mouse and human PZD embryos are altered.[3] The ZP does not thin as it does normally during blastocyst expansion, and hatching occurs earlier and at a higher frequency. Though the sample sizes in the original studies were relatively small, human PZD embryos implanted better than zona-intact embryos.[29] This notion is supported in studies presented here (Table 8.4).

Assisted hatching

Assisted hatching of cleaved embryos was first applied to 99 patients at Reproductive Biology Associates in Atlanta using PZD as the technique to open the ZP.[37,38] Embryos allocated for replacement were micromanipulated in alternate patients. This resulted in an experimental group (patients whose embryos were micromanipulated) and a control group (patients whose embryos had intact ZP). The ZP of a total of 144 fresh two- to eight-cell embryos were thus micromanipulated. All embryos appeared intact following micromanipulation and none of the blastomeres were damaged. Positive βHCG was confirmed in 17/51 (34 per cent) of the control patients who received ZP-intact embryos, and 24/48 (50 per cent) of the assisted hatching patients. The incidence of clinical pregnancy increased from 26 per cent in the control group to 46 per cent per embryo replacement in the experimental group, a significant improvement (P < 0.05; chi-square test). Moreover, embryo implantation increased from 13 per cent to 22 per cent (P < 0.05). Half of the pregnancies in the experimental group were either twin or triplet pregnancies. Based on these experiments we have postulated that approximately one quarter of all

IVF embryos have the ability to implant, that a substantial number of IVF embryos are unable to breach the ZP at the time of hatching and that many can be rescued by opening their ZP several days earlier. It is as yet unclear whether assisted hatching using PZD should be applied as part of the standard IVF procedure. The PZD technique may have some disadvantages, some of which are discussed below.

Only 7 per cent of human embryos treated with assisted hatching implanted when we applied PZD in 20 couples at the IVF programme at Cornell in 1989. This series of investigations was not performed as part of a prospective randomised trial. However, the implantation rate of zona-intact embryos in this programme normally exceeds 10 per cent, indicating that PZD holes in the ZP may also have an adverse effect on implantation.

This may be due to differences between culture methods and replacement procedures between the two IVF programmes at the time. It is also possible that variations in follicular stimulation methods cause the ZP to be physically different in subgroups of patients. Though the hatching process may be inhibited following IVF (or perhaps even following natural fertilisation), it may not always be advantageous to perform assisted hatching on an embryo using the PZD technique two days after egg collection. Zona hardening alters the resilience of the ZP to the PZD technique; the incisions are easier to make and may be smaller than those made prior to fertilisation. Such embryos may only partially hatch.

The absence of zona thinning and expansion during expulsion of the blastocyst through the narrow artificial PZD opening may cause constriction of the trophoblast and the inner cell mass. Indeed, trophoblast tissue may be lost when the blastocyst squeezes through the narrow gap. At least one of the twins obtained following assisted hatching was monozygotic and miscarried in the second trimester of gestation. An animal model for assessing abnormalities of hatching after application of techniques like SZI and PZD has recently been developed in our laboratory.[50] Two types of distinctively different holes were made in 1190 eight-cell mouse embryos. Limited PZD was applied to produce small narrow incisions, and zona drilling with acidic Tyrode's (AT) across a larger area in the ZP was exercised to produce sizable round holes. Some embryos were only micromanipulated once, others were micromanipulated several times in order to simulate repetitive ZP breaching techniques occasionally applied in human IVF (for instance multiple stabbings of the ZP during subzonal sperm insertion). Blastocysts preferred to hatch through the artificial gaps, but completion of hatching was entirely dependent on the size of the hole. Only 16 per cent (26/167) of hatching PZD embryos migrating through narrow holes hatched completely, the remainder of them becoming trapped in a typical figure-of-eight shape. Seventy two per cent (43/60) of those migrating through larger PZD holes hatched. However, trophoblast outgrowth was not observed in any of the hatched PZD embryos. Significantly (P < 0.001) more AT blastocysts hatched (248/270; 92 per cent) and 176/248 (70 per cent) showed trophoblast outgrowth. Hatching through several openings simultaneously was rarely observed in AT embryos (14/167; 8 per cent), but occurred in 36 per cent (73/201) of the PZD embryos. The occurrence of trapped PZD embryos could be almost entirely avoided by performing zona drilling with AT elsewhere on the ZP following the PZD procedure(s) (Table 8.8). Only 3 per cent (4/158) of PZD embryos also drilled with AT became trapped during hatching. This compares favourably with micromanipulated PZD controls in which 77 per cent (104/136) became trapped (P < 0.0001). Embryos with multiple holes in their zonae preferentially hatched through the

largest opening. It is suggested that practitioners of human IVF carefully (re)assess the ability of micromanipulated embryos to fully hatch *in vitro*, prior to application of clinical micromanipulation systems. Micromanipulated embryos with small holes in their zonae may be rescued by performing an additional more aggressive opening procedure elsewhere on the ZP.

Another disadvantage of the clinical PZD procedure may be the loss of blastomeres or even the whole embryo during the replacement procedure.[32] Results may improve by enlarging the artificial hole and patching it with a self-digesting biological gel to improve its strength during embryo replacement and reduce intra-uterine immune invasion. Alternatively, embryos may be micromanipulated with acidic medium, a laser or a more vigorous mechanical procedure, to increase the size of the opening after the formation of constructional junctions between the blastomeres. This may avoid the hazards imposed on the embryos during replacement and would facilitate trophoblast expulsion during hatching. Recently it was demonstrated that desmosomes and gap junctions occur during the third cleavage division in the human.[51] Thus, biopsy techniques applied to eight-cell embryos with the use of acidic medium apparently facilitate hatching[52](c.f. Chapter 17). These issues are considered in a fully randomised trial we are currently conducting in consenting patients. Embryos from 30 couples were micromanipulated with AT to produce a large hole and replacements were performed at least 70 hours following egg collection. Preliminary results are very promising

Table 8.8 Abnormal hatching and trophoblast outgrowth following the introduction of narrow holes in the zonae of 8-cell mouse embryos and attempts to rescue such embryos by drilling larger holes elsewhere in the zonae

Experimental group		*Trapped hatching embryos*	*Hatched 8-cell embryos*	*Trophoblast outgrowth*
A	Zona-intact control	0/78 (0%)	78/91 (86%)	74/78 (95%)
B	Conservative PZD (≤ 5 μm hole)	104/136 (77%)	33/149 (22%)	0/33 (0%)
C	Agressive AT (11–25 μm hole)	4/75 (5%)	62/76 (83%)	42/62 (68%)
D	Simultaneous PZD and AT (PZD rescue)	4/158 (3%)	135/158 (85%)	123/135 (91%)
Chi-squares between group B versus A, C and D		P < 0.0001	P < 0.0001	P < 0.0001

since 31 per cent (31/103) of the micromanipulated embryos implanted (fetal heart activity). This compares favourably to randomised zona-intact embryos (from consenting control patients) of which 19 per cent (19/98) implanted. This trial is still continuing due to the relatively high P value (0.06) caused by the small sample sizes.

Acknowledgements

Janet Trowbridge is gratefully acknowledged for editing the manuscript and Adrienne Reing, Alexis Adler, Michael Bedford, Michael Tucker, Alan Berkeley, Owen Davis, Margaret Graf, and Helen Liu are thanked for their support of these studies.

References

1. Gordon JW, Talansky B. Assisted fertilization by zona drilling: a mouse model for correction of oligospermia. *Journal of Experimental Zoology*. 1986; **239**: 347–54.

2. Talansky BE, Gordon JW. Cleavage characteristics of mouse embryos inseminated and cultured after zona pellucida drilling. *Gamete Research*. 1988; **21**: 277–87.

3. Malter H, Cohen J. Blastocyst formation and hatching in vitro following zona drilling of mouse and human embryos. *Gamete Research*. 1989; **24**: 67–80.

4. Talansky BE, Barg PE, Gordon JW. Ion pump ATPase inhibitors block the fertilization of zona-free oocytes by acrosome-reacted spermatozoa. *Journal of Reproductive Fertility*. 1987; **79**: 447–55.

5. Conover JC, Gwatkin RBL. Fertilization of zona-drilled mouse oocytes treated with monoclonal antibody to the zona glycoprotein, ZP3. *Journal of Experimental Zoology*. 1988; **247**: 113–18.

6. Talansky BE, Malter HE, Cohen J. A preferential site for sperm–egg fusion in mammals. *Molecular Reproduction and Development*. 1991 (in press).

7. Gordon J, Grunfeld L, Garrisi GJ, Talansky BE, Richards C, Laufer N. Fertilization of human oocytes by sperm from infertile males after zona drilling. *Fertility and Sterility*. 1988; **50**: 68–73.

8. Malter HE, Cohen J. Partial zona dissection of the human oocytes: a nontraumatic method using micromanipulation to assist zona pellucida penetration. *Fertility and Sterility*. 1989; **51**: 139–48.

9. Garrisi GJ, Talansky BE, Grunfeld L, Sapira V, Gordon JW. Clinical evaluation of three approaches to micromanipulation-assisted fertilization. *Fertility and Sterility*. 1990; **54**: 671–7.

10. Depypere HT, McLaughlin FJ, Seamark RF, Warnes GM, Mathews CD. Comparison of zona cutting and zona drilling as techniques for assisted fertilization in the mouse. *Journal of Reproductive Fertility*. 1988; **84**: 205–11.

11. Odawara Y, Lopata A. A zona opening procedure for improving in vitro fertilization at low sperm concentrations: a mouse model. *Fertility and Sterility*. 1989; **51**: 699–704.

12. Cohen J, Malter H, Fehilly C, Wright G, Elsner C, Kort H, Massay J. Implantation of embryos after partial opening of oocyte zona pellucida to facilitate sperm penetration. *Lancet*. 1988; **2**: 162.

13. Cohen J, Weber RFA, van der Vijver JCM, Zeilmaker GH. In vitro fertilizing capacity of human spermatozoa with the use of zona-free hamster ova: interassay variation and prognostic value. *Fertility and Sterility*. 1982; **37**: 565–72.

14. Aitken RJ, Ross A, Lees MM. Analysis of sperm function in Kartagener's syndrome. *Fertility and Sterility*. 1983; **40**: 696–8.

15. Bronson RA, Cooper GW, Rosenfeld DL. Sperm antibodies: their role in infertility. *Fertility and Sterility*. 1984; **42**: 171–83.

16. DeFelici M, Siracusa G. 'Spontaneous' hardening of the zona pellucida of mouse oocytes during in vitro culture. *Gamete Research*. 1982; **6**: 107.

17. DeFelici M, Salustri A, Siracusa G. 'Spontaneous' hardening of the zona pellucida of mouse oocytes during in vitro culture II. The effect of follicular fluid and glycosaminoglycans. *Gamete Research*. 1985; **12**: 227.

18. Barg PE, Wahrman MZ, Talansky BE, Gordon JW. Capacitated, acrosome-reacted but immotile sperm when microinjected under the mouse zona pellucida, will not fertilize the oocyte. *Journal of Experimental Zoology*. 1986; **237**: 365–74.

19. Yamada K, Stevenson AFG, Mettler L. Fertilisation through spermatozoal microinjection: Significance of acrosome reaction. *Human Reproduction*. 1988; **3**: 657–61.

20. Mann JR. Full term development of mouse eggs fertilized by a spermatozoon microinjected under the zona pellucida. *Biology Reproduction* 1988; **38**: 1077–83.

21. Lacham O, Trounson A, Holden C, Mann J, Sathananthan H. Fertilization and development of mouse eggs injected under the zona pellucida with single spermatozoa treated to induce the acrosome reaction. *Gamete Research*. 1989; **23**: 233–43.

22. Mortimer D, Curtis EF, Dravland JE. The use of strontium-substituted media for capacitating human spermatozoa – An improved sperm preparation method for the zona-free hamster egg penetration

test. *Fertility and Sterility*. 1986; **46**: 97–103.

23. Laws-King A, Trounson A, Sathananthan H, Kola I. Fertilisation of human oocytes by micro-injection of a single spermatozoon under the zona pellucida. *Fertility and Sterility*. 1987; **48**: 637–42.

24. Ng SC, Bongso A, Ratnam SS, Sathananthan H, Chan CLK, Wong PC, et al. Pregnancy after transfer of sperm under zona. *Lancet*. 1988; **2**: 790.

25. Fishel S, Jackson P, Antinori S, Johnson J, Grossi S, Versaci C. Subzonal insemination for the alleviation of infertility. *Fertility and Sterility*. 1990; **54**: 828–35.

26. Fishel S, Antinori S, Jackson P, Johnson J, Lisi F, Chiariello F, Versaci C. Twin birth after subzonal insemination. *Lancet*. 1990; **335**: 722–23.

27. Bongso TA, Sathananthan AH, Wong PC, Ratnam SS, Ng SC, Anandakumar C, Ganatra S. Human fertilization by micro-injection of immotile spermatozoa. *Human Reproduction*. 1989; **4**: 175–9.

28. Cohen J, Alikani M, Malter HE, Adler A, Talansky BE, Rosenwaks Z. Partial zona dissection or subzonal sperm insertion: microsurgical fertilisation alternatives based on evaluation of sperm and embryo morphology. *Fertility and Sterility*. 1991; **56**: 696–706.

29. Cohen J, Malter H, Wright G, Kort H, Massey J, Mitchell D. Partial zona dissection of human oocytes when failure of zona pellucida penetration is anticipated. *Human Reproduction*. 1989; **4**: 435–42.

30. Wolf DP. The block to sperm penetration in zona-free mouse eggs. *Developmental Biology* 1978; **64**: 1–10.

31. Cohen J, Talansky BE, Malter HM, Alikani M, Adler A, Reing A, Berkeley A, Graf M, Davis O, Liu H, Bedford JM, Rosenwaks Z. Microsurgical fertilization and teratozoospermia. *Human Reproduction*. (In press.)

32. Cohen J, Malter HE, Talansky BE. Microsurgical fertilization. In: Brinsden P, Rainsbury P, Yovich J (eds.) *Assisted Reproduction*. (In press.)

33. Malter H, Talansky BE, Gordon JW, Cohen J. Monospermy and polyspermy after partial zona dissection of reinseminated human oocytes. *Gamete Research*. 1989; **23**: 377–86.

34. Yanagimachi R. Mammalian fertilization. In: Knobil E, Neill J (eds.) *The Physiology of Reproduction*. New York: Raven Press, 1988.

35. Cohen J, Edwards R, Fehilly C, Fishel S, Hewitt J, Purdy J, Rowland G, Steptoe P, Webster J. In vitro fertilization: a treatment for male infertility. *Fertility and Sterility*. 1985; **43**: 422–32.

36. Tucker MJ, Bishop FM, Cohen J, Wiker SR, Wright G. Routine application of partial zona dissection for male factor infertility. *Human Reproduction*. 1991, (in press).

37. Cohen J, Wright G, Malter H, Elsner C, Kort H, Massey J, Mayer MP, Wiemer KE. Impairment of the hatching process following in vitro fertilization

in the human and improvement of implantation by assisting hatching using micromanipulation. *Human Reproduction*. 1990; **5**: 7–13.

38. Cohen J, Malter H, Talansky B, Tucker M, Wright G. Gamete and embryo micromanipulation. In: Mars RP, Speroff L (eds.) *The Impact of IVF on the Infertile Couple*. New York: Thieme Inc., 1990, p. 290.

39. Janzen R. Personal communication – Sydney IVF, Sydney, Australia.

40. Pike I. Personal communication – Royal North Shore Hospital, Human Reproduction Unit, St Leonards, Sydney, Australia.

41. Kruger TF, Acosta AA, Simmons KF, Swanson RJ, Matta JF, Oehninger S. Predictive value of abnormal sperm morphology in in vitro fertilization. *Fertility and Sterility*. 1988; **49**: 112–21.

42. Malter HE, Cohen J. Embryonic development after microsurgical repair of polyspermic human zygotes. *Fertility and Sterility*. 1989; **52**: 373–80.

43. Kane MT. Variability in different lots of commercial bovine serum albumin affects cell multiplication and hatching of rabbit blastocysts in culture. *Journal of Reproductive Fertility*. 1983; **69**: 555–8.

44. Boatman DE. In vitro growth of non-human primate pre- and peri-implantation embryos. In: Bavister BD (ed.) *The Mammalian Pre-Implantation Embryo*. New York and London: Plenum Press, 1987.

45. Fehilly CB, Cohen J, Simons FR, Fishel SB, Edwards RG. Cryopreservation of cleaving embryos and expanded blastocysts in the human: a comparative study. *Fertility and Sterility*. 1985; **44**: 638–44.

46. Lindenberg S, Hyttel P, Sjogren A, Greve T. A comparative study of attachment of human, bovine and mouse blastocysts to uterine epithelial monolayer. *Human Reproduction*. 1989; **4**: 446–56.

47. Wiemer KE, Cohen J, Wiker SR, Malter HE, Wright G, Godke RA. Coculture of human zygotes on fetal bovine uterine fibroblasts: embryonic morphology and implantation. *Fertility and Sterility*. 1989; **52**: 503–8.

48. Willadsen SM. A method for culture of micromanipulated sheep embryos and its use to produce monozygotic twins. *Nature*. 1979; **77**: 298–301.

49. Cohen J, Malter H, Elsner C, Kort H, Massey J, Mayer MP. Immunosuppression supports implantation of zona pellucida dissected human embryos. *Fertility and Sterility* 1990; **53**: 662–5.

50. Cohen J, Fedlberg D. Unpublished observations.

51. Dale B, Gualtieri R, Talevi R, Tosti E, Santella L, Elder K. Intercellular communication in the early human embryo. *Molecular Reproduction and Development*. (In press.)

52. Handyside AH, Kontogianni EH, Hardy K, Winston RML. Pregnancies from biopsied human preimplantation embryos sexed by Y-specific DNA amplification. *Nature*. 1990; **344**: 378–80.

Chapter 9

Partial zona pellucida dissection as an assisted fertilisation technique in subfertile males

Alex Simon

Introduction

In our studies we have attempted to evaluate the mechanical partial zona dissection (PZD) procedure and to assess the effect of sperm morphology on its efficacy in treating male infertility.

Material and methods

Twenty-two couples who had documented infertility associated with a male factor were included in the study. All cases had failed at least one previous *in vitro* fertilisation (IVF) attempt due to lack of oocyte fertilisation. Prior to PZD cycles, sperm was evaluated by transmission electron microscope (TEM). Specific internal malformations were observed quantitatively in three major cell organelles: acrosome, tail and nucleus. Chromatin abnormalities were defined when subcondensation, disorganisation because of huge vacuoles, or degradation of chromatin fibres mass were observed. Acrosomal malformations were defined as atretic

and partial or complete loss of the acrosome mass. Tail malformations were defined as coiling, multiplicity, or axonemal disorganisation.

The minimal criterion for inclusion in this trial was a sperm count in excess of three million total motile sperm cells. Sperm morphology defects, even when affirmed by TEM, were not used as a limiting criterion for inclusion in the trial.

All retrieved oocytes were incubated for six to eight hours before micromanipulation and insemination. After that period all oocytes were placed in a serum-free Ham's F-10 medium supplemented with 0.1 per cent hyaluronidase (Sigma Chemical Company, bovine testes type 1- S, St Louis, MO) for two to three minutes to remove the cumulus cells. Following cumulus dispersal, all eggs were washed and scored for maturity. Whenever possible, denuded oocytes were divided into three treatment groups; micromanipulated and inseminated with the husband's sperm (Group A), inseminated with the husband's sperm without undergoing PZD (Group B), not micromanipulated and inseminated with donor sperm (Group C). Donor sperm as well as homologous sperm specimens were collected in the morning of follicular aspiration and prepared through a discontinuous Percoll gradient.[1] Just before insemination, the prepared sperm were counted to calculate the motile sperm concentration. Each egg was inseminated with 200 000 to 500 000 motile sperm.

The micromanipulation entailed the creation of a slit in the zona pellucida performed in two steps. First, the sharp microneedle pierced the zona from one side to another near the area of the polar body. In the second step, the holding pipette was placed on top of the piercing pipette and rubbed to and fro until the zona was incised and the oocyte released. After zona slitting, the oocytes were transferred to an insemination medium and immediately inseminated. Sixteen hours after insemination, all oocytes were examined for the presence of pronuclei. Fertilised oocytes were moved to fresh medium and cultured until embryo transfer.

Data were analysed employing the chi-square test in all instances unless the expected frequency was < 5, in which the Fisher's exact test was used.

Results

Twenty-two patients were treated by the PZD procedure. Fertilisation of at least one oocyte subjected to PZD occurred in 13 (59 per cent) patients. Normal cleavage and embryo development followed by embryo transfer was completed in 16 (73 per cent) patients. In seven patients, embryos generated exclusively from PZD procedure were transferred. In seven patients, embryos from a conventional

IVF only were replaced, and in another two patients, both micromanipulated and conventional embryos were transferred. The average total motile sperm count was 67 ± 17 million (mean ± standard error), ranging from three million to 210 million. After sperm preparation for insemination, the mean sperm concentration was 10.3 ± 1.8 million/ml, ranging between 0.2–22 million/ml. When the sperm concentration after preparation was ≥ 5 million/ml (16 patients), fertilisation of at least one oocyte undergoing the PZD procedure was achieved in 69 per cent (11) of the patients. In contrast, when the sperm count was < 5 million/ml (six patients), fertilisation was obtained in only 33 per cent (two) of the patients.

The analyses of sperm morphology revealed that fertilisation occurred mainly if the morphology was normal or if defects were localised in the acrosome and tail regions only. Of 13 patients in that category, ten (77 per cent) had oocytes fertilised after the PZD procedure. Normal cleavage followed by ET was accomplished in seven (70 per cent) of these patients. When chromatin abnormalities were noted (nine patients), fertilisation occurred in only three (33 per cent), and in two cases ET was performed.

A total of 245 oocytes were retrieved and inseminated in three different modes (Table 9.1). One hundred and fifty-one oocytes were subjected to micromanipulation; two of them were damaged during the PZD procedure. The remaining 149 oocytes were inseminated by the husband's sperm after PZD (Group A). Group B served as a control, and included 55 oocytes which were not manipulated but inseminated also with the

Table 9.1 Results of fertilisation in 22 patients' oocytes undergoing partial zona dissection (PZD)

	Group A: husband's sperm PZD (+)	Group B: husband's sperm PZD (−)	Group C: donor sperm PZD (−)
Oocytes	149	55	39
Fertilisation	40 (26.8%)*,†	3 (5.5%)*	21 (53.8%)†
Polyspermic fertilisation	5 (3.3%)	0	1 (2.6%)
Cleaved zygotes	17 (48.6%)=	2 (67%)	18 (90%)=

Notes: * $P < 0.01$.
　　　† $P < 0.01$.
　　　= $P < 0.01$.

husband's sperm. Another 39 oocytes were not manipulated and inseminated with donor sperm.

When PZD was used, 26.8 per cent of the oocytes were fertilised. This rate was significantly higher than the fertilisation rate of 5.5 per cent in Group B (p < 0.01). The polyspermic fertilisation rate was low and similar between Group A and Group C. The cleavage rate was significantly lower after PZD and insemination with husband's sperm compared with the use of donor sperm (p < 0.01).

Discussion

Our work demonstrates that mechanical zona slitting is capable of enhancing fertilisation in a population of strictly selected patients who failed previous IVF attempts. In this unique subfertile population the fertilisation rate achieved by the procedure was 26.8 per cent and was significantly higher than that obtained in untreated oocytes (5.5 per cent). The fertilisation rate obtained by micromanipulation was lower than that observed when donor sperm was used (53.8 per cent) and demonstrated the relatively low efficacy of the procedure. Higher fertilisation rates of 79 per cent were reported by Malter and Cohen[2] employing a similar method (see Chapter 8). However, these authors used less stringent criteria for patient selection and therefore had a fertilisation rate of 53 per cent with conventional IVF. In a group of seven patients with a selection criteria similar to ours, Ng et al.[3] employed a subzonal sperm insertion method and found that fertilisation failed to occur in all candidates. They concluded that transfer of sperm from men with previously failed IVF was ineffective. This failure may have resulted from either the use of an acid solution to drill the zona prior to sperm insertion or from the use of non acrosome reacted sperm cells (see Chapter 6 for comparison).

The cleavage rate following successful fertilisa-tion of micromanipulated oocytes in our work was relatively low (48.6 per cent) and may have resulted either from damage to the oocytes incurred by the procedure or because of fertilisation by defective sperm. The possibility of subtle damage to the oocytes due to the micromanipulative procedure is negated by the fact that the morphological electron microscopic observations in this study (data unpublished) demonstrated that micromanipulation in itself did not induce a premature cortical granule reaction or any other structural injury to the oocyte or its organelles. This has been confirmed in other studies.[4,5] The fact that the cleavage rate following homologous insemination was significantly lower than that following donor insemination strongly suggests that a factor associated with the sperm quality contributed to the phenomenon. It may be that some subfertile sperm cells lack factors conducive to normal oocyte cleavage.

The results of this work may be helpful in selecting potential candidates for the procedure. We found that fertilisation following micromanipulation occurred mostly in patients with a motile sperm count following preparation exceeding 5×10^6/ml and consider this value now as a lower limit for inclusion in the programme of PZD. Our preliminary results suggest that the PZD technique was mostly effective in patients whose sperm morphology was normal or in which morphologic defects were localised to the acrosome and tail regions. Although the number of cases were small, it seemed that when a chromatin morphological defect existed, fertilisation was not expected to occur in most of the patients. It is concluded that the PZD technique enhances fertilisation of severely subfertile sperm. Total motile sperm count and sperm morphology should be taken into consideration in selecting candidates for the procedure.

References

1. Gorus FK, Pipeleers DJ. A rapid method for the fractionization of human spermatozoa according to their progressive motility. *Fertility and Sterility*. 1981; **35**: 662–5.

2. Malter HE, Cohen J. Partial zona dissection of human oocytes: a non-traumatic method using micromanipulation to assist zona pellucida penetration. *Fertility and Sterility*. 1989; **51**: 139–48.

3. Ng SC, Bongso A, Chang SI, Sathananthan H, Ratnam S. Transfer of human sperm into the perivitelline space of human oocytes after zona drilling or zona puncture. *Fertility and Sterility.* 1989; **52**: 73–8.

4. Cummins JM, Edirisinghe WR, Odawara Y, Wales RG, Yovich JL. Ultrastructural observations on gamete interactions using micromanipulated mouse oocytes. *Gamete Research.* 1989; **24**: 461–9.

5. Depypere HT, McLaughlin KJ, Seamark RF, Warnes GM, Matthews CD. Comparison of zona cutting and zona drilling as techniques for assisted fertilization in the mouse. *Journal of Reproductive Fertility.* 1988; **84**: 205–11.

Chapter 10

Preliminary studies with partial zona dissection and clinical pregnancies

G Calderon and A Veiga

Introduction

In the last four years many studies have been published demonstrating that oocyte micromanipulation substantially increases fertilisation rate in *in vitro* fertilisation IVF with male factor infertility (see previous Chapters 1, 6, 7 and 8).

After co-operating with one of the pioneering groups in partial zona dissection, we began using this technique in our Reproductive Medicine Service and present here our first results.

Material and methods

Partial zona dissection (PZD) (see Chapters 7 and 8) is used in our IVF programme for two indications:

Group 1: In cases of male factor IVF with an apparently low or zero fertilisation rate. The PZD technique was applied before proceeding to conventional insemination, that is on the same day as the oocyte retrieval.

Group 2: Partial zona dissection was also used in cases with low or no fertilisation immediately after routine IVF, i.e. approximately 20 hours after the first insemination of the oocytes.

Treatment of the oocyte-cumulus complexes

The cumulus cells were removed via enzymatic action using hyaluronidase 0.1 per cent (w/v) (Sigma), followed by the mechanical action of pipetting with a fire-sharpened pipette. The polar body must be evident in order to confirm metaphase II.

The oocyte cytoplasm was shrunk in a sucrose solution (0.1 M) to facilitate needle penetration through the widened perivitelline space.

The shape of oocytes after sucrose exposure can be of different types:

1. The oocyte shrinks evenly overall: regular spherical shrinkage.

2. The oocyte shrinks in some zones but not in others, leaving some membrane 'bridges' attached to the zona pellucida: irregular shrinkage.

3. The oocyte shrinks only at one of its poles, ending up in a 'pear' shape.

The micromanipulation of the oocytes was done in a glass well slide in 20–30 μl of culture medium, under mineral oil.

The equipment used was an inverted Olympus microscope with Nomarski optics, to which two Narishige micromanipulators have been attached. The instruments for the dissection of the zona pellucida (a holding pipette and a dissection pipette) were made with the aid of the Narishige pipette puller and microforge.

The oocyte to be manipulated was held by suction in such a way that the area of greatest perivitelline space is on top since this is where the needle or dissecting pipette pierces. After penetration, the oocyte is released from the suction and the pierced area is rubbed against the holding pipette so as to enlarge the hole created (Figure 10.1).

Longitudinal incisions, often irregular, are visible through the microscope immediately after manipulation.

Results

The technique has been performed on 131 patients: 60 per cent of them in Group 1, and 40 per cent in Group 2. In the latter group, the same sperm sample was employed in 45 per cent of the cases and a new sample was requested in the others. In all cases, Mini-Percoll gradients have been used[1,2] to prepare the sperm sample.

The total number of oocytes manipulated was

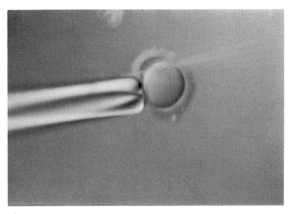

a)

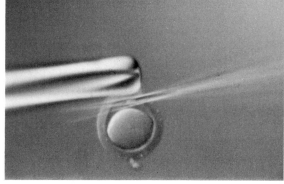

b)

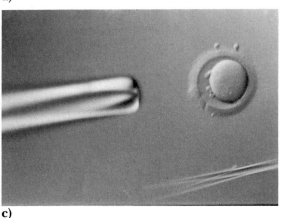

c)

Figure 10.1a The human oocyte held on to a holding pipette under negative pressure

Figure 10.1b The approach of the microneedle piercing two opposing sides of the zona pellucida

Figure 10.1c A large breach is visible in the zona pellucida after the oocyte had been rubbed against the holding pipette to effect the tear

851; 4.3 per cent of them were damaged at some stage in the procedure.

The type of oocyte shrinkage was spherical in 88 per cent, irregular in 4 per cent and 'pear shaped' in 4 per cent.

Fertilisation was achieved in 51.2 per cent of the patients and in 141 oocytes, representing 16.3 per cent of the total. However, 8.5 per cent of the fertilised oocytes had two pronuclei, and 7.8 per cent had three or more pronuclei (polyspermia). Parthenogenetic activation occurred in 1.3 per cent of oocytes.

Eighty-five per cent of the oocytes with two pronuclei cleaved and the morphology of these embryos was similar to that observed in embryos after routine IVF.

Twenty-five replacements were carried out exclusively with embryos achieved after PZD on day 0, i.e. Group 1. Three clinical pregnancies were obtained (12 per cent pregnancy rate per replacement).

In 11 patients, mixed replacements of embryos coming from PZD and embryos from traditional IVF were carried out. Two pregnancies resulted. One of these was an interrupted gestation with four gestational sacs. This patient received four embryos, two of which had been achieved by PZD. It is probable in this case that there was implantation of one or two of the micromanipulated embryos.

The first pregnancy was achieved in a 36 year old woman with two previous IVF cycles with fertilisation failure. Three PZD embryos were replaced and a singleton male delivery resulted. Two other healthy boys have been delivered after PZD embryo replacements.

Recently we have carried out a study to evaluate the efficiency of PZD versus classical IVF in male factors. Patients with male factor were included in the study if the number of spermatozoa was under 10×10^6/ml, the progressive motility was under 15 per cent and the total motility under 35 per cent.

The total number of patients was 29. Approximately half of the oocytes of each patient were inseminated with classical IVF and PZD was performed in the other half. In the former group, the fertilisation rate was 11.5 per cent, and 14.7 per cent after partial zona dissection. Polyspermia was observed only in the latter group of oocytes.

No pregnancy was obtained after six replacements with classical IVF embryos ($\bar{x}$ = 1.6 embryos/replacement). Two pregnancies were obtained after eight replacements of PZD embryos ($\bar{x}$ = 2.1 embryos/replacement). The pregnancy rate was 6.8 per cent per patient and 25 per cent per replacement.

More data are needed to establish conclusions, but it seems that there is a higher implantation rate in PZD embryos as already demonstrated in other studies (see Chapter 8).

Discussion

The dissection of the zona pellucida technique is relatively easy to perform and the percentage of damaged oocytes is relatively low. It is a useful technique in cases of male factor IVF, but if fertilisation fail, re-insemination is not an effective option. Very few pregnancies are obtained with embryos resulting from delayed fertilisation, and only re-insemination with donor sperm seems a viable option in such cases.[3]

Some data with a larger series of cases show that the rate of embryo implantation after PZD is even higher than that of classical IVF (see Chapter 8). It may be that the hatching process of the blastocyst would be enhanced if the zona pellucida has been dissected as described in Chapter 8.

The problem of polyspermia after PZD is still under study. Polyspermia is excessively high with this technique but seems to drop if the interval between the exposure of the oocyte in sucrose and its insemination is longer.[4]

The technique described is useful in failed cases of IVF for male factor. It is necessary, though, to raise the rate of single sperm fertilisation and to reduce that of polyspermia, which will improve the efficacy of the technique.

References

1. Pardo M, Barri PN, Bancells N, Coroleu B, Buxaderas CH, Pomerol JM, Sabater J. Spermatozoa selection in discontinuous Percoll gradients for use in artificial insemination. *Fertility and Sterility.* 1988; **49**: 505–9.

2. Ord T, Patrizio P, Marello E, Balmaceda JP, Asch RH. Mini Percoll: a new method of semen preparation for IVF in severe male factor infertility. *Human Reproduction.* 1990; **5(8)**: 987–9.

3. Pool TB, Martin JE, Ellsworth LK, Perez JB, Atiee SH. Zygote intrafallopian transfer with 'donor rescue': a new option for severe male factor infertility. *Fertility and Sterility.* 1990; **54**: 166–8.

4. Malter H, Talansky B, Gordon J, Cohen J. Monospermy and polyspermy after partial zona dissection of re-insemination human oocytes. *Gamete Research.* 1989; **23**: 377–86.

Section V
New approaches to micro-assisted fertilisation

Chapter 11

From conventional to laser micromanipulation of gametes

Yona Tadir, Benjamin Fisch and Michael W Berns

Introduction

Various methods of gamete micromanipulation have been introduced in recent years. For infertility, two main approaches are aimed at improving fertilisation rates of oocytes *in vitro*; (a) interruption of the integrity of the zona pellucida; and (b) active deposition of spermatozoa beyond the zonal barrier by methods such as subzonal insemination (SUZI) and micro-injection into cytoplasm (see Chapter 1).

Our experience with the subzonal insemination of one, two, three or four sperm cells obtained from severe oligoasthenoteratozoospermic samples yield similar fertilisation rates (Figure 11.1). Likewise, no significant differences in fertilisation rates were observed when the technique was employed using sperm samples with high or low total motile count (Figure 11.2).

The modest results reported with SUZI so far urged us to focus our research on improving the methods for interrupting the integrity of the zona pellucida. The relative inaccuracy and uncontrollable extent of the damage induced on the zona by the mechanical zona breaching methods (see

Chapters 7 and 8) contribute to the high incidence of polyspermic fertilisation (see Chapter 8), and this stimulated us to look at a less conventional technique. The microlaser beam, which offers theoretical advantages due to its precision, seemed to be an ideal tool for this purpose.

LASER beams (the acronym for 'light amplification by stimulated emission of radiation',) were first introduced into gynaecologic surgery by Kaplan and colleagues in 1973[1] for the treatment of uterine cervix erosion, and about a year later by Bellina[2] for intra-abdominal application. Recent advances in endoscopic technology inspired the adaptation of various lasers with suitable delivery systems for reconstructive pelvic surgery. In endoscopic or microsurgery, the effect of the laser beam on tissues is basically of thermal origin, as the absorbed photons are converted into heat. By changing parameters such as power and spot size it is possible to treat a wide variety of lesions in the reproductive tract using the carbon dioxide, neodymium:yttrium-aluminium garnet (Nd:YAG) and the argon lasers. Further developments in optics and laser technology, such as the tunable dye laser microbeam (wavelength range: 217–800

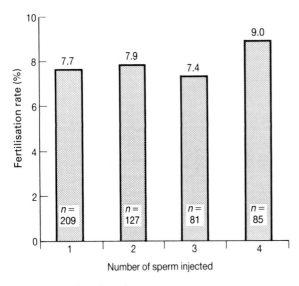

n = number of oocytes

Figure 11.1 Fertilisation rate in relation to number of sperm injected

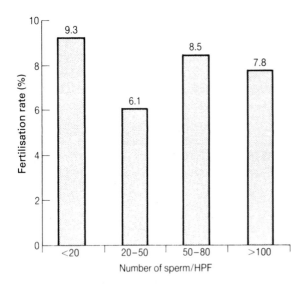

Figure 11.2 Fertilisation rate in relation to sperm count (following swim-up)

developed cellular micromanipulation are summarised in Figure 11.3.

	Reconstructive pelvic surgery and laparoscopy	Cell microsurgery and optical trap
Spot size ∅ Micrometer	300–1000 µm	0.5–5 µm
Wavelength Nanometer	CO₂ 〰〰〰 10.600 nm Nd:YAG 〰〰〰 1.064 nm Frequency doubled Nd:YAG (KTP)　532 nm Argon 〰〰〰 515 nm	1064 nm 532 nm 366 nm 355 nm 266 nm 193 nm
Power ⚡ Watt & milliwatt	5–30 W Continuous Wave	$10^2–10^6$ W** @ 532 nm Pulse width 10–14 ns 10–1000 mW***

*　Typical wavelengths (used in our studies.)
∧　ArF Excimer laser (Ref 9)
**　Peak powers, pulsed mode. Power varies according to wavelengths and application
***　Power range in the optical trap

Figure 11.3 Laser parameters for pelvic, cellular and subcellular surgery

Laser micromanipulation of sperm cells

The zona pellucida of the mammalian egg is a barrier which sperm must penetrate if fertilisation is to proceed. Therefore, the flagellar movement of the spermatozoon is essential for its reproductive capabilities. In order to test sperm force and, if possible, to enhance its penetrating potential, we applied the force generated by radiation pressure of a low power laser beam to induce an optical trap[3] which is capable of manipulating microscopic particles. A single beam gradient force trap consists of a high quality laser beam with a Gaussian energy profile, focused to a spot smaller than the particle being trapped. This trap confines the particle to a spot just below the focal point of the laser beam and centred in the transverse direction. The force generated by the beam of light is greater than all other forces acting on the particle and its magnitude and direction is dominated by the refraction of the laser light through the object. The Nd:YAG laser was

nm) at spot diameters of 1.5 µm, and the gradient force optical trap using a single beam of laser light, opened opportunities for cell microsurgery and micromanipulation. Comparative parameters for the application of lasers in reconstructive pelvic microsurgery, laparoscopic surgery and the newly

directed into a Zeiss photomicroscope and focused into the field of view (Figure 11.4). The power of the laser beam on the target was measured to be 1 Watt ($\pm$ 10 per cent) in a focused spot with a diameter of 2–3 μm.[4] Sperm were placed on a joystick coupled motorised X–Y stage that allows positioning in the optical trap. Remote real-time viewing of the sperm in the trap was performed using a video camera collinear with the path of the trapping beam. A dichroic mirror was used to separate the trapping beam from the image projected onto the video camera, and then recorded on a videotape for later analysis. The recorded images were analysed using a computer assisted image processing system. The image processor was used to measure specific characteristics of sperm movement before and after exposure to the optical trap. In this experiment we demonstrated that there was no significant change in sperm velocity for exposure times of 15 and 20 seconds (33.4 μm/sec and 34 μm/sec before as compared to 32 μm/sec and 31.8 μm/sec after release, respectively). Sperm exposed to the trap for 45 seconds or longer had a statistically significant decrease in velocity when released (36.4 μm/sec before compared to 29.2 μm/sec after exposure [$p < 0.0116$]). In another experiment, the sperm

population was subdivided into two groups based on their initial velocity: slow (1–30 μm/sec) and rapid motile (31–60 μm/sec). In the slow motile group, sperm exposed to 15 seconds in the trap showed a significant 20 per cent increase in linear velocity (from 19.6 μm/sec before to 23.5 μm/sec after exposure). Following 30 and 45 seconds of exposure, there was no significant change of mean velocity in this group. A gradual decrease in sperm velocity was observed following 60, 90 and 120 seconds in the trap. Manipulation of up to three sperm at the same time in the trap was possible. Reduction of the laser power in the range of 50–90 per cent from the highest setting lowered the number of sperm that could be caught and manipulated in the trap. There was a clear power threshold that allowed the sperm to be spontaneously released. Based upon these observations, and assuming that the trap power is proportional to the force generated by the sperm, we measured the relative force generated by each single spermatozoon.[5] This was performed by immobilising and gradually decreasing the trap power to allow for the spontaneous sperm release from the trapping beam. Tabulation of the threshold power level at which each spermatozoon was released enabled determination of the relative force. The sperm patterns were classified as straight and zigzag motile, and linear velocities were subdivided into three groups: slow ($\leq$ 20 μm/sec), medium (21–40 μm/sec) and fast ($\geq$ 41 um/sec). There was a correlation between velocity and power for the entire sperm population. The mean power readings for these groups were 57 mW, 73 mW, and 84 mW, respectively. The analysis of power in the total population demonstrated that zigzag motile sperm had significantly higher mean power readings when compared to straight motile sperm with similar mean linear velocities. In these studies it was demonstrated that optical trapping and micromanipulation of sperm using a low power laser beam is technically feasible. The optical trap may be used as a micromanipulator, permitting sperm traction *in vitro* and combined with other micromanipulating procedures described below. Measurements of sperm force may contribute to better understanding sperm physiology. Such measurements before and after the introduction of drugs that are known to affect sperm motil-

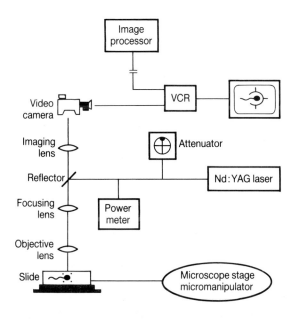

Figure 11.4   The optical trap unit

ity may provide a more accurate determination on the possible effects of such chemicals. From these experiments, the optical trapping of sperm may be developed into a new micromanipulation technique.

Laser zona drilling (LZD)

Mammalian fertilisation is an inefficient process in which only one sperm, of millions initially deposited in the female reproductive tract, penetrates the egg. Even *in vitro*, the ratio of sperm to eggs needed for successful fertilisation is several thousands to one. By drilling a small hole through the zona pellucida of mouse oocytes with acidified Tyrode solution, Gordon and Talansky[6] were able to achieve *in vitro* fertilisation with only 1 per cent of the sperm concentration that otherwise would be required. An increased fertilisation rate of human oocytes in cases of male infertility after partial zona dissection has been observed by Malter and Cohen[7] (see Chapter 8). In order to assess the potential use of laser microbeams for controlled, non-contact zona drilling, a different approach was used on 420 oocytes (231 hamster, 148 mouse and 41 human oocytes). Lasers at 532 nm, 366 nm, 355 nm and 266 nm wavelengths with the power range of five to nine millijoules were applied through an inverted microscope (Zeiss-Axiomat, Thornwood, NY) with a 25X objective. The oocytes, incubated in Ham's F-10 medium, were placed in a specially designed glass container, on the motorised X–Y microscope stage. The laser beams at 10 nanosecond pulse were directed towards the oocyte. Following exposure to the laser light, oocytes were fixed in 4 per cent glutaraldehyde solution and stored in cocodylate buffer. Light and scanning electron microscopy confirmed the laser effects. Our results[8] indicate that the optimal configuration incorporates the use of 366 a nm laser light at spot diameter of 2–4 μm. Better control on the depth of zonal damage is obtained when the beam is directed tangent to the egg sphere rather than orientation towards the lower pole. A well shaped controlled crater in the zona pellucida is performed. Recently, Palanker and colleagues[9] reported on another modification for laser zona drilling (LZD). The essence of their approach was based on high energy deposition of the argon fluoride excimer laser (ArF) operating at 193 nm to remove biological materials without the deposition of heat. They have developed an optical method that could generate holes at the tip as small as 3.5 μm. Special tubes are prepared by drawing glass capillaries under heat, tension and precise cooling.

Intracellular application of laser beams

Polyspermy is a potential complication of human *in vitro* fertilisation with a reported incidence of between 4 to 5 per cent, depending on the hormonal stimulation used for superovulation. Rawlins et al.[10] identified and removed a supernumerary male pronucleus in three tripronuclear (3PN) human zygotes using a fine pipette. They observed syngamy without subsequent cleavage of the resultant diploidised zygotes. In our experiments, nine 3PN oocytes were exposed to laser at 532 nm and 355 nm wavelength with the power setting of five millijoules through the inverted microscope with a 100 × magnification objective. A specially designed quartz glass dish was placed on the X–Y motorised stage and the beam was directed towards one of the extra pronuclei. The high magnification and the marked changes in power density within short distances allowed non-traumatic penetration through the zona pellucida and selective destruction of the pronucleus. Two out of the nine fertilised ova exposed to the laser light cleaved to the six- to eight-cell stage and were further processed for chromosomal analysis. However, technical difficulties limited our knowledge concerning selective inactivation of the extra male pronucleus (see Chapter 8). This experiment demonstrated that this selective, 'non-touch' procedure is technically feasible. More experience is needed to assess its effectiveness.

Concluding remarks

The field of reproductive technologies has rapidly developed since the introduction of *in vitro* fertilisation as a clinical service more than a decade ago.

Various procedures especially in the field of male infertility may require micromanipulating manoeuvres. Laser beams have already been added to the armamentarium of the reproductive surgeon. In our recent experiments we have demonstrated that a single beam gradient force optical trap is capable of manipulating sperm and chromosomes. For the first time, based upon simple principles, it was possible to measure the force generated by a single spermatozoon. Such sperm parameters are accurately compared to linear velocity determined in μm/second. It was also demonstrated that sperm with different motility patterns generate more force than straight moving sperm. Superficial damage to the zona pellucida and precise dissection of chromosomes with laser microbeams are technically feasible.[9] It is too early to predict which is the preferred micromanipulation procedure that may significantly improve fertilisation and pregnancy rate in the presence of severe male factor infertility. However, the simplicity and special accuracy of laser beams as 'light scalpels' in the non-contact mode are clinically applicable for breaching the zona pellucida. The selectivity of the laser in targeting the active focal point towards intracellular structures can be used to inactivate an extra pronucleus following polyspermic fertilisation or other surgical corrections of the pre-embryos. Further progress in these technologies may clarify more physiologic phenomena and may possibly be integrated into clinical services in reproductive medicine.

References

1. Kaplan I, Goldman J, Ger R. The treatment of erosion of the uterine cervix by means of CO_2 laser. *Obstetrics and Gynaecology*. 1973; **41**: 795–6.
2. Bellina JH. Gynaecology and the laser. *Contemporary Obstetrics and Gynaecology*. 1974; **4**: 24–9.
3. Ashkin A, Dziedzic JM, Bjorkholm JE, Chu S. Observation of a single beam gradient force optical trap for dielectric particules. *Optics Letters*. 1986; **11**: 288–90.
4. Tadir Y, Wright WH, Vafa O, Ord T, Asch R, Berns MW. Micromanipulation of sperm by a laser generated optical trap. *Fertility and Sterility*. 1989; **52**: 870–3.
5. Tadir Y, Wright WH, Vafa O, Ord T, Asch R, Berns MW. Force generated by human sperm correlated to velocity and determined using a laser trap. *Fertility and Sterility*. 1990; **53**: 944–7.
6. Gordon JW, Talansky BE. Assisted fertilization by zona drilling: a mouse model for correction of oligospermia. *Journal of Experimental Zoology*. 1986; **239**: 347–54.
7. Malter EH, Cohen J. Partial zona dissection of the human oocytes: a non-traumatic method using micromanipulation to assist zona pellucida penetration. *Fertility and Sterility*. 1989; **51**: 139–48.
8. Tadir Y, Wright WH, Vafa O, Liaw L-H, Asch R, Berns MW. Micromanipulation of gametes using laser microbeams. *Human Reproduction*. 1991; **6**: 1011–16.
9. Palanker D, Laufer N, Ohad S, Lewis A. Technique for cellular microsurgery using the 193 nm Excimer laser. *Laser in Surgery and Medicine*. 1991; **11**: 580–6.
10. Rawlins RG, Binor Z, Radwanska E, Dmowski WP. Microsurgical enucleation of tripronuclear human zygotes. *Fertility and Sterility*. 1988; **50**: 266–72.

Chapter 12

New advances in micromanipulation: applications for treatment of the severe male factor patient

SC Ng, TA Bongso, SL Liow, M Montag, V Tok and SS Ratnam

Introduction

Micromanipulation is a technique in which very fine instruments, usually glass capillaries, are used to manipulate cells. It has been used for many decades in experimental embryology. This volume has documented its recent application to human *in vitro* fertilisation (IVF) to assist fertilisation, especially for severe male factor patients.

Since the first report of Metka in 1985,[1] there has been much progress in trying to optimise the technique. Despite the progress made, the pregnancy rates have been appallingly low.[2] Hence, there have been efforts directed at new and novel ways to increase the fertilisation rates and possibly the pregnancy rates (see Chapter 1). In this review, we shall discuss four possible methods: electrofusion, laser fusion, transfer of spermatids into oocytes, and development of the sperm nucleus in an amphibian cell-free system into a pronucleus before its transfer into an activated oocyte.

Electrofusion

Electrofusion (EF) is a technique in which a current of short duration is passed through adjacent cells in contact with each other. The resulting transient and reversible cell membrane breakdown results in fusion of the cells.[3] This concept can also be applied to the fusion of an oocyte with a sperm. However, there are physical constraints in terms of size, as the two adjacent cells should be of similar size.

To overcome this, we have resorted to developing very fine micro-electrodes with our collaborator, Dr U. Zimmermann, University of Wurzburg. These electrodes must be brought into the manipulated field by micromanipulators. Immediately after the transfer of a sperm into the perivitelline space the sperm is usually in a small 'pocket' of invaginated oolemma, and it is usually swimming against the membrane (Figure 12.1). Hence, if the micro-electrodes are brought in at this point and the current pulsed through, it may be possible to achieve fusion.

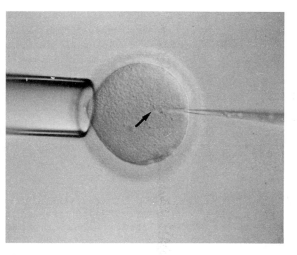

Figure 12.1 Sperm seen in the pocket of invaginated oolemma (arrow) immediately after the subzonal insemination procedure. Direct interference (contrast optics using the Zeiss Axiovert, with a 35 X plan-achromat objective lens × 350)

In an experiment where we studied the efficiency of EF with the use of micro-electrodes, we found that EF may allow sperm–oocyte fusion and that it may have application in micro-injection procedures to increase fertilisation rates.[4] There were two experiments: (a) single EF pulse and (b) double EF pulses at 30 minute interval between the first and second pulses. Pulse strength of 100V and a single pulse duration of 35 μsec were used in these two experiments. Subzonal sperm transfer was done in 23 and 40 murine oocytes for single and double EF respectively with uncapacitated murine sperm. In transmission electron microscopic (TEM) studies, there was evidence of ultrastructural damage in oocytes exposed to double EF. Moreover, sperm exposed to the double EF did not survive.

There was also no decondensing sperm head seen in these oocytes when a DNA-specific dye Hoechst 33342 was used to stain them three hours after the last EF pulse. On the contrary, of the 327 sperm injected into 23 oocytes in the first experiment, only 18 developed into decondensed sperm heads (5.5 per cent) three hours after a single EF pulse.

Laser fusion

It is now possible to induce fusion of cells with a laser beam. This will help to overcome the difficulties with electrofusion. A combination of the single beam gradient optical trap with a pulsed ultraviolet laser microbeam has been used to induce cell fusion.[5] However, this area is new and has applications in assisted reproductive technologies[6] (see also Chapter 12). The optical trap can be generated from an Nd-YAG laser, while the ultraviolet laser can be used to induce fusion (Dr Greulich, personal communication, 1992). Technical problems include possible damage of sperm chromatin from direct laser contact or via heat generation as the spot size can be focused only to 0.5 μm, while the sperm head is about 5.0 μm broad.

Spermatid transfer

As part of our studies to determine the ability of the male genome to fuse with eggs, Ng and Solter[7] transferred murine Golgi-phase spermatids into metaphase II murine oocytes.[7] The electrofusion to induce fusion was not successful in the majority of cases. In those that did fuse, some continued development, but they did not progress beyond the morula stage.

Development of sperm nuclei in cell-free systems

Selection of sperm occurs at every stage. Hence, it is logical to try to select sperm that are able to continue development after they penetrate the oocyte. This strategy is particularly useful for patients with very severe male factor subfertility. It is possible to incubate sperm nuclei in a cell-free system using the eggs of the South African clawed frog *(Xenopus laevis)*. Katagiri and co-workers[8] have demonstrated that it is possible for human sperm to develop into a male pronucleus in such a system.

Our group is now working to develop this system further. Much work needs to be done, but preliminary results have shown that the human sperm nuclei are able to undergo decondensation, take up histones, nuclear lamins and initiate replication in such a system.[9]

Acknowledgements

We wish to thank our collaborators in the various areas described: Professor U. Zimmermann of Wurzburg; Dr H. Spring, Professor M. F. Trendenlenburg and Dr K. Greulich of Heidelberg. We are also grateful to Carl Zeiss, the National Science and Technology Board, Singapore, the Totaliser Board and the National University of Singapore, for their funding and support.

References

1. Metka M, Haromy T, Huber J. Mikromanipulatorische Spermainjektion – ein neuer Weg in der Behandlung infertiler Manner? [Micromanipulatory sperm injection – a new method in the treatment of infertile males] *Wiener Medizinische Wochenzeitshrift.* 1985; **135**: 55–9.
2. Ng SC, Liow SL, Bongso TA, Montag M, Tok V, Sathananthan AH, Ratnam SS. Micromanipulation and possible new approaches to help the severe male factor patient. *Journal of In Vitro Fertilisation and Embryo Transfer.* 1992, (in press).
3. Zimmermann U. Electrical breakdown, electropermeabilisation and electrofusion. *Reviews in Physiology and Biochemical Pharmacology.* 1986; **105**: 175–256.
4. Ng SC, Liow SL, Sathananthan AH, Bongso TA, Ratnam SS, Zimmermann U. Decondensation of mouse sperm in mouse oocytes after electrofusion. (In preparation.)
5. Wiegand-Steubing R, Cheng S, Wright WH, Numajiri Y, Berns MW. Single beam optical trapping and micromanipulation of mammalian cells. *The International Society of Optical Engineering, Society for Photo-optical Instrumentation Engineers.* 1990; **1202**: 272–80.
6. Tadir Y, Wright WH, Vafa O, Liaw LH, Asch RH, Berns MW. Micromanipulation of gametes using laser microbeams. *Human Reproduction.* 1991; **6**: 1011–16.
7. Ng SC, Solter D. Fusion of male germ cells (from male pronucleus to pachytene spermatocyte) with the metaphase II oocytes in the mouse. *Mol Andrology,* 1992; **4**: 263–76.
8. Ohsumi K, Katagiri C, Yanagimachi R. Development of pronuclei from human spermatozoa injected microsurgically into frog (*Xenopus*) eggs. *Journal of Experimental Zoology.* 1986; **237**: 319–25.
9. Montag M, Tou V, Liow SL, Bongso A, Ng SC. In vitro decondensation of pronuclei-like structures for micromanipulation. *Mol Reprod Dev.* 1992; **33**: 338–46.

Chapter 13

Micro-assisted reproduction: is it the treatment of choice after fertilisation failure?

Shlomo Mashiach, David Bider, Izhan Ben Shlomo Lipitz, Zion Ben-Rafael, David Levran and Jehoshua Dor

Introduction

Micromanipulation has been practised for almost a century in invertebrates and lower animals[1-4]. However it is only in the last two decades that many micromanipulation procedures have been initiated for use with human and mouse embryos.[5] These include: removing of the zona pellucida; dissociation of blastomeres; aggregation of denuded embryos can also be subjected to micromanipulation. Micromanipulation in the human will and insertion of isolated blastomeres into foreign zona pellucida[5] (see Chapter 1).

With the advent of human *in vitro* fertilisation (IVF) human oocytes and pre-implantation embryos can also be subjected to micromanipulation. Micromanipulation in the human will probably be limited to diagnosis, correction of genetic diseases and chromosomal disorders and assisting fertilisation in male related infertility.

In vitro fertilisation (IVF) has been used with variable degrees of success to treat male infertility.[6,7] However, the expectation of pregnancy after IVF with compromised sperm is lower than that for other causes of infertility. Since embryos that result from fertilisation with suboptimal sperm

samples develop normally, the low pregnancy rate found in male factor patients is probably due solely to a low fertilisation rate.[8] Recently, several micromanipulation procedures have been developed to increase the rate of fertilisation in human IVF, in cases of abnormal sperm function.

The zona pellucida is thought to be the main barrier or block to sperm penetration. Hence, in situations where the ability of sperm to penetrate the zona is reduced, such as oligozoospermia, teratozoospermia or asthenozoospermia, procedures to assist the sperm to pass through the zona may be of assistance. Complete removal of the zona will result in polyspermy and reduced developmental ability. For further successful cleavage, if the zygote were diploid, the embryo would require a zona pellucida to maintain the correct blastomere geometry until the formation of cell junctions around the eight- to 16-cell stage.

Approaches to micro-assisted fertilisation

Basically, three methods, each with its own advantages and disadvantages, have been proposed.

133

Chronologically, the first method involved opening the zona pellucida to facilitate sperm passage. It has yielded offspring in several species, including the human. Several variations of this technique have been proposed.[8] The clinical disadvantage of this method is that it requires relatively large numbers of motile spermatozoa, since they have to find the artificial gaps in the zona themselves. This may result in several sperm being incorporated into the perivitelline space, and since the human oolemma lacks a rapid block to polyspermy, multiple fertilisation can occur. The most promising variation of this method so far appears to be partial zona dissection (PZD) (see Chapter 7 and 8).

The second method involves insertion of spermatozoa under the zona pellucida (subzonal insemination – SUZI), a method which has produced normal healthy babies[9] (see Chapter 7). This technique requires only a simple puncture of the zona pellucida and may be the least traumatic approach (see Chapters 1, 7 and 8). In this procedure, the cumulus and zona barriers are bypassed, but the sperm fuse with the oocyte membrane by natural means. Although it may require some sperm motility, subzonal insemination can be applied to men with very low sperm counts and in the ideal situation, a single sperm can be inserted. Some cases exhibiting only immotile sperm may succeed with this technique (see Chapter 6).

The third method is sperm micro-injection, directly into the ooplasm. It is the most invasive alternative, entailing the greatest risk to the oocyte. Establishment of a reliable micro-injection method using a single acrosome-reacted sperm cell would be the ideal procedure for severest cases of male infertility. Pregnancies following the use of this method have not yet been reported in the human.

Evaluation of micro-assisted fertilisation

Although these methods are used by a continuously growing number of IVF programmes throughout the world, they still bear a pioneering character. It is one of the main assignments of practitioners to deal with the criteria or the indications for patient allocation to such treatments, bearing in mind the possible disadvantages and potential risks of these new methods. Moreover, and of more importance, we must define the true benefit of these methods, namely, what is their true success rate, and against what 'background' success rate should the results be evaluated.

There are two indications for admission of patients to a method of micro-assisted fertilisation: failure to fertilise (or a very low fertilisation rate [< 20 per cent]) in previous IVF attempts; or severe male factor infertility.

What results have currently been achieved by the most advanced groups involved in micromanipulation?[9,10] (See Chapters 6, 7 and 8.) Zona drilling (ZD), partial zona dissection (PZD) and subzonal micro-insemination (SUZI) have all been performed in cases of moderate or severe male factor patients who had failed previous fertilisation using zona intact oocytes[8,9,10,11] (see Chapters 5, 7 and 8).

Garrisi et al.[8] used three different micromanipulation procedures to assist human fertilisation in cases of severe male infertility. Zona drilling was performed: (i) with acid Tyrode's solution, or (ii) mechanically introducing a hole with a microneedle following zona softening with chymotrypsin, or (iii) by partial zona dissection. The fertilisation rate was lowest in the zona drilling/acid Tyrode's group (17.5 per cent) although the differences between groups (zona drilling/chymotrypsin: 25 per cent, partial zona dissection: 21.7 per cent) were not significant. The fertilisation rate was significantly increased relative to untreated eggs from the same patients only in the partial zona dissection group (21.7 per cent versus 3.9 per cent). Oocyte damage occurred at a high rate as a result of zona drilling with acid Tyrode's solution (37 per cent). Embryonic development was compromised after zona drilling with chymotrypsin: only 7/12 (58.3 per cent) of the fertilised oocytes cleaved, and the morphology of many of the cleaved embryos was abnormal. Sixty one per cent of the diploid embryos resulting from partial zona dissection cleaved and the embryonic morphology of these embryos was comparable with controls. No pregnancies resulted from the transfer of manipulated embryos. They concluded that although zona manipulation increases the fertilisa-

Table 13.1 Results of micromanipulation after failure of fertilisation in male factor infertility

Procedures	Authors	Patients	Oocyte	Fertilisation	
				Per patient %	Per oocyte %
PZD	J Cohen	44	?	59	30
	J Gordon	16	143		21.7
SUZI	Lippi	67	585	49	16.2
	Fishel	130	539	32	12.8
	Gianaroli	13	114		22

tion rate, losses due to oocyte trauma, low rates of diploid fertilisation, low rates of cleavage, and a high frequency of abnormal cleavage reduce the number of embryos available for transfer.

Subzonal micro-insemination (SUZI) seems to yield better results. Table 13.1 summarises the data presented in three studies. With subzonal sperm injection, the fertilisation rate was 32–49 per cent per patient and 12.8–16.2 per cent per oocyte. There was a high rate of polypronuclear embryos except for the study by Fishel. The pregnancy rate was only 4.3 per cent. One must also take into account the potential complications of micromanipulation, namely that 25–30 per cent of the oocytes show signs of trauma; in 8–43 per cent more than one sperm penetrated the cell membrane; there is a relatively low cleavage rate and reduced number of embryos for transfer.[10,12,13,14]

We attempted to find the 'background' success rate after failure of fertilisation in cases of male infertility treated with IVF. In addition, while analysing our results, we aimed to establish the prognosis for future fertilisation in couples with male factor infertility who had an IVF cycle during which no fertilisation occurred.

We have analysed the results of our programme and identified 76 couples, with male factor infertility, in whom no fertilisation occurred during at least one IVF cycle. Of these, 44 couples had additional treatment in our programme, with the husband's semen (Table 13.2). Of the 44 couples, 36 (82 per cent) fertilised at least one of their wives' eggs and 48 per cent of the eggs were fertilised. Nine pregnancies were achieved (20.5 per cent).

A special subgroup of couples were those in whom there were two previous cycles without fertilisation. There were ten such couples, of which six (60 per cent) had fertilised in an additional cycle and one pregnancy resulted. An interesting case is that of a couple who had two cycles without fertilisation, but half a year later achieved a spontaneous pregnancy.

A group of 37 couples with unexplained infertility, with failure of fertilisation in the first IVF attempt, were also evaluated. The results are summarised in Table 13.3.

In the second IVF attempt, 49 per cent of the couples achieved fertilisation and 38 per cent of the eggs were fertilised. Four pregnancies (or 11 per cent) resulted.

Table 13.2 Results of repeated IVF treatment after failure of fertilisation in a previous IVF cycle (male factor)

	Number of patients	Per patient %	Per oocyte %	Number of pregnancies %
Second attempt	44	82	48	9 (20.5)
Third attempt	10	60	33	1 (10)*

Note: * one spontaneous pregnancy.

Table 13.3 Results of repeated IVF treatment after failure of fertilisation in a previous IVF cycle (unexplained infertility)

	Number of patients	Per patient %	Per oocyte %	Number of pregnancies %
Second attempt	37	49	38	4 (11)
Third attempt	19	47	33	3 (15.8)
Fourth attempt	3	33	35	0

Nineteen couples failed fertilisation twice and attempted a third IVF cycle. Again, the fertilisation rate was high – 47 per cent per patient and 33 per cent per oocyte. Another three pregnancies (15.8 per cent) resulted.

Even after three failures of fertilisation, one of the three couples fertilised on the fourth attempt. There were also spontaneous pregnancies after one, two and even after three failures of fertilisation. Emphasis should be placed on the fact that there is no data available in the literature for such couples.

In summary, we conclude that 60–82 per cent of patients with severe male factor infertility will fertilise at an additional IVF attempt after failure to fertilise in the first IVF attempt.

Patients with unexplained infertility, and a failure to fertilise in the first IVF attempt, have a 50 per cent chance to fertilise in the second IVF cycle and another 50 per cent chance to fertilise in the third IVF attempt after two successive failures.

We suggest that after failure of fertilisation, routine IVF and micro-assisted fertilisation achieve similar results. Until micro-assisted fertilisation achieves better success rates, routine IVF is the preferred procedure in cases of one or two failures of fertilisation. Micro-assisted fertilisation should be reserved as an adjunctive technique of treatment.

References

1. Uehara T, Yanagimachi R. Microsurgical injection of spermatozoa into hamster eggs with subsequent transformations of sperm nuclei into male pronuclei. *Biology of Reproduction*. 1976; **15**: 467–70.
2. Markert CL. Fertilisation of mammalian eggs by sperm injection. *Journal of Experimental Zoology*. 1983; **228**: 195–201.
3. Gordon JW, Talansky BE. Assisted fertilisation by zona drilling; a mouse model for correction of oligospermia. *Journal of Experimental Zoology*. 1988; **239**: 347–54.
4. Mann J. Full term development of mouse eggs fertilised by a spermatozoon micro-injected under the zona pellucida. *Biology of Reproduction*. 1988; **38**: 1077–83.
5. Malter HE, Cohen J. Blastocyst formation and hatching in vitro following zona drilling of mouse and human embryos. *Gamete Research*. 1984; **24**: 67–80.
6. Mahadevan AM, Trounson AO. The influence of seminal characteristics on the success rate of human in vitro fertilization. *Fertility and Sterility*. 1984; **42**: 400–5.
7. Cohen J, Rowland G, Steptoe P, Webster J. In vitro fertilization: a treatment for male infertility. *Fertility and Sterility*. 1985; **43**: 422–32.
8. Garrisi GJ, Talansky BE, Grunfeld L, Sapira V, Navot D, Gordon JW. Clinical evaluation of three approaches to micromanipulation assisted fertilization. *Fertility and Sterility*. 1990; **54**: 671–7.
9. Fishel SB, Antinori S, Jackson P, Johnson J, Rinaldi L. Presentation of six pregnancies established by subzonal insemination (SUZI). *Human Reproduction*. 1991; **6**: 124–30.
10. Fishel SB, Timson J, Lisi F, Rinaldi L. Evaluation of 225 patients undergoing subzonal insemination for the procurement of fertilization in vitro. *Fertility and Sterility*. 1992; **57**: in press.
11. Cohen J. Assisted fertilisation by partial zona dissection (Personal communication.)
12. Malter HF, Cohen J. Partial zona dissection of the human oocyte: a non-traumatic method using micromanipulation to assist zona pellucida penetration. *Fertility and Sterility*. 1989; **51**: 139–48.
13. Lippi J, Turner M, Jansen RPS. Pregnancies after in vitro fertilization by sperm micro-injection in the

perivitelline space. Abstract: Fertility and Sterility Society, 1990.

14. Gianaroli L, Sakkar D, Diotallevi L, Fenaretti AP, Mengoli N, Trounson A. The successful use of subzonal sperm injection in human in vitro fertilization. Abstract of the II Joint ESCO/ESHRE Meeting, Milan, 1990.

Section VI
Embryo micromanipulation

Chapter 14

Prelude to pre-implantation diagnosis in the human

Simon Fishel

Cell division and the transference of inherited information

Mitosis is a process that replicates a cell's genome (genetic information) to transfer an identical copy to each daughter cell after division of the parental cell. It occupies a small portion of the cell cycle which includes: gap one (G1), synthesis (S), gap two (G2) and mitosis (M). Before S, the stage at which DNA synthesis and eventual doubling of the genetic information occur, each chromosome will consist of a single chromatid. After S each chromosome will consist of two sister chromatids joined at the single centromere (the body holding together the paired chromatids). Mitosis is traditionally divided into four stages: prophase, metaphase, anaphase and telophase (Figure 14.1). At prophase each chromosome, consisting of its sister chromatids, is elongated before becoming shorter and more compact. At the end of prophase the centriole (paired, cylindrical structures composed of nine sets of microtubule triplets involved in the formation of the spindle) divides into two daughter centrioles and each migrates to opposite poles of the cell. At metaphase a mitotic spindle forms between the centrioles and the nuclear membrane disappears. The chromosomes, which consist of the paired sister chromatids, are orien-

tated for division on the spindle, which is made up of protein fibres. The centromere divides along the longitudinal axis of the chromosome and the sister chromatids pass to opposite poles (Figure 14.1). It is usually at this stage, at metaphase, that the chromosomes are analysed, as agents can be used which disrupt the spindle. The following two phases, anaphase and telophase, represent the stages at which the chromosomes, now single chromatids, move to opposite poles, the mitotic spindle disappears and new nuclear membranes form. The cytoplasm cleaves (cytokinesis) and two complete cells result, each with a full complement of the parental genome.

Therefore, in mitosis the diploid number of chromosomes, 2n, is maintained. In the process of meiosis, however, a unique cell division occurs in which the diploid chromosome number, 2n, is reduced to n, the haploid number. Each gamete, the oocyte and spermatozoon have an haploid (n) number of chromosomes. This meiotic process not only ensures the correct number of chromosomes are provided during the fusion of the gametes, it also serves as a mechanism to generate genetic variability which provides the basis of natural selection.

Meiosis has two divisions, meiosis I and meiosis II. It is during meiosis I that the chromosome

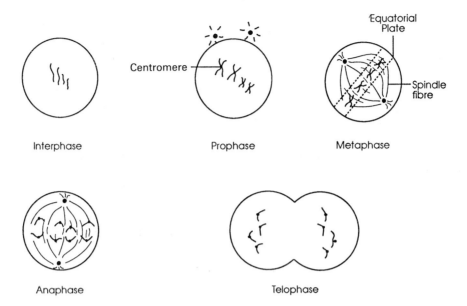

Figure 14.1 Diagrammatic representation of the passage of genetic information by mitosis, from a cell to its daughter cells

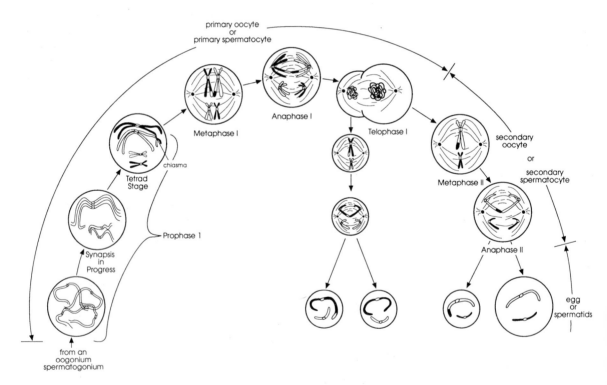

Figure 14.2 Diagrammatic representation of the halving of a cell's chromosome complement, in the germ cells, by meiosis; resulting in four haploid cells from a single diploid parent cell. The process of crossing over, i.e. the exchange of genetic material in non-sister chromatids, is represented by the black/white linkage; the site of the chiasmata

number is reduced from 2n to n in the resulting two germ cells. During meiosis II, each of these haploid germ cells divides resulting in a total of four haploid cells from a single diploid germ cell (Figure 14.2). Meiosis I has four stages, prophase, metaphase, anaphase and telophase, each analogous to the four stages of mitosis. Briefly, the meiotic prophase can be described as longer and more complex than its mitotic counterpart. It is divided into four subdivisions called leptotene, zygotene, pachytene and diplotene. During zygotene the homologous pairs of chromosomes, i.e. autosomes, pair longitudinally with each other. Each gene within the chromosome has an alternative form or allele. Synapsis, or pairing, is highly specific between allelic forms, even to the extent that if these allelic forms are not directly opposite each other the homologous autosomes of the chromosome will contort into a form that aligns them gene by gene. As pairing proceeds the autosomes seem to zip up forming a synaptinemal complex consisting of proteins and RNA.

An event unique to meiosis takes place during synapsis and is called 'crossing over'. This is a normal process of breakage and exchange of parts between homologous chromatids, or autosomes. Viewed at the light microscope, at the pachytene stage, each chromosome is seen to consist of two sister chromatids, with the synapsed pair becoming a four stranded structure called a tetrad (Figure 14.2). The autosomes actually persist in forms of tetrads because of the crossing over in which portions of non-sister chromatids are exchanged. The sites at which these exchanges take place are known as chiasmata and this process of genetic exchange is more properly termed 'recombination'. During the next phase, diplotene, chromosomes shorten and each tetrad moves apart, as if mutually repelled, moving towards the edge of the cell. This orderly separation of homologous chromosomes is called 'disjunction'.

Meiosis and the unique event of chiasmata facilitates the exchange of genes between autosomes providing a source for genetic variability, and it is this that is the basis for natural selection. Chiasmata also prevent the homologous chromosomes from separating prematurely which would cause non-disjunction, a condition giving rise to

aberrations in the overall structure of chromosomes affecting the future developmental potential of the embryo. During the next three phases, metaphase, anaphase and telophase, the nuclear membrane disappears and the chromosomes are orientated equatorially along the spindle. The autosomes then repulse one another and move toward opposite poles (anaphase). However, the centromeres do not divide in meiosis I as they do in mitosis.

At the time of a female's birth her full complement of oocytes have been formed in the ovarian tissue, each having progressed to prophase I (prophase of meiosis I). They will remain arrested at the tetrad stage for up to five decades with their chromosomes still paired but in a diffuse and much extended state. It is only at puberty, when one or a few of these oocytes begin maturation, that they progress through meiosis I to meiosis II. It is at the metaphase stage of meiosis II, i.e. metaphase II, when they are released from the ovarian follicle, at ovulation.

Meiosis I therefore reduces the chromosome number; it is meiosis II which produces additional gametes. Meiosis II is analogous to mitosis (Figure 14.2). Meiosis II lacks the well defined prophase of meiosis I and the chromosomes move directly into metaphase II. Completion of meiosis II results in a single diploid cell dividing into four haploid cells, with the possibility, if recombination has occurred, that no two haploid cells will be genetically identical; that is, no two of the four chromatids of a given chromosome pair are genetically identical. It is apparent in humans that recombination usually occurs twice as frequently in females as males.

In the oocyte during meiosis I, and specifically at telophase I, a remarkable and unique process of cell division occurs. The chromosomes at one pole of the oocyte, together with a tiny fraction of the cytoplasm, are extruded and pinched off to form the minute first polar body (Figure 14.3). The remaining chromosomes remain within the bulk of the cytoplasm. Therefore homologous chromosomes separate with an asymmetric cleavage of the ooplasm with one half of the original chromosome complement residing with the majority of the cytoplasm. The polar body chromosomes, which are chromosomes produced by meiosis I, may be fractionally different from the chromosomes residing in the main body of the cytoplasm due to recombination events. These chromosomes also begin to degenerate in late telophase I. The oocyte continues its development through meiosis II and rests at metaphase II until fertilisation (or parthenogenetic activation).

Each species has its own characteristic number of chromosomes; in humans there are 46 chromosomes in the diploid somatic cells (2n), and 23 in the haploid germ cells (n). There are 22 pairs of autosomes and one pair of sex chromosomes, the XX in females and XY in males. They are recognised and numbered according to size and the position of the centromere (Figure 14.4). Chromosomes are divided by the centromere into the short arm (designated p) or the long arm (q). Chromosomes are classified according to the relative position of the centromere:

metacentric	– p and q are of equal length
submetacentric	– q slightly longer than p
acrocentric	– q much longer than p, the centromere is almost terminal
telocentric	– when the centromere is terminal (Figure 14.4)

Before the early 1970s, few chromosomes could be identified, primarily numbers 1, 2, 3, 16 and Y. The other chromosomes were placed into several groups: A (1–3), B (4–5), C (6–12 and X), D (13–15), E (16–18), F (19–20) and G (21–22).

Structural chromosomal abnormalities

Major structural alterations in the chromosomes cause phenotypic abnormalities, presumably as a result of defective, duplicated or deficient genes. The position of a gene with respect to its neighbours can also affect its transcription. Various forms of structural abnormalities are deficiency, translocation, inversion, isochromosomes, dicentric chromosomes, ring chromosomes and duplication.

Deficiency

The loss of a portion of one chromosome, either terminal or interstitial, results in deficiency. This can arise as a result of breakage and loss of an acentric fragment. Autosome deficiency generally leads to

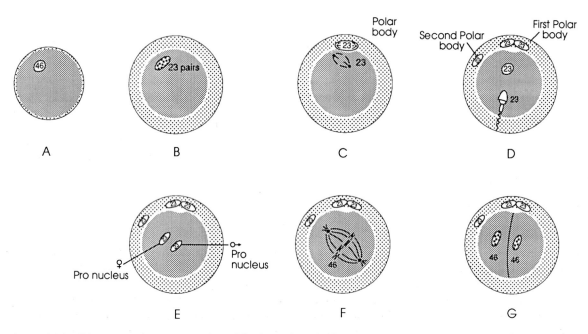

Figure 14.3 Diagrammatic representation of the formation of the polar bodies from the primary oocyte through meiosis, metaphase I and II, and fertilisation

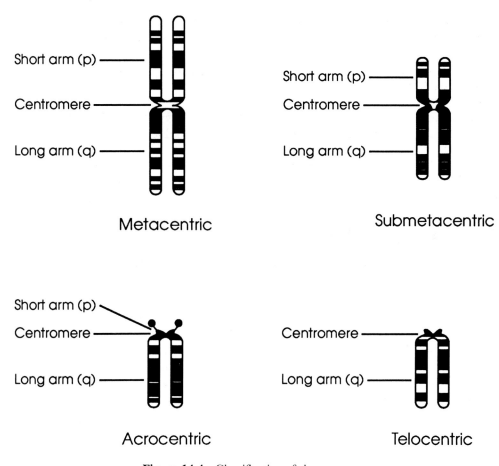

Figure 14.4 Classification of chromosomes

embryonic death or malformation. Deficiency in a sex chromosome is not always deleterious.

Isochromosomes

Isochromosomes are chromosomes with identical arms. They occur if the centromere divides horizontally rather than longitudinally. One result is telocentric which can replicate itself during the following S phase to form a metacentric chromosome. The other product is acentric and is lost at the following cell division. Therefore the isochromosome consists of a complete duplication of one arm and the complete deficiency of the other arm. Both parts of this chromosome are structurally and genetically

identical (isologous). Both identical long arms or identical short arms can arise.

The most common structural abnormality associated with gonadal dysgenesis is the isochromosome for the X long arm [i(xq)].

Duplication

Duplication can arise following meiotic segregation in a parent having a chromosomal translocation (see below). Duplications are generally associated with other deficiencies but the origin of 'pure' duplications may be due to unequal crossing over at meiosis, or in tandem duplication during replication.

Individuals with deletions or duplications affecting large chromosomal regions often have severe phenotypic abnormalities and are usually sterile. Isolated deletions or duplications would theoretically yield 50 per cent gametes with the parental abnormality.

Translocations

Sometimes following chromosome breakage, chromosomal material is exchanged between two or more chromosomal arms resulting in a translocation. Should genes be conserved, neither lost nor gained, the re-arrangement of these may not necessarily be deleterious. If no genetic material is lost and the individual is phenotypically normal, this is termed a balanced translocation. If a translocation leads to deficiency or excess of genetic material, the re-arrangement is said to be unbalanced.

Translocations are said to be either reciprocal or Robertsonian. In the former, breaks and re-arrangements occur in two or more chromosomes, but do not involve centromeres. Therefore heterozygotes will have 46 chromosomes although one or more pairs will differ in morphology and composition from one another. The Robertsonian translocation arises in the acrocentric chromosomes (13, 14, 15, 21, 22) when they fuse at their centromere. No single acrocentric short arm is essential, therefore heterozygotes are phenotypically normal even though they have 45 chromosomes (centromeres). Certain Robertsonian translocations are more common than would be predicted on the basis of chance, either because the acrocentric chromosomes are more breakable or because such re-arrangements are more viable. These are re-arrangements involving the non-acrocentric chromosomes. The most important single translocations involve chromosomes 14 and 21. Two to 3 per cent of individuals with Down syndrome are affected by this translocation. The segregation of unbalanced chromosomes is interesting in that it is theoretically calculated that one third of viable offspring of translocation heterozygotes should have Down syndrome, but empirical data show that only 10 per cent of female heterozygotes and only 2 to 3 per cent offspring of male heterozygotes have

the syndrome. This deficiency of expected versus observed outcomes may be due to preferential segregation of unbalanced products into polar bodies, an increased loss of unbalanced zygotes or early embryos, an increase in the unrecognised loss of unbalanced fetuses late in gestation, or a decrease in the fertilisation of unbalanced oocytes or the fertilisation ability of unbalanced sperm.

A Robertsonian translocation involving homologous chromosomes has a poor prognosis. Translocations involving both chromosome 13 or 21 would yield abnormal live borns, all other conceptions would terminate in spontaneous abortions. Translocations for 14, 15 and 22 almost always result in miscarriage. Females with homologous translocations are often informed about sterilisation or alternative techniques using assisted reproductive technology. Male heterozygotes are often advised to utilise artificial insemination with donor sperm (AID).

Many different reciprocal translocations exist, and have been described for all chromosomes. During meiosis I the two translocation chromosomes involved in the reciprocal translocation and the two structurally normal chromosomes may segregate in several ways with a number of different outcomes.

Dicentric chromosomes

This is a chromosome which has two centromeres. The two centromeres confirm mitotic instability as they may migrate to opposite poles during telophase. This dicentric stretch may cause a break followed by either loss of chromosomal material or secondary re-arrangements. Not infrequently a dicentric Y is detected in 45,X/46,XY mosaicism which results in gonadal dysgenesis predisposing to germ cell neoplasia (gonadoblastoma or dysgerminoma).

Ring chromosomes

This arises following a break in both the long and short arms with subsequent fusion of the chromosomal regions adjacent with the centromeres. Telometric regions of each arm are acentric, lost, and therefore deficient. Such ring chromosomes are unstable because at each replication the ring must open and the site of opening is not necessarily identical each time. This often results in different sized rings, dicentric rings or loss of the entire chromosome.

Inversion

An inversion is when two breaks occur in a single chromosome and the intervening segment becomes inverted before the broken ends rejoin. If the reversed segment includes the centromere, the inversion is pericentric. If it does not include the centromere, the inversion is paracentric. Heterozygotes for either type may be normal if genes are neither lost, gained, altered nor placed next to neighbouring genes which alter their expression. Individuals with inversions may be abnormal due to crossing over during meiosis. A range of problems can exist with the various types of pericentric or paracentric inversions. As the production of acentric and dicentric gametes arise with paracentric inversions the probable outcome would be disorders of reproduction, and it is not uncommon for prenatal diagnosis to be offered to couples in which one parent has a paracentric inversion. Numerous pericentric inversions have now been encountered although, generally, inversions are less common than translocations. Still only limited data exists on the risks of pericentric inversions in humans.

Structural chromosomal re-arrangements account for approximately 5 per cent of all chromosomally abnormal abortuses. Of these, 50 per cent are balanced Robertsonian translocations.

Abnormalities of chromosome numbers

When the full numerical complement of chromosomes (n or 2n) is lacking, aneuploidy exists. If there exists an additional chromosome in the cell (2n+1) this is termed 'trisomy'. Should these arise in an additional sex chromosome (e.g. 47 XXX or 47 XXY) polysomy exists. Approximately one of every 160 live births results in a chromoso-

mal abnormality, most of which are a result of numerical aberrations (Table 14.1).

Trisomy

There are three distinct trisomies: primary, secondary and tertiary. Primary trisomy occurs when the normal complement of chromosomes includes an extra chromosome. When the extra chromosome is an isochromosome for a single chromosome arm, this is secondary trisomy. If the extra chromosome consists of two arms of non-homologous chromo-

Table 14.1 Incidence of chromosomal abnormalities in liveborn infants

Numerical aberrations		
Polysomy:		
47,XYY	1/1000	MB
47,XXY	1/1000	MB
Other males	1/1350	MB
45,X	1/10000	FB
47,XXX	1/1000	FB
Other females	1/2700	FB
Autosomes:		
Trisomies:		
13–15 (D group)	1/20000	LB
16–18 (E group)	1/8000	LB
21–22 (G group)	1/800	LB
Others	1/50000	LB
Structural aberrations		
Balanced:		
Robertsonian:		
t (Dq; Dq)	1/1500	LB
t (Dq; Gq)	1/5000	LB
Reciprocal translocation and interstitial inversions (RTII)	1/7000	LB
Unbalanced		
Robertsonian	1/14000	LB
RTII	1/8000	LB
Inversions	1/50000	LB
Deletions	1/10000	LB
Supernumeraries	1/5000	LB
Others	1/8000	LB
Total	1/160	LB

Notes: t   translocation.
        MB   male birth.
        FB   female birth.
        LB   live births.

Source: Hook and Hamerton, 1977.[1]

somes, this is called tertiary trisomy.

Primary trisomy may be derived from several causes, but it usually arises *de novo* after meiotic or mitotic non-disjunction. Non-disjunction may be the result of the failure of homologous chromosomes to disjoin in meiosis I, or it may originate after the failure of sister chromatids to disjoin in either meiosis II or mitosis. The former is most common in humans. Non-disjunction in meiosis I can be a result of the failure of synapsis, premature terminalisation or absence of chiasmata. Should non-disjunction arise during mitosis the products are two or more cell lines (mosaicism – see below). But if non-disjunction arises during meiosis, aneuploid gametes are produced with any resulting zygote giving rise to an identical chromosome constitution in all descendent cells.

A rare cause for primary trisomy is after normal meiotic segregation in a trisomic parent. A trisomic parent would theoretically produce gametes with n or n+1 chromosomes in equal numbers. Should fertilisation of the n+1 gamete occur this would produce a trisomic zygote, 2n+1. This process is secondary non-disjunction.

Secondary and tertiary trisomies can arise after complicated chromosomal interactions arising during structural aberration. For example, a Robertsonian translocation involving homologous chromosomes, such as both 13 or both 21, could yield abnormal live borns with trisomy 13 or trisomy 21 and therefore the prognosis is extremely poor. Invariably all other conceptions would terminate in spontaneous abortions, for example, translocations for 14, 15 and 22. Generally females with homologous translocations are informed about sterilisation or gamete donation. Male heterozygotes are often offered artificial insemination with donor sperm.

If there is the presence of an additional normal chromosome coupled with two chromosomes involved in a balanced translocation, and the two arms (short and long) of the additional chromosome are derived from non-homologous chromosomes, this is called tertiary trisomy. In this condition the remaining 46 chromosomes are morphologically normal.

Autosomal trisomy accounts for approximately 50 per cent of chromosomally abnormal miscar-

riages, or 25 per cent of all clinically recognised first trimester abortuses. Trisomy for every chromosome has been detected although trisomy I has been observed in an eight-cell embryo.[2] Many trisomies are incompatible with life as they have only been detected with abortuses.

Monosomy

This condition, which is the omission of a chromosome from a normal complement, 2n–1, is usually a result of mechanisms similar to those yielding trisomy. Almost invariably meiotic non-disjunction which results in a disomic gamete also produces a complementary gamete lacking that particular chromosome. Secondary non-disjunction, i.e. normal segregation in a monosomic parent, may also give rise to monosomy. This is only possible in humans 45,X, as autosomal monosomy is lethal. Monosomy may also result from the lagging behind of a chromosome during anaphase, and its failure to pass on to the daughter cells; this is called anaphase lag. Chromosomes lacking a centromere, i.e. acentric chromosomes, in particular, are inevitably eliminated.

Monosomy (45,X) is lethal in the vast majority of cases. Those individuals who survive usually have gonadal and somatic abnormalities, and fertility is very rare. Monosomy X accounts for approximately 15–20 per cent of chromosomally abnormal abortuses with 45,X the most common single complement among them.

Polyploidy

Polyploidy is the occurrence of more than two haploid sets of chromosomes, i.e. 3n, 4n, etc. For example, in the human, 3n = 69 chromosomes. Polyploidy is a frequent occurrence in human abortuses, and is seen at an incidence of between 3 and 8 per cent of all fertilised eggs after *in vitro* fertilisation. Polyploidy is rarely detected in neonates. The most common form of polyploidy is triploidy, 3n, and it arises as a result of either two paternal or two maternal haploid sets of chromosomes.

Causes of polyploidy may be a result of fertilisation of the single haploid egg by two spermatozoa (dispermy). The fertilisation of an egg by more than one sperm is given the general term of polyspermy.

Although the latter is probably the main cause of polyploidy, other possible mechanisms are the fertilisation of the egg with a single diploid spermatozoon, or the fertilisation of a single diploid oocyte that failed to undergo chromosome reduction in meiosis I, re-incorporation or suppression of the expulsion of one of the polar bodies (digny), or a mitotic error involving either the male or female pronucleus at syngamy. In humans tetraploidy, 4n, i.e. 92 chromosomes, is not rare among abortuses although much less common than triploidy. It is quite normal to often detect tetraploid amniotic fluid cells. Approximately 20 per cent of chromosomally abnormal abortuses are polyploid, representing 10 per cent of all clinically recognised first trimester abortions. The placenta of a triploid fetus may be associated with hydropic degeneration, and the hydatiform mole may arise from the triploid condition.

Mosaicism

In this condition the particular individual has two or more genotypes, i.e. specifically two distinct cell lines derived from the same zygote. If non-disjunction or anaphase lag occurs during mitosis, with the survival of at least two lines having different complements, this will result in chromosomal mosaicism. A single non-disjunctional event can result in as many as three cell lines. Generally, some distinct daughter cells fail to survive and this results in less complicated mosaicism.

Chimaerism

Chimaerism, like mosaicism, is the appearance of a single individual with two or more genotypes. However, with chimaerism each genotype is derived from different zygotes which fuse very early in development. Chimaerism accounts for some true hermaphrodites, and is, therefore, distinct from mosaicism. Embryos may fuse once they have hatched from the zona pellucida prior to the implantation stage or early in postimplantation. It is also possible that a biovular zona pellucida, two oocytes contained in a single zona, may be ovulated and each fertilised individually. There may be

a very thin wall of zona pellucida separating the two oocytes initially; dissolution of this during cleavage with subsequent fusion of the zygotes or embryos is feasible. The biovular zona pellucida has been reported in humans[3] (Figure 14.5).

The incidence of chromosome abnormalities in liveborns, and specifically trisomy 21, increases with maternal age (Table 14.2).

Chromosome banding

Hitherto we have discussed the gross anomalies of chromosome number and structure, which depicts

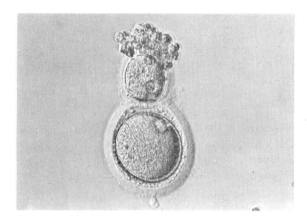

Figure 14.5a Original magnification × 200

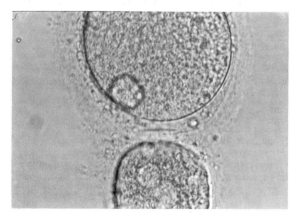

Figure 14.5b Original magnification × 400

Figure 14.5 A human biovular oocyte, as recovered from the follicle

the chromosomal basis of the more common syndromes. However, there are many smaller deletions which are responsible for other syndromes and it was not until the early 1970s that a major advance was made in the study of human cytogenetics. Caspersson et al.[4] used quinacrine mustard, a fluorescent DNA binding compound, and demonstrated that it produced a characteristic banding pattern (Q bands) along the chromosomes when examined using ultraviolet incident light. Using this method the bands rapidly faded. In the same year, 1971, Seabright[5] reported on a rapid banding technique which was permanent and had an almost identical banding pattern using the stain Giemsa (G bands) after the chromosomes had been treated with trypsin. The chromosomes could then be examined using transmitted light. Each pair of homologous chromosomes had a unique banding pattern, which was consistent throughout the species. Therefore, each chromosome can be identified unambiguously with a relatively detailed analysis of its structure (Figure 14.6).

Further additional specialised binding techniques were developed over the next seven years. Thereafter there followed the identification of a range of structural chromosome abnormalities including the duplications, deletions, insertions, ring chromosomes, peri and paracentric inversions and translocations, together with their duplication or deficient recombinant and derivative products.

A variety of methods was used to block the cell cycle in culture, followed by timed release and further arrest which synchronised cells at the metaphase stage where chromosomes could be examined more readily. Under these conditions chromosome preparations with more than 1000 bands per haploid genome were produced

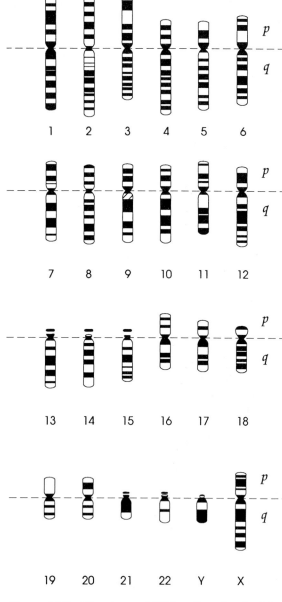

Table 14.2 The incidence of chromosomal abnormalities in liveborns according to maternal age[‡]

Maternal age	Risk of trisomy 21	Total risk for chromosome abnormalities
20	1/1667	1/526*
25	1/1250	1/476*
30	1/952	1/385*
35	1/385	1/164
40	1/106	1/51
45	1/30	1/15
48	1/14	1/7

Sources: [‡] Hook, 1981,[14] and Hook et al., 1983.[15]
Note: * Data for 47,XXX not available for inclusion.

Figure 14.6 The observed 'G' banding of each of the human chromosomes

routinely, and in special circumstances with high resolution techniques, up to 2000 can be identified. Combinations of these techniques provided the essential physical markers for the development of detailed gene localisation studies. These banding techniques laid the foundation for the more detailed location of genes by techniques such as deletion mapping. It would not be in the scope of this introduction to discuss the more powerful tools associated with cytogenetic analysis but the technique of deletion mapping is extremely powerful when combined with techniques such as somatic cell hybridisation and gene dosage studies. With these techniques correlation could be made with the presence or absence of specific chromosome regions and quantitative studies of gene products.

Molecular cytogenetics

It was less than 50 years ago (1944) when it was established that genetic information was stored in DNA and not in the protein of the cell. The structure of the DNA molecule, with its two strands spiralling round each other (the double helix), and its implications for self-replication were established in 1953. The substances, or bases, and therefore the base pair sequence creating the two spiralling strands of DNA were the essence of the genetic code. This genetic code, carried in the base pair sequence, was broken in 1961. In the 1970s DNA probes were developed. These probes were radio-active, single strands of DNA which were capable of finding and hybridising with particular DNA fragments. Using various techniques these probes were first used in prenatal diagnosis of common disorders in the 1970s.

In situ hybridisation

By utilising the direct hybridising of nucleic acid sequences, or base pairs (probes), to their complementary DNA on routinely prepared chromosome preparations, individual genes can be localised to specific chromosome regions. The probe may be labelled using radio-active or non-radio-active techniques. If chromosome banding procedures

are used in conjunction with *in situ* techniques, unambiguous assignments to chromosome regions can be achieved. For example, the immunoglobulin kapa light chain gene was assigned to the short arm of chromosome II[6] and this proved valuable in the precise location of the gene for cystic fibrosis.

A combination of these techniques, *in situ* hybridisation and cytogenic analysis, has been invaluable in defining the break points of certain chromosome re-arrangements, particularly in leukaemic and other cancer related studies. It has also found application in the study of XXX males where the use of Y chromosome short arm probes has depicted a translocation of material from the Y short arm to the short arm of the X chromosome.

The integration of molecular and cytogenic techniques for the analysis of chromosome abnormalities and their related syndromes has led to the development of chromosome 'painting'. A preparation containing the DNA marker is labelled with a fluorochrome and hyridised to prometaphase chromosome preparations. The site of hybridisation on the chromosome can be visualised using fluorescent microscopy. Libraries of probes, covering the whole genome, can be established. Careful use of appropriate probes and fluorochromes should enable different parts of various chromosomes to be seen in contrasting colours, enabling precise identification of structural chromosome abnormalities, opening a new era for clinical cytogenetics.

Flow cytometry and chromosome sorting

A fluorescent activated cell sorter (FACS) is being examined for its ability to separate chromosomes on the basis of size and base per ratio from a fluid suspension of metaphase chromosomes. Two fluorescent dyes are used to stain the chromosomes and the latter are passed sequentially at a speed of up to 2000 per second through two lasers which excite the fluorescent emission from each dye. A flow karyotype of two types is created in which large numbers of individual chromosomes form discreet clusters in characteristic relationship to one another. Using computer programmes, small pieces of chromosome can be analysed and may be useful for detecting deletions and duplications in abnormal chromosomes.

The FACS has the potential to sort and collect large numbers of the same chromosome and offers a very exciting prospect to molecular cytogeneticists. Fluorescent *in situ* hybridisation (FISH) and FACS can be used in conjunction in one of the major problems of cytogenetics, to determine the origins of non-inherited unbalanced chromosomal re-arrangements. FACS can be used to sort the 'unknown' chromosome and a paint probe produced from the sorting material. By painting the probe on to normal chromosomes by FISH, the origin of the abnormality can be determined. This is called the 'FISH FACS approach'.

DNA sequences and the diagnosis of human genetic disease

Within the last ten years rapid progress has been made in the area of prenatal diagnosis and detection of carriers. This is due to the dramatic development of recombinant DNA technology. It is possible to use DNA markers, that is the short DNA sequences, to follow the inheritance of a disease without understanding the biochemical defect or identifying the defective gene responsible for the phenotype. DNA markers can be used to localise a mutation to a chromosomal region – linkage analysis – which is the first step in isolating defective genes and characterisation of the protein involved.

DNA markers

The technique for detecting DNA markers is known as Southern blotting.[7] Briefly, the human DNA is digested with particular enzymes, restriction enzymes, into more than a million fragments and these are separated according to their size by agarose gel electrophoresis. The separated gel fragments are chemically denatured to separate the DNA into single strands. The resulting DNA produced by the restriction enzyme can then be incubated with the single strand radio-active probe. The single strand radio-active DNA would search out and hybridise to its complementary DNA strand. The position of the gene is then observed by autoradiography.

This technique of Southern blotting can be used to detect differences in restriction enzyme fragment length between individuals. Generally two members of a chromosome pair (homologues) will have largely the same restriction patterns at any one point. However, sometimes, a random base-pair change can create or destroy a particular restriction site. Therefore one of the homologues will produce a different restriction pattern for one enzyme compared with its homologue. These differences in restriction pattern are inherited and are known as polymorphisms. In other words, if there is a mutant chromosome in which there is a site missing there will exist a different restriction of fragment length although the same restriction enzyme was used. This is restriction fragment length polymorphism (RFLP). Abnormalities such as gene deletions, mutations or duplication can be detected as size variations in the hybridised DNA bands or as the total absence of a band. Figure 14.7 is a schematic representation of a restriction fragment length polymorphism. RFLP analysis is now used extensively to map diseased genes to chromosomal regions, and it is particularly successful for Duchenne muscular dystrophy where prenatal diagnosis and carrier detection are now routine using DNA probes.

Polymerase chain reaction

Within the last seven years, a new technique has been devised which has dramatically improved the application of DNA recombinant technology to the analysis of human genetic disease.[8] This technique has been called the polymerase chain reaction (PCR). Essentially, a single segment of DNA consisting of a few hundred base pairs (oligonucleotides), which is present in the background of the human genome consisting of three billion base pairs, can be selectively amplified. If the sequence of DNA flanking the region of interest is known the latter can be amplified for analysis, as described in Figure 14.8. Priming molecules of base pairs – oligonucleotide primers – which correspond to the two flanking sequences, are annealed to the genomic DNA being analysed. These primers are

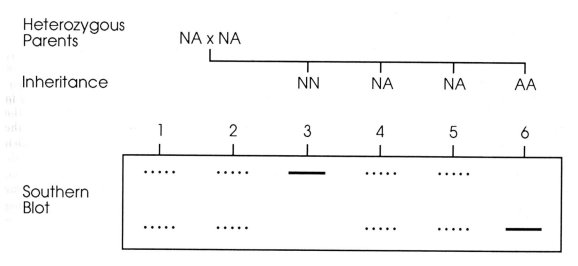

Heterozygous
Parents

NA x NA

Inheritance

NN   NA   NA   AA

1   2   3   4   5   6

Southern
Blot

Figure 14.7 Inheritance and detection of RFLP. Parents, 1 and 2, are heterozygous for the polymorphism. One chromosome has a normal fragment (N), the other abnormal (A). Fifty per cent of the gametes will have one type of chromosome. At fertilisation, four types of inheritance in their children are possible, namely: 3, 4, 5 or 6. Two (4 and 5) will be heterozygous for the polymorphosis, one (3) homozygous for the normal and the other (6) homozygous for the abnormal. If the gene for the recessive disorder resides in the abnormal fragment the embryo (or fetus) homozygous for A will be affected. Fetuses heterozygous for the polymorphism (4 and 5) will not be affected by the disease

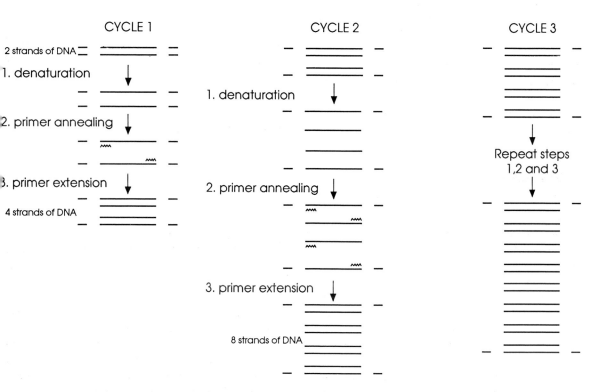

CYCLE 1   CYCLE 2   CYCLE 3

2 strands of DNA

1. denaturation

                  1. denaturation

2. primer annealing

                  Repeat steps
                  1,2 and 3

3. primer extension

4 strands of DNA   2. primer annealing

                  3. primer extension

                8 strands of DNA

Figure 14.8 Diagrammatic representation of the polymerase chain reaction

153

then extended by a polymerase enzyme thereby synthesising the copies of the region of interest between the primers. The DNA is then denatured and allowed to re-anneal. In this process, the second cycle, the primers will anneal to the newly synthesised sequences as well as the original DNA and, therefore, twice as many molecules can be synthesised. This amplification process is repeated to the eventual amplification of more than one million times within three hours. Using fluorescence or direct staining of the DNA with ethidium bromide, the specific region of interest can be visualised. PCR is therefore rapid analysis of a sequence within hours, and allows genetic diagnosis

to be performed the same day as the sampling. This compares with the conventional Southern blotting technique which takes up to two weeks.

The exquisitely sensitive PCR technique encouraged researchers to study DNA sequences in a single haploid or diploid cell[9–11], and led to the idea that genetic disease could be diagnosed in the human embryo.[9,12,13] It is this technique which has become so important for screening genetic mutations in the embryo prior to implantation, the oocyte after fertilisation or perhaps in the polar body of the unfertilised zygote itself. The following chapters give precise examples of the value of these techniques in pre-implantation diagnosis.

References

1. Hook EB, Hamerton JL. The frequency of chromosome abnormalities detected in corrective newborn studies – differences between studies – results by sex and by severity of phenotypic involvement. In: Hook EB, Porters IH (eds.) *Population Cytogenic Studies in Humans*. New York: Academic Press, 1977, pp. 63–79.

2. Watt JL, Templeton AA, Messinis I, Bell L, Cunningham P, Duncan RO. Trisomy I in an 8-cell human pre-embryo. *Journal of Medical Genetics*. 1987; **24**: 60–4.

3. Fishel SB, Kaufman MH, Jackson P, Webster J, Faratian B. Recovery of two human oocytes surrounded by a single zona pellucida. *Fertility and Sterility*. 1989; **52**: 325–7.

4. Caspersson T, Lomakka G, Finch L. The 24 fluorescence patterns of the human metaphase chromosomes – distinguishing characteristics and variability. *Hereditas*. 1971; **67**: 89–102.

5. Seabright M. A rapid banding technique for demonstrating centromeric heterochromatin. *Experimental Cell Research*. 1971; **75**: 302–6.

6. Malcolm S, Barton P, Murphy C, Ferguson-Smith MA, Bently DL, Rabbitts TH. Localisation of human immunoglobulin kappa light chain variable region genes to the short arms of chromosome 2 by in situ hybridisation. *Proceedings of the National Academy of Sciences (USA)*. 1982; **79**: 4957–61.

7. Southern EM. Detection of specific sequences among DNA fragments separated by gel electrophoresis. *Journal of Molecular Biology*. 1975; **98**: 503–17.

8. Saiki R, Scharf S, Faloona F, Mullis K, Horn G, Erlich H, Arnheim N. Amplification of beta-globin genomic sequences and restriction site analysis for diagnosis of sickle cell anaemia. *Science*. 1985; **230**: 1350–4.

9. Li H, Gyllensten U, Cui X, Saiki R, Erlich H, Arnheim N. Enzymatic amplification and analysis of DNA sequences in single human sperm. *Nature*. 1988; **335**: 414–17.

10. Cui X, Li H, Goradia TM, Lange K, Kazazian HH, Galas DJ, Arnheim N. Single sperm typing: determination of genetic distance between the G-gamma globin and parathyroid hormone loci. *Proceedings of the National Academy of Sciences (USA)*. 1989; **86**: 9389–93.

11. Jeffreys AJ, Wilson V, Neumann R, Keyte J. Amplification of human minisatellites by the polymerase chain reaction: towards DNA fingerprinting of single cells. *Nucleic Acids Research*. 1988; **16**: 10953–71.

12. Handyside AH, Pattinson JK, Penketh RJA, Delhanty JDA, Winston RML, Tuddenham EGD. Biopsy of human preimplantation embryos and sexing by DNA amplification. *Lancet*. 1989; **i**: 347–9.

13. Coutelle C, Williams C, Handyside A, Hardy K, Winston R, Williamson R. Genetic analysis from DNA from single human oocytes: a model for preimplantation diagnosis of cystic fibrosis. *British Medical Journal*. 1989; **299**: 22–4.

14. Hook EB. Rates of chromosomal abnormalities of different maternal ages. *Obstetrics and Gynaecology*. 1981; **58**: 282–5.

15. Hook EB, Cross PK, Schreinemachers DM. Chromosomal abnormality rates in amniocentesis and in live born infants. *Journal of the American Medical Association*. 1983; **249**: 2043.

Chapter 15

Embryo microsurgery for large animals

Robert A Godke and Rick W Rorie

Introduction

Embryo micromanipulation has recently generated a great deal of interest among researchers and commercial livestock producers. It was thought in the 1970s that, unlike laboratory animal embryos, the embryos of farm animals would not survive to produce transplant young following micromanipulation procedures. Studies in the early 1980s, however, showed that morulae and blastocysts of farm animal species were able to survive following microsurgery, develop normally *in utero* and produce viable offspring from surrogate females. As procedures for embryo micromanipulation became more efficient, commercial animal transplant units began incorporating this new methodology into their offerings to livestock producers in North America. Today, new embryo microsurgical procedures are being developed such as partial zona dissection for *in vitro* fertilisation (IVF), inner cell mass transfer and the production of chimaeric embryos for possible use in animal reproduction management schemes for the future.

Development of animal micromanipulation techniques

Early studies in mammalian embryo micromanipulation involved evaluation of the developmental potential of single blastomeres isolated from early stage embryos of the rabbit,[1–4] rat[5] and mouse.[6] These studies provided evidence that individual blastomeres of early stage mammalian embryos ($\leq$ 8-cells) were totipotent and the potential existed for the production of multiple offspring from a single embryo. A major obstacle to the production of multiple offspring from early stage embryos was the inability of precompaction stage embryos to survive *in vivo* without an intact or near-intact zona pellucida (ZP). Evidence to the effect has been shown in the rabbit[4], the mouse,[7,8] the pig[9] and the sheep.[10] The obstacle was later overcome by the development of an agar embedding technique for micromanipulated mammalian embryos.[11,12]

Willadsen's technique involved the separation of blastomeres of early stage embryos by microsurgery and the transfer of one or more blastomeres from one embryo to one or more evacuated ZP. The separated blastomeres contained within surrogate ZP were then embedded in agar chips.[12] The agar-embedded blastomeres were transferred to the ligated oviducts of either diestrous or anestrous ewes for subsequent development *in vivo*. After development to the morula or blastocyst stage, the micromanipulated embryos were recovered from the intermediate host, carefully removed from the agar and transferred to respective recipients. This procedure was used to produce the first sets of identical twin lambs from eight-cell embryos.[11] This approach was later used to produce the first identical twin calves and one set of triplet calves,[13] twin foals[12] and to produce twin calves from non-surgically collected day-five to day-six bovine embryos.[14]

Embryo bisection to produce twins

Although the agar embedding technique has been shown to be an excellent method for the micromanipulation and culture of early stage embryos, this procedure is generally considered by most not to be practical enough for routine use by embryo transplant stations. To address a more practical need, procedures for bisecting embryos were required that could be executed with non-surgically collected day-six to day-eight embryos, and that would allow for efficient dissection and immediate transfer of split embryos into recipient animals. In 1982, three independent research groups then reported new micromanipulation techniques for use on non-surgically collected later stage bovine embryos.[15,16,17]

Ozil et al.,[15] from INRA in France, described a technique to produce split embryos in which two glass microneedles were used to open the ZP and a glass transfer pipette was used to remove the embryonic cell mass from the zona cavity. The ZP-free embryo was bisected with a microscalpel, and the halves were replaced into evacuated ZP with the transfer pipette. Using this micromanipulation procedure, 14 early blastocysts were bisected and transferred non-surgically to 14 recipients, resulting in a pregnancy rate of 64.2 per cent and a twinning rate of 66.6 per cent.

Also in 1982, researchers at Louisiana State University (LSU) described an embryo bisection procedure for non-surgically collected bovine embryos.[16] With this method, a fine glass needle

was used to make a rent in the ZP. The embryonic cell mass was removed with the same flexible glass needle and bisected on a vertical plane while resting on the bottom of the petri dish. A glass transfer pipette was used to transfer each 'half' embryo (demi-embryo) to a separate evacuated ZP. In this study, eight demi-embryo pairs and six individual demi-embryos were transferred non-surgically to 14 beef recipients. The twin demi-embryo transfers resulted in a pregnancy rate of 62.5 per cent and the single demi-embryo transfers resulted in a pregnancy rate of 16.6 per cent.

In the same year, Williams et al.[17] from Colorado State University (CSU) in Colorado reported a procedure for splitting the bovine embryo while remaining within the ZP. This method uses a razor blade chip mounted with super glue on a small glass capillary pipette to bisect the intact embryo (Figure 15.1). A fine glass pipette was then used to transfer each of the demi-embryos to evacuated ZP. In this study, 20 good quality bovine embryos (morula to early blastocyst stage) were bisected and transferred as demi-embryo pairs either surgically or non-surgically to 20 recipient cattle. Fourteen surgical and six non-surgical demi-embryo transfers resulted in pregnancy rates of 64 per cent and 17 per cent, respectively.

At present, the more simplified CSU method described by Williams et al.[17] has become more widely adapted for use by commercial embryo transplant units than the other procedures. However in a comparative study, Mertes and Bondioli[18] have suggested there may be an advantage to the LSU procedure,[17] which has been shown to cause less cell damage while bisecting the embryonic cell mass with a fine glass needle outside of the ZP. With practice and patience at the laboratory bench, all three microsurgery procedures can be used effectively to bisect farm animal embryos and produce viable split embryo offspring.

A simplified method for bisecting morula to hatched blastocyst stage ovine embryos has been reported,[19] which is readily adaptable for bovine embryos. This procedure uses a fine glass needle to penetrate and to bisect ZP intact morulae or blastocysts and ZP free hatched blastocysts (Figure 15.2). It was reported that the overall transfer pregnancy rate in sheep using this procedure was 89 per cent.

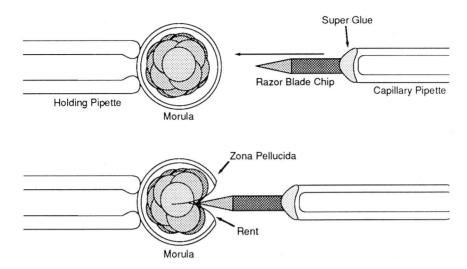

Figure 15.1 An early stage embryo (morula) is bisected into two portions using a razor blade chip attached to glass capillary pipette with super glue (CSU procedure). A fire-polished, glass suction pipette is used to hold the embryo in place during splitting procedure

More recently, a simplified technique for bisecting later stage farm animal embryos was reported by Rorie et al.[20,21] from the LSU laboratory. This technique allows for rapid bisection of intact embryos without the use of a commercial micromanipulation unit. With this method, an intact embryo is placed in a small microdrop of holding medium on a microscope slide, and a razor blade held by a pair of hemostats is used to bisect the embryo. In these studies, 98 per cent of the intact bovine embryos were successfully bisected using this razor blade method. Transplant pregnancy rates have not been different when the standard laboratory glass needle bisection procedure[22] was compared with that of the hand held razor blade procedure on similar stage bovine embryos. This new method is simple to execute, inexpensive and easy to learn.

Pregnancy rates from bisected embryos

In recent years, research efforts have been directed toward identifying factors that contribute to optimal pregnancy rates from bisected embryos.

Experience has shown that, with proper technique, excellent and good quality embryos (quality grades 1 = excellent and 2 = good) are suitable for embryo bisection. The transfer of demi-embryos produced from either excellent or good quality embryos has been shown to result in pregnancy rates similar to those obtained with intact embryos of the same embryo quality grades.[23–26] Pregnancy rates expected from single demi-embryos non-surgically

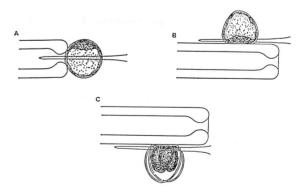

Figure 15.2 An early stage embryo (blastocyst) is bisected into two portions using a fine glass needle to cut through the inner mass cell using the outside wall of the glass suction pipette[19]

157

transplanted to individual bovine recipient females usually range from 45–65 per cent.

Efforts have been made to evaluate the optimal stage of morphological development to bisect bovine embryos for transfer. Similar results have been reported for bovine demi-embryos produced from late morula and blastocyst stage embryos.[26,27] However, pregnancy rates from demi-embryos produced from early morulae have been reported to be significantly lower than pregnancy rates resulting from demi-embryos produced from early blastocysts.[27] These findings suggest that early stage bovine morulae are less suitable for bisection than those at the blastocyst stage of development.

The zona pellucida appears to have little effect on the *in vivo* survival of demi-embryos produced from late morula to blastocyst-stage bovine embryos. Studies have shown that the number of pregnancies produced from bovine demi-embryos placed into the original ZP were similar to those placed in foreign ZP prior to transfer.[26,27] In contrast, Baker and Shea[28] have reported a lower pregnancy rate from bovine demi-embryos placed into surrogate ZP than for demi-embryos left in the original ZP (58 per cent versus 74 per cent). It was suggested that the lower pregnancy rate was probably due to injury to the 'half' embryos during their transfer into the foreign ZP. It is important to note that other studies using bovine embryos have shown that later stage ZP-free demi-embryos survive *in vivo* as well as demi-embryos encased in a ZP prior to transfer.[23,29]

The highest pregnancy and twinning rates have been obtained when demi-embryo pairs are transferred to a recipient rather than a single demi-embryo.[22,28,30] Pregnancy rates have been reported to be similar when demi-embryo pairs are transferred to the same uterine horn or when one demi-embryo is transferred to each uterine horn of recipient cattle.[28]

Studies have shown that when bovine embryos are bisected into 'quarter' embryos from precompaction[14] or postcompaction stage embryos[31,32] lower uterine survival is to be expected. It has been suggested that a single 'quarter' embryo is less likely to produce a sufficient luteotrophic signal *in utero* to prevent luteal regression in the recipient female.[14] Correspondingly, the reduced size of the developing blastocyst from a quarter embryo may lack sufficient embryonic cells in the inner cell mass to form a viable conceptus. Recently Voelkel et al.[32] bisected cultured bovine blastocysts that had been derived from demi-embryos. In this case, only 17.6 per cent of the 'quarter' embryos derived from cultured demi-embryos produced a second blastocyst during *in vitro* culture.

Freezing bisected embryos

Embryos are now routinely bisected as soon as possible after collection and then transferred to recipient animals. Efforts have been made to evaluate the possibility of bisecting frozen/thawed embryos and/or the frozen storage of bisected embryos. Lehn-Jensen and Willadsen[33] reported on the first attempts to cryopreserve 'half' and 'quarter' bovine embryos produced by blastomere separation, agar embedding and *in vivo* culture (ligated oviducts of ewes) prior to freezing. The results from this study indicated frozen/thawed 'half' embryos were less viable than fresh 'half' embryos, and their results indicated that it would probably not be feasible to freeze 'quarter' embryos.

Niemann et al.[34] have investigated the effects of the ZP on the survival of frozen/thawed demi-embryos. Sixteen demi-embryos were placed into two overlapping ZP to produce an 'intact' ZP, and 11 demi-embryos were each placed into a single ZP prior to freezing. Demi-embryos frozen in two ZP or a single ZP (graded as excellent or good postthaw) resulted in six pregnancies (46.2 per cent) and one pregnancy (25 per cent) after transfer, respectively. Transferred 'fresh' demi-embryos resulted in nine pregnancies (47.4 per cent), while frozen/thawed intact embryos produced eight pregnancies (53.3 per cent). Eight demi-embryos produced from frozen/thawed embryos were transferred but resulted in no pregnancies. It was suggested that it may be preferable to freeze bisected bovine embryos rather than bisecting frozen/thawed embryos. Also, it was proposed that freezing demi-embryos in two overlapping ZP (to produce a resemblance of an 'intact' ZP) could enhance postthaw survival.

Rorie et al.[35] have compared the *in vitro* survival of bovine demi-embryos produced either before or after freezing in liquid nitrogen in a controlled study. The results of this experiment indicated that there was no advantage to either producing demi-embryos before or after freezing/thawing and, in either case, the number of transferable quality (excellent to good quality) demi-embryos was considered low (20 per cent versus 21.3 per cent) when compared with intact frozen/thawed control embryos (67.5 per cent). Freezing bisected embryos in liquid nitrogen apparently destroys enough of the embryonic cells that the demi-embryos (each with fewer total number of cells) are unable to recover during the postthaw culture interval.

Heyman[36] bisected frozen/thawed day-eight bovine blastocysts and reported pregnancy rates of 20 per cent at 90 days of gestation for 20 demi-embryos as compared with a 36 per cent pregnancy rate for 11 demi-embryos produced from fresh blastocysts. It was indicated that the lower pregnancy rate for the demi-embryos produced from frozen/thawed embryos may be attributed to a reduction in the luteotrophic signal of the bisected frozen/thawed embryos. It was suggested that co-transfer of trophoblastic vesicles with demi-embryos might improve transfer pregnancy rates. Previously, Voelkel et al.[37] have reported that co-culture of 'fresh' demi-embryos on an uterine cell monolayer enhanced *in vitro* survival of the bovine demi-embryos. An embryo co-culture system would probably be of value during short term culture by allowing demi-embryos to recover from bisection prior to freezing or could be used to aid in evaluating postthaw viability of embryos prior to recipient transfer.

In a preliminary report, Suzuki and Shimohira[38] suggested that bisecting frozen/thawed bovine embryos in sucrose rather than in a standard phosphate-buffered saline medium could improve *in vitro* survival and transfer pregnancy rates. In this study, *in vitro* survival of frozen/thawed day-seven embryos bisected in sucrose was 82.5 per cent (18/22) compared with 53 per cent (9/17) for embryos bisected in a standard phosphate-buffered saline medium. A 50 per cent pregnancy rate was obtained from the embryos bisected in sucrose and transferred within the same ZP (twin transfers). These more recent studies suggest that the use of cell monolayer co-culture systems and bisection of embryos in a sucrose medium are worthy of further

investigation.

Embryo bisection has potential uses other than increasing the number of offspring from a single embryo. An example of this is embryo sexing, where half of the embryo is sexed and the remaining half is transferred to a recipient female.[39] In a recent study, White et al.[40] bisected bovine embryos and sexed one demi-embryo of the pair using an H-Y antibody procedure. Then each demi-embryo of the pair was transferred to a different recipient animal. The success rate for sexing was 90 per cent, and there was no significant difference in pregnancy rates between the sexed and control demi-embryos (47 per cent versus 44 per cent). These and other studies with animal embryos suggest there is an opportunity for embryo biopsy techniques to be used as a tool for embryo sexing and/or genetic disease diagnosis, without reducing postbiopsy transfer pregnancy rates.

Inner cell mass (ICM) transfer

In terms of saving endangered species, one important embryo transfer procedure is the ability to transfer embryos between closely related species.[41] During the 1980s, some success was reported with the transfer of embryos from one exotic species to another more abundant surrogate species.[42,43] This technique has the potential for rapidly expanding small animal populations by using the rare animals only as embryo donors, while animals from a more plentiful species could serve as recipients. In cases where a closely related species will not carry the donor's embryo to term, due to differences in placental morphology and/or maternal–conceptus immuno-compatibility problems, a microsurgical embryo reconstruction technique known as inner cell mass (ICM) transfer could be used with some of these cases in the future.

A microsurgical embryonic cell transfer technique was first developed for farm animals in Cambridge, England, early in the 1980s. This approach involves blastomere separation and the transfer of a cell or cells from one embryo to an asynchronous embryo of that species.[12,44] If this is successfully completed (by microsurgery or micro-injection), the donor embryo derived from one or more of the advanced blastomeres will usually develop normally *in utero* when transferred to a recipient female. The beauty of this micromanipulation technique is that the surgically altered embryo will have the placental membranes develop from the trophectoderm of the second embryo but will have the fetus develop from the more advanced blastomere(s) (inner cell mass) of the first embryo (Figure 15.3). This would allow the reconstructed embryo to be placed in a recipient female of the second embryo's breed type (or species) to enhance an optimal environment for placental membrane attachment; however, the developing fetus would originate from the first embryo.

Another approach to this involves removing the ICM cells from a blastocyst stage embryo of the donor species and placing this ICM into the blastocyst stage embryo of the recipient species, which has had the ICM removed (Figure 15.4). Since the trophoblastic cells develop the fetal placental tissues, this ICM-transfer embryo would have placenta tissue characteristics that match those of the

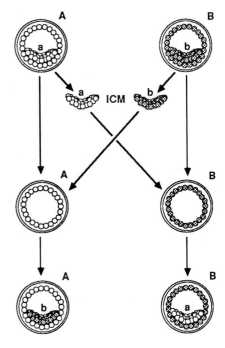

Figure 15.4 The basic inner cell mass (ICM) transfer procedure where two ICM (a and b) from two blastocysts (A and B) are reciprocally changed between the two embryos using a microsurgical technique

recipient animal. The fetus developing within the amnion will be of the donor species, since it originates from the transplanted ICM.

A good example of this would be to use the sheep and goat (two different animal species) as embryo donor females. When a sheep embryo is transferred to a female goat recipient or a goat embryo is transferred to a female sheep recipient the transplanted embryos do not develop to term. If the inner cell mass of the sheep embryo was microsurgically removed and placed in the goat embryo with the ICM removed, the composite embryo could then be transferred to a goat recipient. The chance for an offspring being born from this composite embryo is enhanced, since the placental membranes that develop from this embryo would be derived from the original goat embryo. In this procedure, the goat inner cell mass could then be placed in the remaining trophectoderm cells of the sheep embryo and this composite embryo could be transferred to a female sheep recipient. The end result would be an interspecies transfer of two embryos with the goat

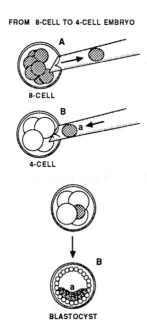

Figure 15.3 The procedure for embryo reconstruction using asynchronous transfer of a blastomere from an eight-cell embryo to a four-cell embryo. The more advanced blastomere contributes to the ICM and the less advanced cells contribute to trophectodermal layers

giving birth to a lamb and the ewe giving birth to a goat offspring. Using this approach, sheep and goat embryos have recently produced ICM transfer offspring.[45] Using a new micromanipulation procedure, Rorie et al.[46] have produced viable lambs from a goat recipient at this laboratory using ICM transfer from the ovine embryos to the caprine embryo.

These asynchronous cell blastomere or ICM transfer techniques could be put to use in saving some of our endangered species, where more abundant recipient species could carry the embryos of endangered species to term. Examples might be rare Indian Gaur cattle embryos placed in domestic cattle, or embryos of the rare Przewalski's horse placed in domestic mare recipients. Requests are being put forth by zoological societies the world over for assistance in developing techniques using the inner cell mass transfer procedures to reconstruct embryos of exotic mammals.

Fertilisation by sperm cell micro-injection

Studies by research groups in many countries have been attempting to develop techniques to produce offspring from micro-injection of sperm cells into unfertilised ova.[47–50] Iritani et al.[51] outlined the procedure for a sperm cell micro-injection method for cattle ova; however, offspring were not produced. One obvious advantage of sperm microinjection would be to fertilise ova with sperm cells from valuable males having subfertile sperm cell concentrations.

With various sperm micro-injection techniques, full term conceptus development and live offspring have been reported in laboratory mice[52] and live offspring has been produced by micro-injection of sperm cells into the ooplasm of rabbit ova.[53] Using improved methodologies, such as hypertonic medium (0.5 M sucrose) to increase the perivitelline space and electrofield induction, the success rate of oocyte activation in the rabbit has been markedly improved.[54–56]

Using a partial zona renting technique (partial zona dissection) to facilitate sperm passage and fresh ejaculated human sperm cells for *in vitro* fertilisation, pregnancies and live births have resulted from human oocytes.[57–59] Also, pregnancies[60] and births[61] have recently resulted from the injection of multiple, acrosome-reacted sperm cells into the perivitelline space of human ova. Using this new subzonal insemination procedure (SUZI) and the transfer of multiple sperm cells into the perivitelline space of human oocytes, six healthy IVF babies were recently reported.[62] In an effort to improve zona renting technology, a laser microbeam from a dye-tuned compact nitrogen laser has been used to make a small opening in the zona pellucida of bovine and murine oocytes and embryos.[63] Although the new approach was successful, at a wavelength of 440 nm, the acridine orange stain used for activating the laser beam for microsurgery at the zona surface was found to be detrimental to subsequent *in vitro* development of the laser treated embryos. Further studies in this area are needed to evaluate the feasibility of this approach. Attempts are being made to use this technology in human infertility (see Chapter 11).

In cattle, success has been reported for *in vitro* fertilisation and normal cleavage of *in vitro* matured oocytes following sperm cell micro-injection of *in vitro* capacitated bovine sperm cells,[64] and more recently sperm cell micro-injection of bovine oocytes resulted in a live transplant offspring in Japan.[65] With recent improvement in oocyte maturation and sperm cell maturation methods, *in vitro* fertilisation rates of bovine oocytes without the use of micro-injection are expected to be > 85 per cent.[66] Identifying appropriate *in vitro* embryo culture systems for IVF-derived embryos seems to be one of the major drawbacks to efficient IVF procedures in farm animals at the present time.

The possibility exists that freeze-dried sperm cells could be used to fertilise farm animal oocytes with micro-injection techniques in the future. It is interesting to note that at least two calves have been born following oocyte fertilisation with previously dried bovine sperm cells.[67,68] Certainly the potential for using this technology with freeze-dried sperm cells or with DNA extracted from preserved cells from extinct animals to produce new embryos merits re-evaluation by the scientific community.

Summary

The bisection methods described by Ozil et al.,[15] Lambeth et al.[16] and Williams et al.[17] have been successfully adapted for use by researchers and the commercial embryo transplant stations. The method of splitting embryos with a hand held razor blade[20] is practical and shows promise for field use application. Research has shown that excellent to good quality, late morula to blastocyst stage bovine embryos can be successfully bisected to produce split embryo offspring. Under optimal conditions, bisected embryos can produce pregnancy rates comparable with those achieved with intact embryos from the same donor collection.

Research has shown that replacement of the bisected embryo into a zona pellucida prior to transfer is not necessary for later stage bovine and ovine embryos. The potential may exist for improving pregnancy rates from bisected embryos by co-culturing them for a short period of time on a uterine, oviduct or possibly granulosa cell monolayer, or by co-transfer of trophoblastic vesicles.

Optimal bovine pregnancy and twinning rates have been achieved thus far by transfer of both halves of a bisected embryo to the same recipient female. In this case, there remains a potential for problems *in utero* during gestation and for complications at the time of parturition. Research is currently underway to develop a procedure for producing transplant offspring from demi-embryos that have been bisected either before or after freezing.

Preliminary results using asynchronous blastomere transfer and inner cell mass transfer techniques to reconstruct early stage farm animal embryos have thus far been encouraging. The potential for using this assisted reproductive technology for rare and exotic species needs to be evaluated by zoologists well before these animals are placed on the endangered species list. Furthermore, this technology should also be evaluated for use in valuable, problem-breeder farm animals by clinical veterinarians. Advances recently made with microsurgically assisting fertilisation in animals are of marked importance and should not be overlooked by human fertility researchers in the years to come.

References

1. Pincus G. In: Pincus G (ed.) *The Eggs of Mammals.* New York: Macmillan, 1936: pp. 75–97.
2. Seidel F. Die entwicklungspotenzen einer isolierten blastomere des zweizellenstadiums in saugetierei. *Naturwissenschaften.* 1952; **39**: 355–6.
3. Daniel JC, Takahashi K. Selective laser destruction of rabbit blastomeres and continued cleavage of survivors in vitro. *Experimental Cell Research.* 1965; **39**: 475–82.
4. Moore NW, Adams CE, Rowson LEA. Development potential of single blastomeres of the rabbit egg. *Journal of Reproduction and Fertility.* 1968; **17**: 527–31.
5. Nicholas JS, Hall BV. Experiments on developing rats. II. The development of isolated blastomeres and fused eggs. *Journal of Experimental Zoology.* 1942; **90**: 441–549.
6. Tarkowski AK. Experiments on the development of isolated blastomeres of mouse eggs. *Nature.* 1959; **184**: 1286–7.
7. Bronson RA, McLaren A. Transfer to the mouse oviduct of eggs with and without the zona pellucida. *Journal of Reproduction and Fertility.* 1970; **22**: 129–37.
8. Modlinski JA. The role of the zona pellucida in the development of mouse eggs in vivo. *Journal of Embryology and Experimental Morphology.* 1970; **23**: 539–647.
9. Moore NW, Polge C, Rowson LEA. The survival of single blastomeres of pig eggs transferred to recipient gilts. *Australian Journal of Biological Science.* 1969; **22**: 979–82.
10. Trounson AO, Moore NW. The survival and development of sheep eggs following complete or partial removal of the zona pellucida. *Journal of Reproduction and Fertility.* 1974; **41**: 97–105.
11. Willadsen SM. A method for culture of micromanipulated sheep embryos and its use to produce monozygotic twins. *Nature.* 1979; **277**: 298–300.
12. Willadsen SM, Micromanipulation of embryos of the large domestic species. In: Adams CE (ed.) *Mammalian Egg Transfer.* Boca Raton, Florida: CRC Press, 1982: pp. 185–210.
13. Willadsen SM, Polge C. Attempts to produce monozygotic quadruplets in cattle by blastomere separation. *Veterinary Record.* 1981; **108**: 211–13.
14. Willadsen SM, Lehn-Jensen H, Fehilly CB, Newcomb R. The production of monozygotic twins of preselected parentage by micromanipulation of non-surgically collected cow embryos. *Theriogenology.* 1981; **14**: 23–9.
15. Ozil JP, Heyman Y, Renard JP. Production of monozygotic twins by micromanipulation and cer-

vical transfer in the cow. *Veterinary Record.* 1982; **110**: 126–7.

16. Lambeth VA, Looney CR, Voelkel SA, Hill KG, Jackson DA, Godke RA. Micromanipulation of bovine morulae to produce identical twin offspring. In: *Proceedings of the 2nd World Congress of Embryo Transfer in Mammals.* Annecy, France: September 20th/22nd, 1982: 5.

17. Williams TJ, Elsden RP, Seidel Jr GE. Identical twin bovine pregnancies derived from bisected embryos. *Theriogenology.* 1982; **17**: 114 (abstract).

18. Mertes PC, Bondioli KR. Effect of splitting technique on pregnancy rate from half embryos. *Theriogenology.* 1985; **23**: 209 (abstract).

19. Willadsen SM, Godke RA. A simplified procedure for the production of identical sheep twins. *Veterinary Record.* 1984; **114**: 240–5.

20. Rorie RW, McFarland CW, Overskei TL, Voelkel SA, Godke RA. A new method of splitting embryos without the use of a commercial micromanipulation unit. *Theriogenology.* 1985; **23**: 224 (abstract).

21. Rorie RW, McFarland CW, Overskei TL, Voelkel SA, Godke RA. A new method of splitting cattle embryos using a simple razor blade technique. *Louisiana Cattleman.* 1986; **19**: 5–6.

22. Lambeth VA, Looney CR, Voelkel SA, Hill KG, Jackson DA, Godke RA. Microsurgery on bovine embryos at the morula stage to produce monozygotic twin calves. *Theriogenology.* 1983; **20**: 85–95.

23. Voelkel SA, Humes PE, Godke RA. Pregnancy rates resulting from non-surgical transfer of micromanipulated bovine embryos. In: *Proceedings of the 10th International Congress on Animal Reproduction and Artificial Insemination.* University of Illinois, Urbana, 10/14 June 1984: **2**: 251.

24. Voelkel SA, Viker SD, Humes PE, Godke RA. Micromanipulation and non-surgical transfer of bovine embryos. *Journal of Animal Science.* 1984; **59**: (suppl. 1), 393 (abstract).

25. Baker RD, Eberhard BE, Leffel BE, Rhoade RE, Henschen TJ. Pregnancy rates following surgical transfer of bovine demi-embryos. *Proceedings of 10th International Congress of Animal Reproduction and Artificial Insemination.* University of Illinois, Urbana, 1984; **2**: 220.

26. Takeda T, Hallowell SA, McCauley AD, Hasler JF. Pregnancy rates with intact and split bovine embryos transferred surgically and non-surgically. *Theriogenology.* 1986; **25**: 204 (abstract).

27. Williams TJ, Elsden RP, Seidel Jr GE. Pregnancy rates with bisected bovine embryos. *Theriogenology.* 1984; **22**: 521–31.

28. Baker RD, Shea BF. Commercial splitting of bovine embryos. *Theriogenology.* 1985; **22**: 3–12.

29. Warfield SJ, Siedel Jr GE, Elsden RP. Transfer of bovine demi-embryos with and without a zona pellucida. *Theriogenology.* 1986; **25**: 212 (abstract).

30. Ozil JP. Production of identical twins by bisection of blastocyts in the cow. *Journal of Reproduction and Fertility.* 1983; **69**: 463–8.

31. Voelkel SA, Viker SD, Johnson CA, Hill KG, Humes PE, Godke RA. Multiple embryo transplant offspring produced from quartering a bovine morulae. *Veterinary Record.* 1985; **117**, 528–30.

32. Voelkel SA, Rorie RW, McFarland CW, Godke RA. An attempt to produce quarter embryos from non-surgically recovered bovine blastocysts. *Theriogenology.* 1986; **25**, 207 (abstract).

33. Lehn-Jensen H, Willadsen SM. Deep freezing of cow 'half' and 'quarter' embryos. *Theriogenology.* 1983; **19**: 49–54.

34. Niemann H, Brem G, Sacher B, Smidt D, Kräusslich H. An approach to successful freezing of demi-embryos derived from day seven bovine embryos. *Theriogenology.* 1986; **25**: 519–24.

35. Rorie RW, Pendleton RJ, Pool SH, Youngs CR, Godke RA. The viability of bovine 'half' embryos produced before and after liquid nitrogen freezing. In: Fiechtinger W, Kemeter P (eds.) *Future Aspects in Human In Vitro Fertilisation.* Heidelberg: Springer-Verlag, 1987, pp. 26–35.

36. Heyman Y. Factors affecting the survival of whole and half-embryos transferred in cattle. *Theriogenology.* 1985; **23**: 63–75.

37. Voelkel SA, Amborski GF, Hill KG, Godke RA. Use of a uterine cell monolayer culture system for micromanipulated bovine embryos. *Theriogenology.* 1984; **21**: 271–81.

38. Suzuki T, Shimohira I. Viability of frozen-thawed bovine embryos bisected in sucrose: A preliminary report. *Theriogenology.* 1986; **26**: 333–9.

39. Nakagawa A, Takahashi Y, Kanagawa H. Sexing of bisected mouse embryos by chromosomal analysis. *Journal of Mammalian Ova Research.* 1985; **2**(1): 79–83.

40. White KL, Anderson GB, BonDurrant RH, Donahue S, Pashen RL. Viability of bisected bovine embryos after detection of H-Y antigen. *Theriogenology.* 1987; **27**: 293 (abstract).

41. Durrant B, Benirschke K. Embryo transfer in exotic animals. *Theriogenology.* 1981; **15**: 77–83.

42. Stover J, Evans J, Dolensek EP. Interspecies embryo transfer from the Gaur to domestic Holstein. *Proceedings of the American Association of Zoological Veterinarians.* Seattle, Washington, 1981: 122–4.

43. Dresser BL, Pope CE, Kramer L, Kuehn G, Dahlhausen RD, Thomas WD. Superovulation of Bongo antelope (*Tragelaphus euryceros*) and interspecies embryo transfer to African eland (*Tragelaphus oryx*). *Theriogenology.* 1984; **21**: 232 (abstract).

44. Willadsen SM, Fehilly CB. The development potential and regulatory capacity of blastomeres from 2-, 4- and 8-cell sheep embryos. In: Bier HM, Lindner HR (eds.) *Fertilisation of the Human Egg In Vitro.*

Heidelberg; Springer-Verlag, 1983: 353–7.

45. Butler JE, Anderson GB, BonDurrant RH, Pashen RL, Penedo MCT. Production of ovine chimeras by inner cell mass transplantation. Journal of Animal Science. 1987; **65**: 317–324.

46. Rorie RW, Pool SH, Prichard JF, Betteridge KJ, Godke RA. Production of chimeric blastocysts comprising sheep ICM and goat trophoblast for intergeneric transfer. *Journal of Animal Science.* 1989; **67**: (suppl. 1), 401–2.

47. Uehara T, Yanagimachi R. Microsurgical injection of spermatozoa into hamster eggs with subsequent transformation of sperm nuclei into male pronuclei. *Biology of Reproduction.* 1976; **15**: 467–72.

48. Thadani VM. A study of heterospecific sperm–egg interactions in the rat, mouse and deer mouse using in vitro fertilisation and sperm injection. *Journal of Experimental Zoology.* 1980; **212**: 435–53.

49. Markert CL. Fertilisation of mammalian eggs by sperm injection. *Journal of Experimental Zoology.* 1983; **228**: 195–201.

50. Shaikh AA, Minhas BS, Bowen MJ, Westhusin JE, Kraemer DC. Pronucleus formation following micro-injection of spermatozoa into baboon ova. *Proceedings of the Society on the Study of Reproduction.* 1984; No. 294 (abstract).

51. Iritani A, Kasai M, Niwa K, Song HB. Fertilisation in vitro of cattle follicular oocytes with injected spermatozoa capacitated in a chemically defined medium. *Journal of Reproduction and Fertility.* 1984; **70**: 487–92.

52. Mann J. Full term development of mouse eggs fertilised by a spermatozoon micro-injected under the zona pellucida. *Biology of Reproduction.* 1988; **38**: 1077–83.

53. Hosoi Y, Miyake M, Utsumi K, Iritani A. Development of oocytes after micro-injection of spermatozoon. *Proceedings of the XIth International Congress on Animal Reproduction and Artificial Insemination.* Dublin, Ireland, 26/30 June 1988, **3**: 331.

54. Yang X, Chen J, Foote RH. Blastocyst development from rabbit ova fertilized by injected sperm. *Journal of Reproduction and Fertility.* 1988; **1**: 13 (abstract).

55. Yang X, Chen J, Chen Y, Foote RH. Improved developmental potential of rabbit oocytes fertilised by sperm micro-injection into the perivitelline space enlarged by hypertonic medium. *Journal of Experimental Zoology.* 1990; **255**: 114–19.

56. Yang X, Jiang S, Kovacs A. Electrofield induced oocyte activation in rabbits. *Proceedings of the 25th Meeting of the Society of the Study of Reproduction.* 1990; **117**: (70) (abstract).

57. Malter H, Cohen J. Partial zona dissection of the human oocyte: A non-traumatic method using micromanipulation to assist zona pellucida penetration. *Fertility and Sterility.* 1989; **51**: 139–48.

58. Malter HE, Cohen J. Blastocyst formation and hatching in vitro following zona drilling of mouse and human embryos. *Gamete Research.* 1989; **24**: 67–80.

59. Cohen J, Malter H, Wright G, Kort H, Massey J, Mitchell D. Partial zona dissection of human oocytes when failure of zona pellucida penetration is anticipated. *Human Reproduction.* 1989; **4**: 435–42.

60. Ng S, Bongso A, Sathananthan H, Ratnam S. Micromanipulation: Its relevance to human in vitro fertilization. *Fertility and Sterility.* 1990; **53**: 203–14.

61. Fishel S, Antinori S, Jackson P, Johnson J, Lisi F, Chiariello F, Versaci C. Twin birth after subzonal insemination. *Lancet.* 1990; **335**: 722.

62. Fishel SB, Antinori S, Jackson P, Johnson J, Rinaldi L. Presentation of six pregnancies established by subzonal insemination (SUZI). *Human Reproduction.* 1991; **6**: 124–30.

63. Godke RA, Beetem DD, Burleigh DW. A method for zona pellucida drilling using a compact nitrogen laser. *Proceedings of the VII World Congress on Human Reproduction.* Helsinki, Finland, 26 June/1 July, 1990, No. 258 (abstract).

64. Younis AI, Keefer CL, Brackett BG. Fertilisation of bovine oocytes by sperm micro-injection. *Theriogenology.* 1989; **31**: 276 (abstract).

65. Goto K, Kinochita A, Takuma Y, Ogawawa K. Fertilisation of bovine oocytes by the injection of immobilised, killed spermatozoa. *Veterinary Record.* 1990; **127**: 519–22.

66. Zhang L, Denniston RS, Godke RA. A simple method for *in vitro* maturation, *in vitro* fertilisation, and co-culture of bovine oocytes. *Journal of Tissue Culture Methods.* 1992; **14**: 107–11.

67. Meryman HT. Drying of living mammalian cells. *Annals of the New York Academy of Sciences.* 1960; **85**: 729.

68. Graham EF, Larson EV, Crabo BG. Freezing and freeze-drying bovine spermatozoa. *Proceedings of the Vth Technical Conference on Artificial Insemination and Reproduction.* 1974.

Chapter 16

An overview of pre-implantation diagnosis

R M L Winston

Introduction

The earliest possible stage of prenatal diagnosis is pre-implantation diagnosis. For about four or so years now various researchers have been examining pre-implantation embryos in detail, learning about their development with the idea of trying to gain information about embryonic health. These studies are potentially important because such studies on embryos may lead to establishing our ability to diagnose genetic defects before implantation. To date, most of these very preliminary studies have been carried out on embryos produced following *in vitro* fertilisation (IVF); a few have been done on embryos flushed from the uterus after *in vivo* fertilisation. Other workers have examined oocytes, by taking biopsies of the first polar body.[1]

Genetic disease

Genetic disease remains fundamentally almost the greatest unsolved medical problem which exists. Basically, a child born with a genetic disease, dies with it; palliation is usually difficult at best. Some treatments for genetic disease are improving, and there is the possibility of somatic cell gene therapy in the future for certain specific diseases, particularly those affecting blood stem cells and possibly cystic fibrosis. However, germ cell gene therapy is certainly not likely to be applicable in the near future, and the risks in altering the human genome make it most unlikely to be a suitable therapy for a long time to come. Most diseases caused by single gene defects have serious prognosis, particularly those which are caused by autosomal recessive inheritance. Overall, genetic disease is now the second commonest cause of infant death. One in 50 babies born in the UK has a major congenital abnormality, one in 100 suffers from a single gene defect and one in 200 has a chromosomal disorder compatible with life. Far more embryos with chromosomal disorders abort. Emory and Rimoin[2] have stated that roughly one quarter of all children in paediatric hospitals are in-patients with what is basically a genetic cause for their disease. Their figures also suggest that up to 12 per cent of adult in-patients are suffering from diseases which are primarily genetic in origin or which have a strong genetic component. Pre-implantation diagnosis is not going to change this pattern but, at the present time, it is the only treatment we can offer couples apart from prenatal diagnosis, followed by abortion of an affected fetus. We, in our group, were also attracted to this line of research because many of the investigations into the feasibility of pre-implantation diagnosis involve improvement of our understanding of the genesis of early embryonic defects.

Most gene defects, of course, do not seem to cause serious embryonic damage, probably because most of the single gene defects do not cause such disturbance as to prevent early viability. This is not true of chromosomal abnormalities, which occur very often and are most disruptive. There are many reasons why human embryos are so frequently genetically abnormal. Some workers estimate that up to 50 per cent of all human conceptuses show severe abnormalities incompatible with life.[3] Most frequently these abnormalities end in early pregnancy loss; few serious abnormalities escape the net of miscarriage.

Reproductive proclivity

Human reproductive ability declines sharply with age. It is not entirely certain why this should be; certainly this trend is not so clear cut in other mammals. Very fertile women, such as those who have already had babies and have had simple tubal sterilisation, followed by surgical reversal, show a remarkably sharp decline in fertility after the age of 40 years (Figure 16.1). These data are interesting because these women are a highly selected group, who actively want more children and who, before

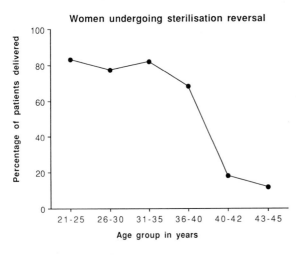

Figure 16.1 Reproductive proclivity in women undergoing sterilisation reversal

undergoing tubal anastomosis, had both their fertility and that of their male partner very carefully checked. Approximately 80 per cent of these women conceived successfully if they had a reversal attempt before their fortieth birthday; less than 15 per cent if they had their operation after 40 years of age. These data confirm those of Trussel and Wilson and also various studies of different racial and ethnic groups which confirm the sharp decline in female fertility in Hutterite women, as well as women from most other parts of the world.[4]

The decline in female fertility with age is paralleled by a rise in the incidence of miscarriage and an increase in Down syndrome.[4] It is likely that trisomy 21 is not the only trisomy associated with maternal age and this may explain why miscarriage is so frequent in older women. It is well documented that trisomy 16[5] and X-monosomy are frequently associated with miscarriage and more studies are needed to see whether these problems are more common when conception occurs late in reproductive life. It is very likely indeed that they are and this has important implications for applying pre-implantation diagnosis.

IVF and pre-implantation diagnosis (PD)

If pre-implantation diagnosis (PD) using IVF is to be a reality, then two prerequisites are necessary. First, the currently rather poor success rates of IVF need considerable improvement. At present, in Britain only 11 per cent of treatment cycles result in a successful delivery.[6] There are, however, encouraging indications that some large well funded units are doing better than average. At Hammersmith we run two IVF programmes treating a total of 1500 patients each year. Our figures confirm that it is possible to get acceptable pregnancy rates, with each IVF treatment cycle giving probably better than the natural chance of conception (Figure 16.2).

Secondly, another problem is the question of multiple birth. This, in Britain, has become a prominent issue, not least because high order multiple births have resulted in a considerable increase in perinatal mortality. In order to increase the chance of pregnancy, many units frequently resort to the practice of transferring up to four embryos simultaneously. In January 1987 we became very concerned at the high chance of triplet pregnancy in our own programme. In the year that followed there were 21 cases of triplets in about 400 pregnancies, and it was this phenomenon which influenced us to routinely transfer no more than two embryos simultaneously. The overall recent figures reported to the Human Fertilisation and Embryology Authority from Hammersmith (Table 16.1), and our figures for limiting embryo transfer[7] demonstrate that the transfer of two embryos only can give at least 45 per cent chance of at least one embryo implanting successfully. Where at least 60 per cent of oocytes have fertilised, particularly in women under the age of 38 years, or in those with only pure tubal disease as a cause of infertility, two embryo transfers are quite sufficient. More than this gives an unacceptable risk of triplets.

Triplet pregnancy must be avoided because of the high obstetric risk and the social implications. Above all, a triplet pregnancy would be a serious problem for a woman carrying a gene defect who is undergoing PD. This is because such women

Table 16.1 Recent figures of the Hammersmith IVF results, since 1990*

Patients treated	971
Treated cycles	1434
Egg collections	1223
Embryo transfers	1093
Clinical pregnancies	401
Live births per cycle	24%
Live birth per patient	32%

Note: * All patients had only two embryos transferred unless there were exceptional circumstances.

are usually only identified when they have already given birth to one affected child; a large order multiple birth would be quite a serious imposition in such a family, when so much care and attention will be needed by the existing child. Secondly, at the present time, it is essential that all attempts at PD are accompanied by subsequent prenatal diagnosis, either by chorion villus sampling, or by amniocentesis. This is not easy in triplet pregnancies and would be accompanied by a high risk of miscarriage as well. The Hammersmith record shows that limited embryo transfer still gives an adequate change of pregnancy, and this therefore is the strategy we have followed.

Apart from its expense, IVF is demanding and emotionally fraught. One question therefore in many clinicians' minds is whether PD with IVF is likely to be an acceptable alternative to prenatal diagnosis with termination of pregnancy where the fetus is thought to be affected. I am indebted to Dr Gene Pergament of Chicago who has supplied me with details of a study he recently completed.[8] Using a questionnaire directed to women at risk of producing a seriously affected child, he showed that most were very concerned indeed at the prospect of an abortion. It seems quite clear that we have tended to trivialise the serious impact that terminating a much wanted pregnancy involves. The couples he questioned were mostly prepared to go to quite marked extremes to avoid termination. Forty per cent were more worried that the IVF would simply be unsuccessful. Many were also worried that the biopsy procedure might carry a risk of damage to an embryo. Surprisingly few patients

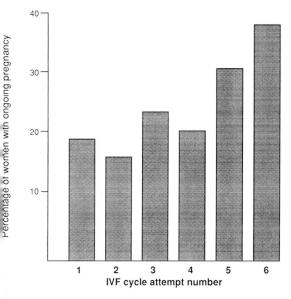

Figure 16.2 Incidence of pregnancy in women undergoing repeated IVF cycle attempts at the Hammersmith Hospital

seemed very concerned at the expense that might possibly be involved in avoiding termination of pregnancy by undergoing the complex procedures required for pre-implantation diagnosis.

Our experience with British couples has been very similar. We have consistently found that most women are very anxious to avoid abnormal pregnancy and that they readily offer spare embryos to serious research programmes designed to reduce this complication in other patients' pregnancies. One particular concern that carriers of X-linked disorders such as Duchenne muscular dystrophy have is that parents are worried that, in terminating a male pregnancy, they would be destroying a normal child on average 50 per cent of the time.

Embryo biopsy

A major concern, particularly when PD is accomplished by gene amplification after embryo biopsy of one or two blastomeres, is that the biopsy procedure might itself cause embryonic damage. Alan Handyside (Chapter 17) has led a scientific team which has examined these risks carefully. There is, of course, considerable evidence already that surgical damage of a cleavage embryo with removal of blastomeres is safe, at least in various animal models. Apart from Handyside's own work in the mouse[9], various workers have taken biopsies from the embryos of the rabbit, or dissected cattle, sheep and pig embryos without inducing malformations. Summers[10] biopsied trophectoderm of the marmoset monkey and normal offspring were born. Perhaps more significantly, most workers freezing human embryos have transferred thawed zygotes which are missing at least one, and often many more, blastomeres, without observing any fetal abnormalities.

In our laboratories work has continued on the effects of biopsy on subsequent human development. In conjunction with Dr Henry Leese, of York University, we have shown that the energy substrate requirements, in particular pyruvate and glucose utilisation and lactate production, do not substantially change after biopsy. Hardy et al.[11] have examined embryos after biopsy and showed that removal of a blastomere at the eight-cell stage

does not alter development to the blastocyst stage; nor does it affect the number of cells dying or the mitotic index. Differentiation into inner and outer cell mass is unaffected.

All the observations on biopsied human embryos have been reassuring. Certainly, our own ethics committee and the committee of the Licensing Authority felt satisfied with these data. Once they had reviewed these data independently, they agreed that it would be appropriate to attempt uterine transfer of biopsied embryos after PD.

There are three stages (Table 16.2) when embryo biopsy might be contemplated. Biopsy of a polar body, removal of cleavage stage cells, and excision of a piece of trophectoderm from the blastocyst have all been mooted (see Chapter 17). However, it is relevant to consider in a little detail the prospect for recovering *in vivo* fertilised blastocysts by uterine flushing, and performing a biopsy on these.

Embryo lavage

Recovery of *in vivo* fertilised blastocysts is an attractive option for PD because it avoids the need for IVF. Secondly, biopsy of a blastocyst would yield many more cells than the single cell obtained from a cleavage embryo. Finally, there is preliminary evidence that individual *in vivo* fertilised blastocysts have a much higher chance of implantation than do embryos transferred to the uterus at earlier stages of development. Buster et al.[12] were remarkably successful in establishing normal pregnancy after transfer of *in vivo* fertilised oocytes. In their series, blastocysts were flushed from the uterus of normal female donors after a timed LH peak and normal intercourse. The resulting embryo was transferred to the uterus of an infertile recipient approximately 92 to 130 hours after ovulation. A total of 25 fertilised eggs were recovered; three intra-uterine pregnancies occurred after individual transfer of a total of five blastocysts. Only one other pregnancy occurred, an ectopic after transfer of a cleavage stage embryo. This high implantation rate following blastocyst transfer, confirmed in a somewhat larger study by Formigli et al.[13], raises interesting questions. Very few authors have reported successful pregnancies after transferring *in vitro* fertilised

Table 16.2 Advantages and disadvantages of pre-implantation biopsy at different stages

	Advantages	Disadvantages
Unfertilised egg	• No ethical problem as not an embryo • No removal of specialised or differentiated cells • No mechanical disruption of an embryo	• Smallest amount of available genetic material • No assessment of paternal allele • Diagnosis of healthy egg depends on assumption that affected gene is in polar body, risking failed diagnosis • Inefficient as many eggs, which will not subsequently fertilise, need biopsy • Risk of damage to cytoskeleton during biopsy procedure
Cleavage stage embryo	• Biopsy involves unspecialised totipotential cells only • Signal from both maternal and paternal cells • Embryo can be transferred in cycle of biopsy avoiding the need for frozen storage	• Smallest amount of genetic material, but can take two cells in biopsy • Removal of cells may reduce developmental potential • Difficult to do once compaction started • Some blastomeres anucleate etc., risking failed diagnosis
IVF blastocysts	• Several cells can be biopsied giving more DNA • Biopsy procedure may assist hatching	• Some trophectoderm cells may be mosaic • Biopsy procedure may collapse blastocyst • IVF blastocysts currently have poor implantation rate after embryo transfer • Inner cell mass may be inadvertently damaged • By the time diagnosis available, may be necessary to transfer embryo after storage in subsequent cycle
Flushed blastocyst	• Avoids need for IVF • Perhaps best pregnancy rate after *in vivo* fertilisation	• So far been impossible to harvest blastocysts reliably after superovulation • Risk of lost genetically affected blastocyst • Risk of ectopic pregnancy

blastocysts, apart from Bolton et al.[14] In our unit, where the implantation rate (sac with fetal heart seen on ultrasound) per single embryo transferred is 23 per cent, we have only had a sole biochemical pregnancy after the transfer of 18 *in vitro* fertilised blastocysts. While it is just possible that these differences are due to uterine factors leading to implantation failures in stimulated cycles, these data suggest that *in vivo* fertilised blastocysts may be more viable than those obtained after IVF; this may be because of deficiencies in the various culture media used.

Buster has more recently used HMG to stimulate the ovaries of potential embryo donors. Rather unexpectedly, uterine flushing after ovarian stimulation resulted in relatively fewer zygotes being recovered. Other workers have confirmed this effect, but the reason for the failure of recovery is unclear. It has been suggested, probably incorrectly, that the epithelium of the tube or uterus may be more 'sticky' after gonadotrophin treatment, leading to the embryos being adherent to the mucosa. For the time being then, relying on *in vivo* fertilisation looks like being an unlikely strategy for PD.

Clearly, there are several problems with embryo lavage if it were to be used for PD. First, inadequate uterine flushing could lead to an embryo being lost in the genital tract. An ectopic pregnancy could occur as a result (indeed, one of Buster's own patients suffered an ectopic pregnancy after uterine flushing). An ectopic pregnancy would obviously have serious consequences for a woman, a known carrier, who was simply undergoing screening to ensure that a second term pregnancy would be healthy. Moreover, the 'lost' embryo could implant normally, but be affected with the disease for which screening was intended. Uterine flushing may also lead to other problems such as endometritis. Apart from the complications caused by flushing, another major difficulty is that recovery is more difficult after superovulation. PD really requires the availability of multiple embryos. The act of biopsy invariably means that some embryos are inadvertently damaged and cannot be transferred. Multiple embryos are also needed partly to ensure that at least one or two screened embryos are free from the defect being screened, partly to ensure the

best pregnancy rate, but most of all so that, after recovery, each screened embryo can act as a control for the other screened embryos during the difficulties of adequate gene amplification with such small amounts of DNA.

In view of all these difficulties, we felt that perhaps the best option was to undertake embryo biopsy during the cleavage stage, preferably before compaction. Biopsy of an 8-cell embryo is relatively easy, and up to two cells can be removed with relative impunity. This strategy means that, with rapid diagnosis offered by gene amplification by the polymerase chain reaction (PCR), embryo transfer can be accomplished late on day two or on day three after fertilisation. This avoids the need for storing embryos into a subsequent cycle. Recently, in collaboration with Leeanda Wilton at the Institute of Zoology, London, and Joy Delhanty at University College, London, a rapid method of fluorescent *in situ* hybridisation (FISH) has been largely perfected, and we have started to use these highly promising techniques to establish the diagnosis of the sex of the embryo. This seems to be an effective technique in women carrying serious X-linked disorders.

Measuring gene expression

The possibility still remains that, in certain cases in addition to using PCR and FISH, one might employ biochemical methods to measure products of gene expression as a method of establishing embryonic health. For example, enzymes such as hexoamidase-A and hypoxanthine guanine phosphoribosyl transferase (HPRT)[15] have the potential of being used as markers for Tay-Sachs disease and Lesch-Nyhan syndrome, respectively. Although no attempts have been made as yet to diagnose Tay-Sachs in pre-implantation embryos, HPRT assays have been used by a few workers both experimentally and in preliminary clinical trials. At present such markers do not seem to give reliable results, because it is not clear where maternal expression ends and embryonic expression begins. Nevertheless, there is hope still that rapid microassays of such compounds may be a useful tool for certain specific disorders, where the gene involved is expressed very early during human development.

Pre-implantation diagnosis has been used in our unit to sex embryos in families at risk for Duchenne muscular dystrophy, adrenoleukodystrophy, and X-linked mental retardation. So far, six babies have been born, with an overall pregnancy rate of 30 per cent per cycle. We have also recently used PCR to screen embryos for the specific defect in Lesch-Nyhan syndrome and cystic fibrosis, and one patient has recently delivered a healthy baby after screening for the δF508 mutation in cystic fibrosis. Progress is not rapid; pre-implantation diagnosis is not easy, requiring meticulous embryo handling, good molecular biology and, not least, a really reliable IVF service. There is a general impression given that pre-implantation diagnosis is relatively routine to establish and this is undoubtedly not the case. Nevertheless, the indications are that these techniques hold considerable promise, not only for the management of patients at risk of giving birth to children with genetic defects, but also for women who habitually abort, and those who experience pregnancy failure in late reproductive life.

Some time ago[16] I pointed out that these techniques held not only promise, but also ethical and clinical risks. A parallel was drawn with the sixteenth century when alchemists were attempting to transmute base metals into gold. They subsumed everything in the futile pursuit of a technology which ultimately could not benefit society. Peter Brueghel the Elder drew an elegant woodcut (1555) now in the Künst Museum in Berlin, 'Alghemiste', depicting the alchemist neglecting his family, the next generation, in frivolous technological endeavours. It is incumbent on us as scientists and clinicians to ensure that this intriguing and complex work is ultimately used for human good and not for ill.

References

1. Verlinsky Y, Ginsberg N, Lifchez A, Valle J, Moise J, Strom CM. Analysis of the first polar body: pre-conception genetic diagnosis. *Human Reproduction.* 1990; **5**(7): 826–9.
2. Emery AEH, Rimoin DL. In: Emery AEH, Rimoin DL (eds.) *Principles and Practice of Medical Genetics.* Churchill Livingstone, 1990, pp. 3–6.
3. Creasy MR. The cytogenetics of spontaneous abortion in humans. In: Beard RW, Sharp F (eds.) *Early Pregnancy Loss.* New York: Springer-Verlag, 1988, pp. 293–304.
4. Gray RH. Biological and social interactions in the determination of late fertility. *Journal of Biosocial Science.* 1979; suppl. 6, 97–115.
5. Warburton D, Stein Z, Kline J, Susser M. In: Porter IH, Hook EB (eds.) *Human Embryonic and Fetal Death.* New York: Academic Press, 1980, pp. 261–87.
6. Sixth Report of the Interim Licensing Authority (1991) Medical Research Council and Royal College of Obstetricians and Gynaecologists, London.
7. Dawson K, Rutherford AJ, Margara RA, Winston RML. Reducing triplet pregnancies following in vitro fertilisation. *Lancet.* 1991; **337**: 1543–4.
8. Pergament G, 1990, personal communication.
9. Hooper M, Hardy K, Handyside A, Hunter S, Monk M. HPRT-deficient (Lesch-Nyhan) mouse embryos derived from germline colonisation by cultured cells. *Nature.* 1987; **326**: 292–5.
10. Summers, PM, Campbell JM, Miller MW. Normal in vivo development of marmoset monkey embryos after trophectoderm biopsy. *Human Reproduction.* 1988; **3**: 389–93.
11. Hardy K, Winston RML, Handyside AH. Nuclear abnormalities and developmental arrest in human pre-implantation embryos in vitro. *Human Reproduction.* 1991; **6**: 152.
12. Buster J, Bustillo M, Rodi IA, Cohen SW, Hamilton M, Simon JA, Thorneycroft IH, Marshall JR. Biologic and morphologic development of donated human ova recovered by non-surgical uterine lavage. *American Journal of Obstetrics and Gynaecology.* 1985; **153**: 211–17.
13. Formigli L, Roccio C, Belotti G, Stangalini A, Coglitore MT, Formigli G. Non-surgical flushing of the uterus for pre-embryo recovery: possible clinical applications. *Human Reproduction.* 1990; **5**: 329–35.
14. Bolton VN, Wren ME, Parsons JH. Pregnancies after in vitro fertilization and transfer of human blastocysts. *Fertility and Sterility.* 1991; **55**: 830–2.
15. Leese HJ, Humpherson PG, Hardy K, Hooper MA, Winston RML, Handyside AH. Profiles of hypoxanthine guanine phosphoribosyl transferase

and adenine phosphoribosyl transferase activities measured in single pre-implantation human embryos by high performance liquid chromatography. *Journal of Reproduction and Fertility*. 1991; **91**: 197–202.

16. Winston RML. Allocation of resources for infertility treatments. *Bailleres Clinical Obstetrics and Gynaecology*. 1991; **5**: 551–73.

Chapter 17

Pre-implantation diagnosis: strategies for embryo biopsy and genetic analysis

Alan H Handyside

Introduction

Over the last ten years or so, the introduction of chorion villus sampling (CVS) has enabled prenatal diagnosis of many inherited diseases in the first trimester of pregnancy avoiding the possibility of terminating an affected pregnancy at a much later stage after amniocentesis. During the same period, methods of ovarian stimulation, oocyte collection, *in vitro* fertilisation (IVF), embryo culture and transfer have been established for the treatment of infertility. If genetic defects can be reliably identified at these early stages, before implantation, selection and transfer of unaffected embryos would eliminate the possibility of a termination completely.

Strategies for embryo biopsy

Pre-implantation diagnosis requires the biopsy of one or more cells from each embryo obtained either by IVF or by uterine lavage for genetic analysis. The biopsied embryo can then be returned to culture while the biopsied cell is analysed and later unaffected embryos selected for transfer to the uterus. Human embryos have been biopsied at cleavage[1] and blastocyst stages[2] and the first polar body has been biopsied from unfertilised oocytes for the detection of maternal genetic defects before attempting IVF.[3] Each approach has its advantages and disadvantages.

Polar body biopsy

The first polar body is extruded on completion of the first meiotic division during the maturation of the oocyte prior to ovulation and contains a haploid set of bivalent chromosomes. If the woman is heterozygous for a genetic defect, two copies of either the normal or affected allele on one bivalent remain in the oocyte while two copies of the other allele are segregated to the first polar body. Thus diagnosis of maternal genetic defects in the unfertilised oocyte should be possible by inference from the allele present in the first polar body. The main advantages of this approach are that manipulation of gametes may be ethically more acceptable and it allows a maximum time for genetic analysis before transferring the selected embryos. However, there are several significant drawbacks.

First, recombination during the first meiotic division will result in one copy of both alleles being inherited with each bivalent so that the allele inherited by the oocyte will only be determined at fertilisation when the second meiotic division is completed and the second polar body containing a univalent is extruded. The frequency with which recombination occurs is determined by the distance between the centromere and the affected gene but in these cases where both alleles are detected in the first polar body, no diagnosis can be made about the eventual genotype of the fertilised zygote. The problem is that if the frequency of uninformative polar bodies is high the chances of establishing a pregnancy may be reduced since two unaffected embryos need to be transferred to maximise pregnancy rates. Secondly, only maternal defects can be analysed. Thus with an autosomal recessive condition, for example, in which it would be acceptable to transfer carriers, the proportion of embryos available for transfer will be further reduced from three-quarters to a half. Finally, the first polar body cannot divide and therefore any analysis will always be limited to a single set of chromosomes. However, since the majority of trisomies arise during the first meiotic division of the oocyte, polar body analysis may be useful as a screen for aneuploidy.[4]

Blastocyst biopsy

Biopsy of some of the outer trophectoderm (TE) cells of the blastocyst has several advantages. Most importantly, at this stage the embryo reaches a maximum number of cells before implantation. The number of cells in human blastocysts *in vitro* increases from an average of 58 to 126 cells between days five to seven postinsemination and the majority of these are TE cells.[5] Thus, it has been possible to biopsy between ten and 30 TE cells from individual blastocysts on day six.[2] Clearly, the more cells available for analysis the more reliable any diagnosis is likely to be. TE biopsy also has the advantage that these cells are thought, by analogy with detailed lineage studies of rodent embryos, to be extra-embryonic and contribute mainly to the placenta after implantation; the inner cell mass

(ICM) of the blastocyst, from which the fetus is later derived, is not affected. In effect, therefore, this would be the equivalent of an early chorion villus biopsy and may be ethically more acceptable.

The major problem with this approach, however, is the disappointing pregnancy success rate after transfer of blastocysts during routine IVF[6,7] which, coupled with the low proportion of embryos reaching this stage[5], is likely to reduce the number of unaffected embryos available for transfer and the prospects of establishing a pregnancy.

Cleavage stage biopsy

At early cleavage stages, each cell of the mammalian embryo remains totipotent and can contribute to all the tissues of the conceptus. Indeed, single cells from embryos at these stages have been demonstrated, under appropriate conditions, to form blastocysts and to develop into normal offspring following transfer in a number of rodent and domestic species.[8] The proportion developing successfully to term, however, declines rapidly with cells isolated at progressively later stages. This is because cleavage divisions simply subdivide the cytoplasm of the zygote into successively smaller cells and there appears to be a lower limit to the cellular mass of the embryo compatible with implantation and development.

The implications for cleavage stage biopsy of human embryos are that the reduction of cellular mass should be minimised to avoid an increase in biochemical pregnancies and implantation failure. We, therefore, decided to biopsy human embryos early on day three, at the six- to ten-cell stage when the removal of a single cell at the appropriate stage only reduces the cellular mass by one eighth. This is the latest day embryos have been routinely transferred without affecting pregnancy rate. A maximum of about 12 hours is available to biopsy the embryos and carry out the genetic analysis before transfer later the same day. This limitation could be overcome if cryopreservation of biopsied embryos was possible allowing transfer of selected embryos in later cycles. Biopsied four-cell mouse embryos cryopreserved using an ultrarapid protocol developed to term after thawing and transfer.[9] Making a slit or hole in the zona pellucida for human embryo biopsy, however, may increase the proportion of embryos damaged during freezing since the presence of an intact zona is thought to provide protection from mechanical damage caused by ice crystal formation in the medium.

For cleavage stage biopsy, normally fertilised embryos at the appropriate stage are placed in drops of medium under oil and transferred to a dissecting microscope for micromanipulation. The embryo is immobilised by suction on a flame polished holding pipette and a hole drilled in the zona pellucida with a stream of acid Tyrode's from a fine micropipette.[10] A second larger micropipette is then pushed through the hole in the zona to aspirate one or two cells (1/8 or 2/8 cells) (Figure 17.1). Immediately following biopsy, the corresponding 7/8 or 6/8 biopsied embryo is returned to culture and the cell biopsy prepared for analysis. This simple biopsy procedure can be completed in five to ten minutes minimising the time embryos are manipulated at room temperature.

Before transferring biopsied embryos, we examined them carefully for effects on pre-implantation development *in vitro*.[1] The proportion of biopsied embryos developing to the blastocyst stage was similar to non-manipulated embryos. Metabolic activity measured by energy substrate uptake from the medium and cell numbers at the blastocyst

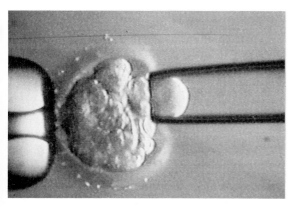

Figure 17.1 Cleavage stage biopsy of a 12-cell polyspermic human embryo on day three. The embryo is immobilised on a flame-polished holding pipette and a sampling pipette pushed through a hole drilled in the zona pellucida to aspirate a single cell

stage were reduced, but only in proportion to the cellular mass removed at biopsy. Hence we conclude that removal of one or two cells at the eight-cell stage does not adversely affect their immediate and subsequent development. Effects on postimplantation development are unlikely since cleavage stage blastomeres of mammalian embryos are totipotent and partially fragmented or degenerate embryos are routinely transferred after IVF without any apparent increase in congenital abnormalities in the resulting pregnancies. Also, one or more blastomeres often lyse when cryopreserved embryos are thawed and the first pregnancy achieved in this way was from an embryo in which only five out of the eight blastomeres remained intact after thawing.[11] Although this patient had a late miscarriage, the fetus was morphologically normal with no detectable defects.

Strategies for detection of genetic defects

Chromosomal defects

The most prevalent genetic defects causing inherited disease involve chromosomal abnormalities. For example trisomies of chromosomes 21, 18, 16 and 13 and aneuploidies of the sex chromosomes are compatible with development to term but cause a variety of clinical syndromes with varying degrees of severity. The risk of some trisomies increases with increasing maternal age; the risk of, for example, trisomy 21 (Down syndrome) rises to about 0.5 per cent at age 40.[4] However, this is probably not high enough to warrant pre-implantation diagnosis. On the other hand, carriers of balanced translocations, especially those who have already had an affected pregnancy, are known to be at very high risk, typically 50 per cent, of having another affected pregnancy. For these patients pre-implantation diagnosis may offer significant advantages.

The most straightforward approach to diagnosing chromosomal defects would be to karyotype metaphase chromosomes (see Chapter 14). Metaphase chromosome spreads of nuclei from whole human embryos have been studied extensively to determine the incidence of chromosome defects after IVF.[12] For identification of each chromosome, however, and for complete karyotype analysis including the detection of deletions, insertions and translocations, etc., it is necessary to stain the chromosomes to reveal one of the well established banding patterns characteristic for each chromosome pair. This has proved universally very difficult with pre-implantion embryos mainly because the chromosomes are short and often clumped. Hence information about chromosome defects has mainly been limited to analysing abnormalities of chromosome number including polyploidy and aneuploidy, sometimes with assignment of the affected chromosome to a particular group based on size and morphology, and more gross defects such as chromosome fragmentation. Alternatively, *in situ* hybridisation with chromosome-specific probes or 'chromosome painting' offer the prospect of diagnosing specific chromosomal abnormalities in either metaphase or interphase nuclei (see Chapter 14).

Single gene defects

Although individually much rarer, about 5000 single gene defects have now been described. Some of the more prevalent diseases include the autosomal recessive conditions cystic fibrosis, Tay-Sachs, sickle cell disease and beta-thalassaemia and the X-linked recessive conditions Duchenne muscular dystrophy and haemophilia. With some diseases identified as single gene defects from pedigree analysis, the molecular basis of the disease is unknown. In others the biochemical basis for the disease has been established allowing prenatal diagnosis by biochemical assay. Finally, an increasing number of specific gene defects has been established at the DNA level allowing specific prenatal diagnosis by DNA analysis.

DNA amplification

The polymerase chain reaction (PCR), first described for the prenatal diagnosis of sickle cell disease from as few as 75 fetal blood cells,[13] allows in excess of a millionfold amplification of short fragments of genomic DNA from cell lysates. This involves, first, denaturing the target DNA,

reducing the temperature to allow annealing of a pair of oligonucleotide primers, generally about twenty- mers, to the sense and antisense strands at the ends of the fragment to be amplified, and finally, raising the temperature to the optimum for a heat stable DNA polymerase to synthesise complementary strands of DNA from the primers. The next cycle is then begun by again raising the temperature to denature the DNA. In this way there is, at least in the initial cycles, an exponential increase in the specific fragment of DNA, usually a few hundred base pairs long, defined by the primers. The optimum annealing temperature and reaction conditions are largely determined by the sequence of the primers. Twenty five to 40 cycles are generally sufficient to produce enough of the amplified fragment to be detected by gel electrophoresis and staining. However, to increase the amount of amplified fragment, re-amplification of the initial product is possible and nested primers are often used for this purpose since the final shorter fragment cannot be amplified by the first primer set and the possibility of carry-over contamination is minimised. Simultaneous amplification of more than one target fragment is possible by modifying the conditions and selecting primers with similar annealing temperatures.[14]

For pre-implantation diagnosis, the most important advantage of PCR, apart from its sensitivity, is that DNA fragments diagnostic of particular genetic defects can be amplified within a few hours and, although further analysis may be necessary, this can often be accomplished within the time available before transfer later the same day.[15] Furthermore, since the original report, a variety of unique sequences have been amplified from single cells including human sperm and fibroblasts[16] and unfertilised oocytes from which the first polar bodies have been removed,[17] demonstrating the potential for pre-implantation diagnosis from one or only a few cells.

Two main strategies for pre-implantation diagnosis of single gene defects by DNA amplification are being investigated. The first involves the amplification of one or more closely linked restriction sites defined by restriction fragment length polymorphisms (RFLPs). In this case, pedigree analysis is necessary beforehand to establish that the RFLPs are informative for the particular couple and the sequence of the restriction site itself must be known to design appropriate oligonucleotide primers. It has the advantage that after amplification of the region containing the restriction site, analysis simply involves digestion of the fragment with the appropriate restriction endonuclease. The second strategy involves amplifying a fragment containing the defect itself. This requires detailed sequence information about the particular defect and the genomic sequence of the gene and also subsequent analysis of the amplified fragment for the defect. This has been achieved with a number of single gene defects including sickle cell disease[18] and more recently, the predominant deletion causing cystic fibrosis has also been successfully detected in single cells.[3,19]

Inherited diseases caused by recessive X-linked genetic defects are characterised by transmission through unaffected female carriers and typically only affect boys. In some of these conditions, the biochemical basis for the disease is known and prenatal diagnosis is possible by biochemical analysis. An example is Lesch-Nyhan syndrome which is caused by deficiency of the X-linked enzyme hypoxanthine phosphoribosyl transferase (HPRT).[20] In others, the defects have been mapped to particular regions of the X chromosome using closely linked markers, usually RFLPs, which in conjunction with pedigree analysis of the family involved can often be used to diagnose the presence of an affected locus by DNA analysis. Finally, in an increasing number of conditions, the genes and specific defects involved have been identified and diagnosis of the defect itself is possible. A notable example is Duchenne muscular dystrophy (DMD) which is caused by defects, often large deletions, in the dystrophin gene.[21] With many other X-linked recessive conditions, however (for example, X-linked mental retardation), the molecular basis is not yet understood. For this reason, we have concentrated initially on establishing reliable methods for identifying the sex of pre-implantation embryos since this approach is equally applicable to all X-linked recessive conditions only affecting boys and to all families with a particular condition irrespective of their particular genetic defect.

Since PCR is essentially not quantitative, the most straightforward way to identify male embryos is to amplify a sequence specific for the Y chromosome. With the majority of unique target sequences which have been examined, however, amplification fails in about 10–20 per cent of single cells irrespective of the cell type or sample preparation.[16,22] If this occurred with single cells biopsied from cleavage stage embryos, this could have the serious consequence of misidentification of a male as a female and result in the transfer of a potentially affected embryo. In an attempt to overcome this problem, therefore, we decided to amplify Y-specific repeated sequences to increase the number of target sequences present in single or small numbers of biopsied cells.

Initially, we amplified a 149 base pair (bp) fragment of a sequence repeated 800 to 5000 times on the long arm of the Y chromosome[23,24] used for identifying the sex of the fetus following CVS.[25] Amplification was consistently achieved with as little as 2pg of male DNA (the equivalent of a diploid cell) and in single cells, and the sex of biopsied embryos, based on the presence or absence of the amplified fragment, was confirmed in a small series of biopsied embryos by labelling metaphase chromosomes with $(CMA)_2S$ – bis-spermidine acridine (a fluorescent label specific for the Y chromosome) – or *in situ* hybridisation (ISH) with a Y-specific probe.[26] More recently, we have also amplified a Y-specific alphoid satellite repeat.[27] The alphoid repeat has the advantage that it is centromeric, whereas the Y-specific long arm repeat can, in rare cases, be deleted in normal men or translocated to autosomes and inherited by women, so that each couple has to be screened beforehand.[28,29]

For each of the repeats, 40 cycles of amplification generated enough of the fragment, from dilutions of genomic DNA down to 2 pg or single embryo cells, to be easily visualised on ethidium bromide stained polyacrylamide gels (Figure 17.2). Sporadic contamination among control blanks was infrequent. However, despite rigid precautions to separate sample preparation and product handling[30] carry-over contamination of the amplified product was sometimes detectable with female cells and control blanks. The level of amplification from this form of contamination was generally low enough, however, to be reliably distinguished from that generated from single cells.

Pregnancies from embryos sexed by DNA amplification

Using PCR for DNA amplification of these Y-specific repeat sequences, the identification and transfer of normal or carrier female embryos was attempted in eight couples known to be at risk of transmitting various X-linked diseases.[31,32] These included X-linked mental retardation, Lesch-Nyhan syndrome, adrenoleukodystrophy, retinitis pigmentosa and hereditary sensory motor neurone disease type II. Also, two couples at risk of Duchenne muscular dystrophy opted for this approach even though a specific DNA diagnosis by conventional methods may have been possible after CVS.

After routine assessment of each couple for IVF, women were induced to superovulate using an established protocol involving an initial period of suppression of ovarian function with a Luteinising hormone releasing hormone (LHRH) agonist followed by stimulation of folliculogenesis and administration of human chorionic gonadotrophin (HCG) to trigger ovulation.[33] The numbers of oocytes recovered and normally fertilised in these predominantly fertile couples were similar to those obtained with infertile couples. Normally fertilised

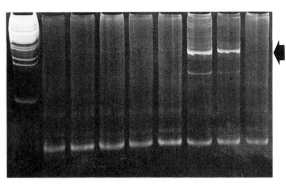

Figure 17.2 Analysis of polymerase chain reaction products from single biopsied blastomeres with oligonucleotide primers for a 149 base pair fragment (arrowed) of a Y-specific repeat sequence by electrophoresis on a 12 per cent polyacrylamide minigel and staining with ethidium bromide. DNA markers first lane on the left. Note the clear amplification of the Y-specific band in two cases. (The lower band in all lanes is an artefact of amplification from dimers of the primers)

embryos developing to the six- to ten-cell stage by the morning of day three were biopsied and 1/8 removed (in one cycle 2/8 cells were biopsied). Since between 5 per cent of cells from embryos with good morphology, and 15 per cent from embryos with poor morphology, are anucleate at the five- to eight-cell stage,[34] each cell was checked for the presence of a single nucleus after disaggregation either by phase contrast microscopy or by vital labelling with a DNA fluorochrome before preparation for PCR. On average, about five embryos were biopsied so that in many treatment cycles at least two female embryos were identified as suitable for transfer even though the probability of an embryo being female is only approximately 50 per cent. This is important because pregnancy rates after the transfer of two embryos are significantly higher than after the transfer of one. On the other hand, two embryos are considered the maximum number safe to transfer because of the risk of multiple pregnancies and the need to confirm the pre-implantation diagnosis by CVS of each fetus, which is feasible with twins but not triplets.

Five out of the eight women became pregnant after a total of 13 treatment cycles, three after one and one each after two and three treatment cycles. The first two were both twin pregnancies and the other three singletons. The sex of each of the seven fetuses was examined by CVS and karyotyping at about ten to 11 weeks. All were female except for one singleton pregnancy in which the karyotype indicated that the fetus was male. Since this couple is at risk of transmitting type II hereditary sensory motor neurone disease and in their case a specific diagnosis to determine whether a male fetus is affected is not possible, the couple took the decision to terminate the pregnancy. Both of the twin pregnancies and the remaining two singleton pregnancies have now gone to term. Apart from the second set of twins which was stillborn, all are apparently normal healthy girls. Detailed post mortem examination failed to reveal any gross abnormality in the stillborn twin and the cause was probably intrapartum anoxia prior to caesarean delivery.

The misidentification of the sex in one out of seven cases highlights the problem of identifying the sex of an embryo on the basis of the presence or absence of a Y-specific fragment alone. In the treatment cycle in which the misidentification occurred, two apparently female embryos were transferred after amplification from single biopsied cells failed to demonstrate the presence of the Y- specific fragment. With each of the four remaining biopsied embryos not transferred, including one male from which two cells had been biopsied and from which the Y-specific fragment had been clearly amplified in both cases, the predicted sex was confirmed by amplification from the biopsied embryos at a later stage. This indicates that the problem was an isolated amplification failure rather than a more general technical failure on this occasion.

Biochemical microassay

Biochemical microassays capable of measuring the activity of several enzymes involved in inherited syndromes at the single cell level are available.[35–37] Indeed, the first successful demonstration of pre-implantation diagnosis in an animal model involved the use of HPRT-deficient mice[38] as a model of Lesch-Nyhan syndrome and the measurement of HPRT activity in single cells biposied at the eight-cell stage.[39] However in the mouse, it had long been established that embryo-coded enzyme predominates over maternally-coded enzyme inherited from the oocyte at these stages since, among other evidence, HPRT activity increases exponentially from the eight-cell stage onwards and is reduced after treatment with transcriptional inhibitors.[35,40]

In contrast, the levels of HPRT activity measured in individual human oocytes and embryos, using the same microassay as in the mouse, were low and variable at all stages and the only change in activity appeared to be a gradual decline towards the blastocyst stage.[41] Also, the transcriptional inhibitor alpha-amanitin, which would be expected to reduce the level of embryo-coded enzyme activity, did not appear to have any consistent effect on enzyme levels. Using a more sensitive high pressure liquid chromotography (HPLC) microassay and higher substrate concentrations, however, higher levels of HPRT activity were measured and there was a significant increase between days two and four and a sharp decline at the blastocyst stage

on day six postinsemination (Figure 17.3).[37] Since the embryonic genome is first expressed at the four- to eight-cell stage on day two to three,[42,43] this increase in activity on day four may result from the synthesis of embryo-coded enzyme which would allow the diagnosis of enzyme deficiencies at this stage. Although the levels of enzyme activity in different embryos and in embryos from different patients were variable, complete enzyme deficiencies may, therefore, be detectable if maternal enzyme activity at this stage is sufficiently low.

Prospects for pre-implantation diagnosis

The prospects for pre-implantation diagnosis will depend on several factors: the accuracy of the diagnosis, the pregnancy rate and the cost of the treatment. Any pre-implantation diagnosis based on the genetic analysis of one or two cells biopsied from cleavage stages or even ten to 30 cells at the blastocyst stage is unlikely to be as reliable

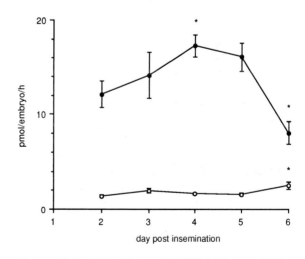

Figure 17.3 HPRT (●) and APRT (○) (± standard error) of normally fertilised human embryos between days two and six after insemination *in vitro*. Only embryos developing at the normal rate were assayed. The number of observations ranged from 8–50 per day with a total of 118 measurements of HPRT activity and 115 for APRT activity

as that available after CVS when relatively large numbers of cells and corresponding quantities of DNA are available. Thus a follow-up CVS may always be necessary to confirm the diagnosis. Pre-implantation diagnosis as a screening process may nevertheless make a valuable contribution, if not completely eliminating the risk of an affected pregnancy, at least significantly reducing it, and may still be preferable to many couples.

The implantation rate of biopsied cleavage stage embryos in the series of eight women carrying X-linked defects was very much higher than commonly achieved following IVF with infertile couples. Ten out of 22 (45 per cent) biopsied embryos implanted as detected by raised HCG levels around day 14. Although three of these embryos, including one 'vanished' twin, failed to develop further, the remaining seven which established clinical pregnancies have resulted in a pregnancy success rate of 32 per cent per embryo transferred. The use of IVF techniques for recovery of large numbers of pre-implantation embryos for biopsy and genetic screening has, therefore, proved to be both reliable and efficient in terms of establishing pregnancies. The reason for this success may be that the majority of these couples are fertile. But it is also possible that the zona drilling which is required for cell biopsy assisted hatching from the zona pellucida and consequently implantation. It has been suggested that zona hardening in culture contributes to implantation failure after IVF.[44]

Although two of the women had two and three cycles of treatment before becoming pregnant, this was achieved in a period of approximately six months. This indicates that a second major advantage of pre-implantation diagnosis may be a substantial reduction in the time necessary to establish an unaffected pregnancy compared with what in many cases would be a series of spontaneous pregnancies followed by conventional post-implantation prenatal diagnosis.

Finally, the availability of resources for IVF and the cost of treatment will also be an important factor, especially in countries like the United States where the expense of pre-implantation diagnosis compared with CVS may discourage many couples. This will provide an added incentive to develop safe and effective methods for uterine lavage as an alternative to the expensive procedure of IVF.

Acknowledgements

I would like to thank my students, Kate Hardy and Helen Kontogianni and also Karen Martin, Dr Henry Leese and Professor Robert Winston for allowing me to discuss our joint work, and Karen Dawson, Joe Conaghan, Dr Jacob Soussis for their help with clinical management and IVF. The work on pre-implantation diagnosis of X-linked disease was supported by the Muscular Dystrophy Group of Great Britain and Northern Ireland and was approved by the research ethics committee of the Royal Postgraduate Medical School and the Interim Licensing Authority for Human Fertilisation and Embryology.

References

1. Hardy K, Martin KL, Leese HJ, Winston RML, Handyside AH. Human pre-implantation development in vitro is not adversely affected by biopsy at the 8-cell stage. *Human Reproduction*. 1990; **5**: 708–14.

2. Dokras A, Sargent IL, Ross C, Gardner RL, Barlow DH. Trophectoderm biopsy in human blastocysts. *Human Reproduction*. 1990; **5**: 821–5.

3. Strom CM, Verlinsky, Y, Milayeva S, Evsikov S, Cieslak J, Lifchez A, Valle J, Moise J, Ginsberg N, Applebaum M. Preconception genetic diagnosis of cystic fibrosis. *Lancet*. 1990; 306–7.

4. Bond DJ, Chandley AC. Aneuploidy. *Oxford Monographs on Medical Genetics*. No. 11. Oxford: Oxford University Press, 1983.

5. Hardy K, Handyside AH, Winston RML. The human blastocyst: cell number, death and allocation during later pre-implantation development in vitro. *Development*. 1989; **107**: 597–604.

6. Dawson KJ, Rutherford AJ, Winston NJ, Subak-Sharpe R, Winston RML. Human blastocyst transfer, is it a feasible proposition? *Human Reproduction*. 1988; suppl. 145, 44–5.

7. Bolton VN, Wren ME, Parsons JH. Pregnancies after in vitro fertilization and transfer of human

blastocysts. *Fertility and Sterility.* 1991; **55**: 830–2.

8. Papaioannou VE, Ebert KM. Comparative aspects of embryo manipulation in mammals. In: Rossant J, Pedersen R (eds.) *Experimental Approaches to Mammalian Embryonic Development.* Cambridge: Cambridge University Press, 1986: 67–96.

9. Wilton LJ, Shaw JM, Trounson AO. Successful single cell biopsy and cryopreservation of pre-implantation mouse embryos. *Fertility and Sterility.* 1989; **51**: 513–17.

10. Gordon J, Talansky BE. Assisted fertilization by zona drilling: a mouse model for correction of oligozoospermia. *Journal of Experimental Zoology.* 1986; **239**: 347–54.

11. Trounson A, Mohr L. Human pregnancy following cryopreservation, thawing and transfer of an 8-cell embryo. *Nature.* 1983; **305**: 707–9.

12. Angell RR, Templeton AA, Aitken RJ. Chromosome studies in human in vitro fertilization. *Human Genetics.* 1986; **72**: 333–9.

13. Saiki RK, Scharf S, Faloona F, Mullis KB, Horn GT, Erlich HA, Arnheim N. Enzymatic amplification of β-globin sequences and restriction site analysis for diagnosis of sickle cell anaemia. *Science.* 1985; **230**: 1350–4.

14. Chamberlain JS, Gibbs RA, Ranier JE, Caskey CT. Multiplex PCR for the diagnosis of Duchenne muscular dystrophy. In: Innis M, Gelfand DH, Sninsky JJ, White TJ (eds.) *PCR Protocols: A Guide to Methods and Applications.* San Diego: Academic Press, 1990: 272–81.

15. Handyside AH. Pre-implantation diagnosis by DNA amplification. In: Chapman M, Grudzinskas G, Chard T, Maxwell D (eds.) *The Embryo: Normal and Abnormal Development and Growth.* London: Springer-Verlag, 1991; 81–90.

16. Li A, Gyllensten UB, Cui X, Saiki RK, Erlich HA, Arnheim N. Amplification and analysis of DNA sequences in single human sperm and diploid cells. *Nature.* 1988; **335**: 414–19.

17. Coutelle C, Williams C, Handyside A, Hardy K, Winston R, Williamson R. Genetic analysis of DNA from single human oocytes – a model for pre-implantation diagnosis of cystic fibrosis. *British Medical Journal.* 1989; **299**: 22–4.

18. Monk M, Holding C. Amplification of a beta-haemoglobin sequence in individual human oocytes and polar bodies. *Lancet.* 1990; 985–8.

19. Lesko J, Snabes M, Handyside A, Hughes M. Amplification of the cystic fibrosis delta F508 mutation from single cells: applications toward genetic diagnosis of the pre-implantation embryo. *American Journal of Human Genetics.* 1991; **49**: 223 (abstract).

20. Lesch M, Nyhan WL. A familial disorder of uric acid metabolism and central nervous system function. *American Journal of Medicine.* 1964; **36**: 561–70.

21. Koenig M, Hoffman EP, Bertelson CJ, Monaco AP, Feener C, Kunkel LM. Complete cloning of the Duchenne muscular dystrophy (DMD) cDNA and preliminary genomic organization of the DMD gene in normal and affected individuals. *Cell.* 1987; **50**: 509–17.

22. Boehnke M, Arnheim N, Li H, Collins FS. Fine structure genetic mapping of human chromosomes using the polymerase chain reaction on single sperm: experimental design considerations. *American Journal of Human Genetics.* 1989; **45**: 21–32.

23. Cooke HJ. Repeated sequences specific to human males. *Nature.* 1976; **262**: 182–6.

24. Cooke JH, Schmidtke J, Gosden JR. Characterisation of a human Y chromosome repeated sequence and related sequences in higher primates. *Chromosoma.* 1982; **87**: 491–502.

25. Kogan SC, Doherty M, Gitschier J. An improved method for prenatal diagnosis of genetic disease by analysis of amplified DNA sequences. *New England Journal of Medicine.* 1987; **317**: 985–90.

26. Handyside AH, Pattinson JK, Penketh RJA, Delhanty JDA, Winston RML, Tuddenham EDG. Biopsy of human pre-implantation embryos and sexing by DNA amplification. *Lancet.* 1989; **I**: 347–9.

27. Witt M, Erickson RP. A rapid method for the detection of Y chromosomal DNA from dried blood specimens by the polymerase chain reaction. *Human Genetics.* 1989; **82**: 271–4.

28. Bobrow M, Pearson PL, Pike MC, El-Alfi OS. Length variation in the quinacrine-binding segment of human Y chromosomes of different sizes. *Cytogenetics.* 1971; **10**: 190–8.

29. Cooke JH, Noel B. Confirmation of Y/autosome translocations using recombinant DNA. *Human Genetics.* 1979; **67**: 222–4.

30. Kwok S, Higuchi R. Avoiding false positives with PCR. *Nature.* 1989; **339**: 237–8.

31. Handyside AH, Kontagianni EH, Hardy K, Winston RML. Pregnancies from biopsied human pre-implantation embryos sexed by Y-specific DNA amplification. *Nature.* 1990; **344**: 768–70.

32. Handyside AH. Biopsy of human cleavage stage embryos and sexing by DNA amplification. In: Verlinsky Y, Strom C (eds.) *Proceedings of the First Symposium on Pre-Implantation Genetics.* New York: Plenum, 1991, pp. 75–83.

33. Rutherford AJ, Subak-Sharpe RJ, Dawson KJ, Margara RA, Franks S, Winston RML. Improvement of in vitro fertilisation after treatment with buserelin, an agonist of luteinising hormone releasing hormone. *British Medical Journal.* 1988; **296**: 1765–8.

34. Hardy K, Winston RML, Handyside AH. Binucleate cells in human pre-implantation embryos in vitro: failure of cytokinesis during early cleavage. *J. Reprod Fert.* In Press.

35. Monk M. Biochemical micro-assays for X-chrom-

osome-linked enzymes HPRT and PGK. In: Monk M (ed.) *Mammalian Development – A Practical Approach.* Oxford: IRL Press, 1987, pp. 139–61.

36. Benson C, Monk M. Micro-assay for adenosine deaminase, the enzyme lacking in some forms of immunodeficiency, in mouse pre-implantation embryos. *Human Reproduction.* 1988; **3**: 1004–9.

37. Leese JH, Humpherson PG, Hardy K, Hooper MAK, Winston RML, Handyside AH. Profiles of hypoxanthine guanine phosphoribosyl transferase and adenine phosphoribosyl transferase activities measured in single pre-implantation human embryos by high performance liquid chromatography. *Journal of Reproduction and Fertility.* 1991; **91**: 197–202.

38. Hooper M, Hardy K, Handyside A, Hunter S, Monk M. HPRT-deficient (Lesch-Nyhan) mouse embryos derived from colonization by cultured cells. *Nature.* 1987; **326**: 292–5.

39. Monk M, Handyside AH, Hardy K, Whittingham DG. Pre-implantation diagnosis of deficiency of hypoxanthine phosphoribosyl transferase in a mouse model for Lesch-Nyhan syndrome. *Lancet.* 1987; **II**: 423–5.

40. Monk M, Harper M. X chromosome activity in pre-implantation mouse embryos from XX and XO mothers. *Journal of Embryology and Experimental Morphology.* 1978; **46**: 53–64.

41. Braude PR, Monk M, Pickering SJ, Cant A, Johnson MH. Measurement of HPRT activity in the human unfertilised oocyte and pre-embryo. *Prenatal Diagnosis.* 1990; 839–50.

42. Braude PR, Bolton V, Moore S. Human gene expression first occurs between the 4- and 8-cell stages of pre-implantation development. *Nature.* 1988; **332**: 459–61.

43. Tesarik J, Kopecny V, Plachot M, Mandelbaum J. Early morphological signs of embryonic genome expression in human pre-implantation development as revealed by quantitative electron microscopy. *Developmental Biology.* 1988; **128**: 15–20.

44. Cohen J, Wright G, Malter H, Elsner C, Kort H, Masssey J, Mayer MP, Wiemer KE. Impairment of the hatching process following in vitro fertilization in the human and improvement of implantation by assisting hatching using micromanipulation. *Human Reproduction.* 1990; **5**: 7–13.

Chapter 18

Pre-implantation cytogenetic diagnosis

Joy Delhanty

Introduction

The ultimate aim of our work is to achieve pre-implantation diagnosis of chromosomal anomalies. This may appear to be unnecessary, since early prenatal diagnosis is available from chorionic villus sampling at eight to ten weeks gestation. As frequently occurs in the field of human genetics, the pressure for pre-implantation diagnosis has come from the families themselves. There are two groups involved, those who have been unfortunate enough to suffer repeated terminations of pregnancy because of recurrent genetic abnormality, and those who are fundamentally opposed to selective abortion. Both groups wish to be able to start a pregnancy knowing that it is free from the genetic defect that occurs in their family.

After fertilisation *in vitro*, selective embryo transfer has two main aims. The first aim is to avoid known genetic anomalies, but secondly to improve the overall success rate of *in vitro* fertilisation (IVF). The simplest situation involves sex linked single gene defects[1] (see Chapter 16). Embryos have been sexed using the polymerase chain reaction (PCR) but an alternative is to use X- or Y-specific probes for *in situ* hybridisation (ISH) to cells fixed on slides.

Autosomal single gene defects may also be diagnosed using the PCR providing sufficient is known about the gene sequence involved, but cytogenetic diagnosis requires an alternative approach. Additional copies of whole chromosomes may be readily detected by ISH,[2] but if there is a chromosomal rearrangement segregating in the family this poses a different problem and the technique known as chromosome painting, using chromosome-specific library probes,[3] will probably be necessary.

A contributory cause of IVF failure must be the naturally occurring high number of zygotes with missing or extra chromosomes. Since IVF is normally offered to women who have been unable to conceive over a period of years, they tend to come in the older age group. Based solely on data from recognised pregnancies, at age 35, 12–20 per cent of oocytes can be expected not to have the normal haploid number of chromosomes.[4,5] At conception the percentage of cytogenetically abnormal embryos would be expected to be much higher than this since no selection has taken place. The ability to screen for the common trisomies before embryo transfer would be of considerable benefit.

Interphase cytogenetics

We use surplus embryos from the IVF programme at the Hammersmith Hospital, London, to develop

183

these techniques. The embryos are disaggregated so that we may work on one or two cells to simulate early cleavage biopsies. The cells are then prepared as for standard chromosome preparations, that is, subjected to hypotonic sodium citrate treatment followed by acetic alcohol fixation and finally spread by being allowed to dry on microscope slides (see also Chapter 14).

If it were possible to reproducibly obtain good quality chromosomes from embryo biopsies there would be no problem in carrying out cytogenetic diagnosis. Technically, this is extremely difficult. What is needed is a method of determining chromosome copy number in non-dividing cells. This approach is known as interphase cytogenetics and depends on the availability of appropriate chromosome-specific repetitive DNA probes. The Y chromosome has a large block of repetitive DNA on the long arm from which numerous Y-specific probes have been derived. For the X chromosome and the autosomes, the probes which lend themselves to this technique have been derived from repetitive sequences of the class known as 'alphoid' which are situated at the centromeres (the site of attachment to the metaphase spindle during cell division). During mitosis, chromosomal DNA is condensed, but during interphase, when gene transcription occurs, it becomes decondensed. It has become evident that even during interphase the DNA from a particular chromosome occupies a specific 'domain' or site within the nucleus. It is this which enables detection of chromosome copy number in interphases when using probes which have sufficiently high numbers of the target sequences present.

Fluorescent *in situ* hybridisation

We are using a technique of fluorescent ISH, with biotin labelled probes and an indirect detection system, with sequential layers of avidin-fluorescein isothiocyanate (FITC) conjugate and biotin-anti-avidin conjugate.[6] As the fluorescent signal fades very quickly it is necessary to mount in an anti-fade medium. A counterstain, such as DAP1 or propidium iodide, either of which stain total DNA, enables location of the cell. The FITC signal, which corresponds to the site of hybridisation of the probe, is then visible as a bright yellow/green spot. Using probes derived from the X or Y chromosome on control material, such as cultured lymphocytes or direct preparations from chorionic villi, we obtain efficiencies of hybridisation of between 95 and 100 per cent.[7] There are technical difficulties associated with applying this technique directly to embryonic cleavage cells. These include the amount of cytoplasm present, frequent occurrence of large, diffuse nuclei and, since they are surplus embryos, degenerating cells. By modifying the technique, we have surmounted these problems to a large extent, and have found that only about 15 per cent of embryonic nuclei fail to hybridise to these probes.[7] The presence of a Y chromosome indicates a male embryo, but a false negative result would mean that absence of signal is erroneously taken to indicate a female embryo. It was for this reason that we commenced work on the use of an X probe for sexing. However, comparison of results with the X probe for several disaggregated cells derived from a single embryo showed a minority with double the expected number of hybridisation signals. In some instances, the enlarged size of these nuclei suggested tetraploidy, but in others the nuclei were no larger than those with the normal number of signals.[7] A chimaeric origin or mitotic non-disjunction of chromosomes are possible explanations for the latter group. In either case, misdiagnosis of sex based on the number of X chromosomes could occur.

Multiple labelling

The best option appears to be double labelling with X and Y probes simultaneously. We are now using this technique. Since it is most important not to miss the Y signal, we are using a combination of two Y probes, pHY2.1[8] and CY98 (provided by Dr J. Wolfe), which together give a large signal. They are labelled with the hapten digoxygenin and detected by FITC. The X probe, pbam X 7[9], is then labelled with biotin which is detected with Texas red. A technical problem is that optimal hybridisation is achieved with the X probe at a different temperature from that required for other probes. A compromise has been achieved with some success, but best results are currently obtained when chromosomes are visible even if they are of poor quality.[10]

Screening for trisomy

Among spontaneously aborted fetuses, trisomies for all the autosomes have been found, with the exception of chromosome 1, and three copies of that chromosome have been seen in a pre-implantation embryo.[11] For practical purposes, the only autosomal trisomies compatible with live birth are those for chromosomes 21, 13 and 18. By far the most common trisomy in the abortion material is that for chromosome 16, which must occur in more than 1 per cent of recognised conceptions. Obviously, there is a limit to the number of trisomies that we could hope to screen for in a single human embryo. The availability of different fluorochromes makes simultaneous detection of three or more probes theoretically possible. Testing for chromosomes 16, 13 and 18 should reduce early fetal loss (trisomy occurs in 8–12 per cent of recognised conceptions at ages 35–39 years[5]). To reduce the likelihood of later terminations, testing for chromosomes 18 and 21 would seem to be the best option. At present, good centromeric probes are available for chromosomes 16 and 18, and we are able to use them successfully in control material. Preliminary results suggest that they will hybridise also to embryonic nuclei. There is no widely available probe specific for chromosome 21, but one that is obtainable hybridises to both chromosomes 13 and 21, which would allow simultaneous testing of copy number for these two important chromosomes. Reciprocal or Robertsonian translocations, which involve exchange of genetic material between non-homologous chromosomes without affecting the phenotype of genetically balanced carriers, may nevertheless result in unbalanced gametes after meiosis. Detection of these unbalanced products in a subsequent zygote will not be possible using centromeric probes unless the rearrangement involves the centromere. The technique of chromosome painting[3] will be required to pick up abnormal copy number of acentric chromosomal segments. For this technique the probe consists of DNA prepared from the appropriate chromosome-specific libraries; after hybridisation the whole chromosome will fluoresce brightly. This enables precise analysis to be undertaken even when the chromosome preparation is of very poor quality, as is likely to be the case with embryonic cleavage cells. It appears that chromosome preparation will be necessary as the use of library probes does not give clear interphase signals.

As centromere specific and library probes are now available for almost all chromosomes it appears that the fluorescent ISH technique has considerable potential for use in both diagnosis and research at the pre-implantation stage of human development.

Acknowledgements

This research is very much a team effort. The ISH is carried out by my research student, Darren Griffin. The IVF embryos are available thanks to the whole IVF team at Hammersmith Hospital, London, headed by Robert Winston. Cytogenetic preparation of the embryos is being done by Leeanda Wilton of the Institute of Zoology, London.

References

1. Handyside AH, Kontogianni EH, Hardy K, Winston RML. Pregnancies from biopsied human pre-implantation embryos sexed by Y-specific DNA amplification. *Nature*. 1990; **344**: 768–70.
2. Cremer T, Landegent J, Bruckner A, Scholl HP, Schardin M, Hager HD, Devilee P. Detection of chromosome aberrations in the human interphase nucleus by visualisation of specific target DNAs with radioactive and non-radioactive in situ hybridisation techniques; diagnosis of trisomy 18 with probe L 1.84. *Human Genetics*. 1986; **76**: 346–52.
3. Pinkel D, Landegent J, Collins C, Fuscoe J, Segraves R, Lucas J, Gray J. Fluorescent in situ hybridisation with human chromosome specific libraries: detection of trisomy 21 and translocations of chromosome 4. *Proceedings of National Academy of Sciences (USA). 1988;* **85**: 9138–42.
4. Warburton D. Reproductive loss: how much is

preventable? *New England Journal of Medicine.* 1987; **316**: 158–60.

5. Hassold T, Chiu D. Maternal age-specific rates of numerical chromosome abnormalities with special reference to trisomy. *Human Genetics.* 1985; **70**: 11–17.

6. Griffin DK, Leigh SEA, Delhanty JDA. Use of fluorescent in situ hybridisation to confirm trisomy of chromosome region 1q 32-qter as the sole karyotypic defect in a colon cancer cell line. *Genes, Chromosomes and Cancer.* 1990; **1**: 281–3.

7. Griffin DK, Handyside AH, Penketh RJA, Winston RML, Delhanty JDA. Fluorescent in situ hybridisation to interphase nuclei of human pre-implantation embryos with X and Y chromosome specific probes. *Human Reproduction.* 1991; **6**: 101–5.

8. Cooke JH, Schmidtke J, Gosden JR. Charac-

terisation of a human Y chromosome repeated sequence and related sequences in higher primates. *Chromosoma.* 1982; **87**: 491–502.

9. Willard HF. Chromosome-specific organisation of human alpha satellite DNA. *American Journal of Human Genetics.* 1985; **37**: 524–32.

10. Griffin DK, Wilton LJ, Handyside AH, Winston RML, Delhanty JDA. Dual fluorescent in situ hybridisation for simultaneous detection of X and Y chromosome-specific probes for the sexing of human pre-implantation embryonic nuclei. *Human Genetics.* 1992; **89**: 18–22.

11. Watt JL, Templeton AA, Messinis I, Bell L, Cunningham P, Duncan RO. Trisomy 1 in an 8-cell human pre-embryo. *Journal of Medical Genetics.* 1987; **24**: 60–4.

Chapter 19

In vitro culture of biopsied blastomeres and diagnosis of aneuploidy

Leeanda J Wilton

Introduction

The techniques of *in vitro* fertilisation (IVF) for treatment of infertility have enabled access to early cleavage stage embryos and it has been reasoned that, for patients who are at risk of transmitting a genetic disease to their offspring, diagnosis of disease in early embryos may circumvent the need for termination of affected fetuses. This could be achieved by biopsying one or two cells from the pre-implantation embryo, testing the biopsied material for the presence of the genetic defect and only transferring embryos predicted to be free of the suspected abnormality.

Micromanipulation

For pre-implantation diagnosis to be feasible it is essential that the biopsy technique has little or no effect on embryo development. We have used the mouse embryo as a model to develop and optimise techniques of micromanipulation, and have demonstrated that a single blastomere can be biopsied from a four-cell embryo.[1] The embryo is held sta-

tionery by suction through a heat polished fine glass pipette while another finer aspiration pipette, bevelled to an angle of 45°, is used to puncture the zona pellucida. A single cell is drawn into the aspiration pipette which is then removed from the embryo and the cell is carefully expelled into the surrounding medium. Embryo transfer experiments have unequivocally demonstrated that, in the mouse, embryo biopsy has no detrimental effect on pre-implantation development, implantation rate or fetal development[2,3] and live young have been born from biopsied embryos (Figure 19.1). Other workers have biopsied one or two cells from eight-cell human embryos and this procedure has no effect on development to the blastocyst stage *in vitro*.[4]

Growth of single blastomeres *in vitro*

One of the major limitations of pre-implantation embryo biopsy is the small amount of material available for diagnosis of the genetic defect.

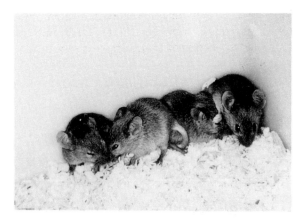

Figure 19.1 Live young at approximately two weeks of age born from mouse embryos biopsied at the four-cell stage

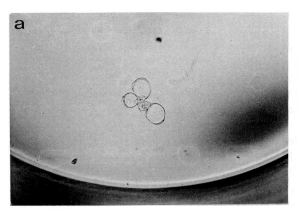

Figure 19.2a A small number of cells with large intracellular fluid-filled cavities derived from culture of a single mouse blastomere in M16 for three days

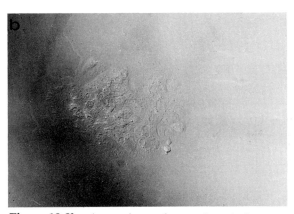

Figure 19.2b A monolayer of approximately forty cells derived from culture of a single mouse blastomere in M16 on a layer of LNC for six days

Consequently we have attempted to grow single embryonic cells *in vitro*.

A single blastomere from a four-cell mouse embryo cultured in medium M16[5] has little proliferative potential and will divide only once or twice. After this time the cells accumulate fluid and form large fluid filled cavities (Figure 19.2a). This behaviour is not unexpected and parallels their behaviour in forming a blastocoelic cavity had they been part of a developing embryo. Other workers have made similar observations and described the formation of false blastocysts, mini blastocysts and trophoblastic vesicles from single blastomeres from four-cell mouse embryos.[6]

We used many different culture media in attempting to increase the replicative potential of single blastomeres. Simple salt solutions such as T6[7] or M16 or more complex media such as DMEM (Dulbecco's Minimum Essential Medium) were ineffective even when supplemented with sera. Also, medium that had been conditioned by cultured mouse oviduct epithelial cells had no effect on the growth of single blastomeres *in vitro*. In some earlier studies[1] we cultured single mouse blastomeres in human amniotic fluid as this had been reported to improve the growth of mouse and human pre-implantation embryos *in vitro*.[8] However, we now believe human amniotic fluid offers no real advantage. Culture on feeder layers of 3T3 fibroblasts did slightly increase the replicative potential of single mouse blastomeres. However,

before a diagnosis using the polymerase chain reaction or DNA isolation could be performed the two different cell types would have to be completely separate. Contamination by even one fibroblast cell could result in misdiagnosis. Consequently this approach was not pursued further.

The *in vitro* growth of many eukaryotic cells is dependent on their ability to adhere to a substratum. We have used a number of different attachment factors to induce single blastomeres to form a monolayer on the floor of the tissue culture well. In particular, fibronectin (F), laminin (LN) and a complex of laminin and nidogen (LNC) induced attachment and significant proliferation of single blastomeres in culture (Table 19.1). Without an extracellular matrix cells divided only once or twice. Single blastomeres cultured on swine skin gelatin (SSG) replicated to an average of 9.5 cells and a mean of more than 20 cells was obtained from single blastomeres grown on FN or LNC (Table 19.1, Figure 19.2b). When this data is presented as a frequency distribution (Figure 19.3) it can be seen that monolayers or more than 30 cells were often obtained on FN or LNC (Figure 19.2b). FN and LNC proved to be more effective than SSG possibly because of greater specificity. Mouse embryos secrete nidogen at the compacted eight-cell stage and fibronectin at the two-cell stage.[9] When grown on any of the attachment factors cells did not cavitate as in Figure 19.2a but formed small sheets of six to eight cells which then attached to the floor of the well. After five or six days when maximum cell number was obtained, the cells had the morphological appearance of trophectodermal outgrowths from whole embryos (Figure 19.2b) although we have not yet established that cells are true trophectoderm.

Table 19.1 *In vitro* growth of single blastomeres from 4-cell embryos on extracellular matrix components. Number of cells per well (mean ± SE) after six days in culture

Control (no matrix)	SSG	FN	LN	LNC
2.2 ± 0.6 (N = 21)	9.5* ± 3.7 (N = 53)	20.7† ± 6.6 (N = 53)	13.8* ± 6.2 (N = 32)	22.1† ± 5.0 (N = 68)

Notes:
* P < 0.005 compared to control.
† P < 0.001 compared to control.

Karyotypic analysis of embryonic biopsies

Other workers have successfully sexed cells biopsied from human pre-implantation embryos for the identification of female embryos not afflicted with X-linked diseases[10] (see Chapter 17). However, many inherited diseases are caused by a chromosome imbalance or aneuploidy and these are currently detected after amniocentesis or CVS

by analysis of metaphase chromosomes from hundreds or thousands of cells. If the small amount of material obtained after pre-implantation biopsy

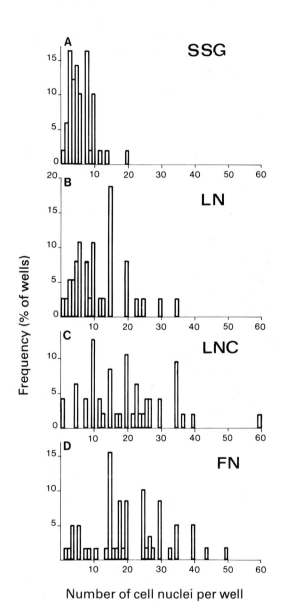

Figure 19.3 Frequency distribution of the mean number of cell nuclei per well after six days of culture of single blastomeres isolated from four-cell mouse embryos. Wells were coated with swine skin gelatin (SSG), laminin (LN), fibronectin (FN) or complexed laminin and nidogen (LNC)

could reliably be karyotyped it may be possible to detect aneuploidic diseases in the early embryo.

We have used the mouse as a model to develop techniques to obtain metaphase chromosomes from a few cells. Preliminary experiments demonstrated that the plaques of cells obtained from culture of single blastomeres were very adhesive and difficult to handle without considerable cell loss. It appeared that analysis of single blastomeres might be more efficient. This had the added advantage that, because cell culture and replication was not required, the diagnosis could be done rapidly and in sufficient time for the embryos to be transferred without requiring storage by cryopreservation.

Aneuploidic embryos were produced by mating male mice heterozygous for a Robertsonian translocation of chromosomes 16 and 17 with normal female mice. This results in a mixed population of euploid, trisomy 16 (Ts16) and monosomy 16 (Ms16) embryos. During the pre-implantation period these embryos are morphologically indistinguishable but Ms16 embryos die around implantation.[11] Ts16 embryos survive to late gestation but have phenotypic abnormalities including stunted growth and craniofacial defects.[11]

In a series of replicate experiments a single blastomere was biopsied from these embryos at the four-cell stage. The individual blastomeres were incubated overnight in colchicine while the remaining embryos were cultured. Metaphase chromosomes were obtained from the blastomeres by briefly exposing them to a hypotonic solution of sodium citrate and then fixing them with a 3:1 methanol:acetic acid solution.[3] With due care this proved to be an efficient technique and analysable chromosomes were obtained from 80 per cent of all cells spread. On the basis of the karyotype predicted

from the single cell the biopsied embryos were grouped into those thought to be euploid, Ms16 and Ts16 and transferred to pseudopregnant recipient mice.

Pregnant recipients were killed on day 15 of pregnancy and the fetuses examined for the morphological abnormalities associated with Ts16. All abnormal and some normal fetuses were karyotyped. As shown in Table 19.2, the fetal morphology and karyotypes correlated exactly with the pre-implantation diagnosis. That is, all five embryos predicted to be Ts16 by analysis of a single cell at the four-cell stage developed into fetuses which were confirmed to be Ts16.[3] Similarly, all embryos predicted to be euploid were morphologically normal and all eight that were karyotyped were confirmed to be euploid. One embryo predicted to be Ms16 did not implant and, although this is not conclusive, the observation is consistent with the embryo actually being Ms16.[3] So the diagnosis of aneuploidy at the four-cell stage was 100 per cent correct.

Cytogenetic analysis of single human blastomeres

Recently I have attempted to karyotype single blastomeres isolated from human embryos. These embryos were surplus from the IVF programme at Hammersmith Hospital and were obtained with patients' permission. Blastomeres were not obtained by embryo biopsy as had been done using the mouse model, but instead whole four- to eight-cell embryos were incubated overnight in colchicine. Cell number was assessed both before and after incubation in colchicine to confirm that

Table 19.2 *In vivo* viability, fetal morphology and fetal karyotype of biopsied embryos after transfer

Predicted genotype	N	Implantation site %	Fetuses %	Correct fetal morphology %	Correct fetal karyotype %
Euploid	27	22 (81)	18 (67)	18 (100)	8* (100)
Ms16	1	0 (0)	0 (0)	–	–
Ts16	5	5 (100)	5 (100)	5 (100)	5 (100)

Note: * only eight fetuses predicted to be euploid were karyotyped.

mitosis was arrested in all cells. The zona pellucida was then removed by brief exposure to acid Tyrodes solution. The individual blastomeres were separated by gentle pipetting through a flame polished pipette and then subjected to hypotonic treatment and fixed in methanol: acetic acid.

Several features of early human development have made it difficult to obtain metaphase chromosomes from single human blastomeres. First, cell division in human embryos is far less synchronous than in mouse embryos and the time of the previous mitosis can only be determined by constant observation. This means that, to obtain a high percentage of cells in metaphase, the cells had to be incubated in colchicine for up to 20 hours. Prolonged exposure to colchicine results in shortened chromosomes which are difficult to differentiate from each other and often inappropriate for routine banding techniques. In order to reduce colchicine exposure, the colchicine concentration was decreased to about 1/100 of that used for mouse blastomeres.

In an initial series of experiments, metaphase chromosomes fixed on the microscope slide could only be obtained from 67 per cent of single cells that were spread (Table 19.3). It was impossible to know whether the cells were being lost during the procedure or whether the cells had not gone into metaphase (interphase DNA from a single cell is extremely difficult to locate on a microscope slide). Consequently, in a second series of experiments each cell was stained with a specific nuclear fluorochrome (Hoechst 33342) after the overnight colchicine incubation and before fixing. As shown in Table 19.3, this demonstrated that only 68 per cent of cells were in fact going into metaphase and when these were fixed, metaphase chromosomes

were obtained from 91 per cent of cells (Table 19.3). Cells that were not in metaphase were in interphase and more than half had nuclear abnormalities. Twenty-one per cent were binucleate, 22 per cent had more than two nuclei (and up to six) and 15 per cent were anucleate. The remaining 41 per cent of cells that did not go into metaphase had one interphase nucleus. It seems probable that the cells that were not in metaphase were severely retarded or arrested.

It was not possible in this small sample to determine whether any correlations could be made between nuclear abnormalities and embryo morphology. Furthermore nuclear abnormalities did not seem to be peculiar to particular patients or embryos. For example, of the nine four-cell embryos which had at least one interphase cell, in one embryo all four cells were in interphase, two embryos had two cells in interphase and six embryos had a single interphase cell. Similarly, of seven embryos which had at least one cell with more than one nucleus, two four-cell embryos each had four multinucleate cells, two embryos had two multinucleate cells and three embryos had one multinucleate cell.

That such a large proportion of cells in four- to eight-cell human embryos may have nuclear abnormalities and/or have ceased mitosis is of grave concern to those attempting pre-implantation diagnosis. The experiments described here utilised only a small number of embryos and it is imperative to investigate the phenomenon more thoroughly and in a larger number of embryos. Such a study may demonstrate that the inability to obtain a diagnosis or risk of misdiagnosis can be considerably reduced if more than one cell is biopsied from the embryo. This should not compromise embryonic viability

Table 19.3 Production of metaphase chromosome spreads from single human blastomeres

	Number of cells	Number of cells in metaphase %	Number of cells spread	Number of metaphases visualised %
Experiment 1	110	?	94	93 (67)
Experiment 2*	104	71 (68)	70	64 (91)

Note: * In experiment 2, cells were stained with a nuclear fluorochrome after colchicine treatment but prior to fixation to determine whether the nucleus contained metaphase chromosomes or was in interphase.

as has previously been demonstrated[4] (see Chapter 17).

Even though it has been demonstrated that spreads of metaphase chromosomes can be obtained from single human blastomeres, the majority of the chromosomes are insufficiently spread for successful g-banding. However, the preparations are remarkably clean and free of cytoplasmic contaminants and so are ideal for fluorescent *in situ* hybridisation with centromere specific DNA probes (see Chapter 18).

In conclusion, single mouse blastomeres can be rapidly and efficiently karyotyped. Some technical problems arise when attempting to karyotype single human blastomeres but these are not insurmountable. It is anticipated that it will soon be possible to identify human aneuploidic diseases by pre-implantation diagnosis.

References

1. Wilton LJ, Trounson AO. Biopsy of pre-implantation mouse embryos: development of micromanipulated embryos and proliferation of single blastomeres in culture. *Biology of Reproduction.* 1989; **40**: 145–52.

2. Wilton LJ, Shaw JM, Trounson AO. Successful single cell biopsy and cryopreservation of pre-implantation mouse embryos. *Fertility and Sterility.* 1989; **51**: 513–17.

3. Kola I, Wilton LJ. Pre-implantation embryo biopsy: detection of trisomy in a single cell biopsied from a 4-cell mouse embryo. *Molecular Reproduction and Development.* 1991; **29**: 16–21.

4. Hardy K, Martin KL, Leese JH, Winston RML, Handyside AH. Human pre-implantation development in vitro is not adversely affected by biopsy at the 8-cell stage. *Human Reproduction.* 1990; **5**: 708–14.

5. Whittingham D. Culture of mouse ova. *Journal of Reproduction and Fertility* (suppl.). 1971; **17**: 7–21.

6. Tarkowski AK, Wroblenska J. Development of blastomeres of mouse eggs isolated at the 4- and 8-cell stage. *Journal of Embryology and Experimental Morphology.* 1967; **18**: 155–80.

7. Quinn P, Barros C, Whittingham DG. Preservation of hamster oocytes to assay the fertilizing capacity of human spermatozoa. *Journal of Reproduction and Fertility.* 1982; **66**: 161–3.

8. Gianaroli L, Serracchioli R, Ferraretti AP, Trounson AO, Flamingi C, Bovicelli L. The successful use of human amniotic fluid for mouse embryo culture and human in vitro fertilization, embryo culture and embryo transfer. *Fertility and Sterility.* 1986; **46**: 907–13.

9. Yohkaichiya T, Hoshiai H, Uehara S, Yajima A. Fibronectin localisation in the mouse embryo from the two cell stage to the morula stage. *Tohoku Journal of Experimental Medicine.* 1988; **154**: 95–100.

10. Handyside AH, Kontogianni EH, Hardy K, Winston RML. Pregnancies from biopsied human pre-implantation embryos sexed by Y-specific DNA amplification. *Nature.* 1990; **344**: 768–70.

11. Epstein CJ. Mouse monosomies and trisomies as experimental systems for studying mammalian aneuploidy. *Trends in Genetics.* 1985; **1**: 129–34.

Chapter 20

Gamete and embryo micromanipulation in human reproduction: perspicacity or opacity?

Simon Fishel

Introduction

The previous pages of this book brought together the experiences of the first practitioners of human gamete and embryo micromanipulation for the purpose of procreation. The manipulation of conception and pre-implantation embryos of our own species has created a confused welter of inconsistencies, often based largely on scientific ignorance or absolute dogma. The following chapters deal with the ethical debate, and the interpretation of such which has resulted in the various legal consequences.

In addition to the important moral arguments, there still remains the 'simple' scientific debate: this includes questions such as efficacy, efficiency, safety, realities and prospects, to consider a few. This chapter attempts to place much of the preceding part of this book into a current perspective.

Micro-assisted fertilisation

It is now incontrovertible that mechanically created breaches in the human zona pellucida and injecting unselected spermatozoa into the perivitelline space can result in normal fertilisation, cleavage, fetal development and the birth of healthy babies. But are these techniques really necessary, does the level of efficiency, both clinically and financially, justify their use and, in the long term, can they be considered safe?

Efficacy

In considering whether these techniques are effective, we must be clear and consistent in our understanding of which patients may benefit from these procedures, and we must evaluate which techniques would be most appropriate for the variety of disorders that present. It has been discussed extensively elsewhere that patients fall into two clearly defined groups. First, those for whom we are absolutely certain that the conventional IVF procedure – including the microdrop IVF procedure – is not indicated. These cases will be due, primarily, to severe seminal defects such as immotile cilia syndrome, or extremely severe asthenozoospermia, globozoospermia, or the presence of very few sperm. Data presented in previous chapters (see Chapters 7 and 13) indicate that even with severe seminal defects fertilisation *in vitro* may occur, particularly if the microdrop IVF technique is used. However, it is sometimes efficiency rather than a low level of fertilisation that may indicate the use of micro-assisted fertilisation, perhaps in conjunction with conventional IVF.

The second group of patients for which the micro-assisted fertilisation techniques may be effective are those in whom fertilisation *in vitro* has been tried repeatedly – at least twice under conditions which are acceptable to the clinic offering micro-assisted fertilisation. Complete failure of fertilisation of all oocytes or an extremely low incidence of fertilisation would indicate micro-assisted fertilisation (MAF).

Patient evaluation is only the first step in defining the efficacy of these procedures. Gamete evaluation is a major factor, and in future years this will probably be the major determinant of the most effective technique to be used. Evaluating the efficacy of these procedures must be performed, first and foremost, in conjunction with control studies. It is common practice in this author's clinic to offer to all patients, even those who have failed to achieve fertilisation on at least two occasions at clinics elsewhere, IVF, with either conventional or microdrop procedures, in at least a proportion of the metaphase II oocytes from the same cohort. Morphological observations under the microscope which relate to the binding of the spermatozoa to the zona pellucida will be of some use as an initial score of sperm–zona interaction. More data is required to evaluate the relationship between sperm zona binding between a couple's own gametes and the future prognosis for conception by either the conventional IVF or MAF techniques. There is also an urgent need to evaluate the initial ejaculate, based on the classification of spermatozoa and, particularly, the morphology, in

relation to prognosis. For example, if an increasing body of data suggests that morphology does not aid in the prognosis of fertilisation with MAF,[1] but does so for IVF,[2,3] it is then acceptable to utilise the morphological parameters as a pointer to MAF procedures rather than IVF.[1] This can only be on the basis that there will be an unequivocal indication of the effect of the particular morphological defect on the outcome of insemination.

Therefore, it is necessary to devise various sperm function assessments which can act as a prognosticator of the various techniques available. These assessments, to be valuable, must provide unequivocal data which can be acted upon. As long as various sperm function tests, such as the addition of drugs, or zona penetration assays with low sperm counts, provide a low correlation with fertilisation, whatever the technique employed, it may be more efficient to go straight to the IVF/MAF controlled procedures. It is still the case that using the couple's own gametes is the ultimate prognosticator!

Computerised movement characteristics may offer some indication of the fertilisation potential of spermatozoa. In an assessment of a number of parameters, Wolf et al.[4] observed that for spermatozoa exhibiting a normal pattern of movement the percentage of acrosome-reacted spermatozoa was highly significantly correlated with the incidence of fertilisation after SUZI. But there was no correlation with density, motility or morphology of the spermatozoa, or with the hamster egg penetration assay.

The acrosome reaction challenge test (ARIC) and the hamster egg penetration (HEP) assay are part of a number of sperm function tests which are currently being assessed for their prognosticative value of fertilisation. The HEP assay will continue to present a problem with ejaculates having a low sperm count as a certain density of motile spermatozoa is required for an efficient and reliable assay.[5] Only by carefully evaluating individual patients, and by assessing the fertilising potential of the particular ejaculate, will the efficiency of MAF be truly apparent.

Recent publications using the MAF procedures throw into confusion the efficacy of these techniques. Few publications offer adequate control studies. Cohen et al.[6] described their experience comparing SUZI with PZD and IVF. However, difficulties arise in interpreting some of their data. For example, patients had been grouped into three categories: those unacceptable for IVF, those who had failed IVF and those who had no previous attempts at IVF. Seminal parameters were divided into < 10 per cent motility, $< 5 \times 10^6$/ml density and < 2 per cent normal morphological forms for the former group. However, these parameters were 'and/or' and therefore not clear-cut. Patients with a density of $< 5 \times 10^6$/ml and a motility of < 10 per cent but with a total volume of 3 or 4 mls could still achieve successful fertilisation *in vitro*, especially if microdrop IVF is used.[7] However, as shown in Tables 20.1 and 20.2, when assessing the percentage fertilisation, no controls with IVF were performed. There were, therefore, a number of difficulties in forming conclusions on the efficacy of these procedures based on the data of Cohen et al.[6] Control studies were performed in only a few patients (Tables 20.1 and 20.2). In the group of patients with severe male infertility, although fertilisation occurred with MAF, no IVF controls were performed. Comparing the results with the group of patients with previous IVF failure, the incidence of fertilisation was not significantly different in the oocytes undergoing IVF. Comparing the results with SUZI/PZD/IVF in patients who had not previously attempted IVF, the incidence of fertilisation per patient or per oocyte was similar. These workers also concluded that with control (sibling) oocytes, PZD had a lower efficiency of fertilisation than SUZI per patient and per oocyte in the group of patients who had previously failed IVF, and in those patients who had semen parameters unacceptable for IVF.

Other published work to date also presents small numbers of patients, creating difficulties for a clear evaluation. Payne et al.[8] had an apparent improvement in the incidence of fertilisation with zona breaching procedures compared with IVF. This study represented 19 patients who had a previous failure of IVF and eight patients who were precluded from an IVF attempt, but no pregnancies were obtained. However, their 'unacceptable' semen parameters (a mean count and motility of 12×10^6/ml and 29 per cent, respectively) would be considered acceptable by other groups. Sibling oocytes used for conventional IVF would have served as useful controls. Schmutzler et al.[9]

Table 20.1 Comparison between SUZI, PZD and IVF in sibling oocytes: patients*

Group	Total number	Fertilisation		
		SUZI	PZD	IVF
Unacceptable for IVF	7	3/7 (43%)	1/7 (14%)	Not done
Failed IVF	5	4/5 (80%)	1/5 (20%)	1/7 (40%)
No previous IVF	11	6/11 (55%)	7/11 (64%)	7/11 (64%)

* From reference 6.

Table 20.2 Comparison between SUZI, PZD and IVF in sibling oocytes: oocytes*

Group	Total number	Fertilisation		
		SUZI	PZD	IVF
Unacceptable for IVF	81	7/50 (14%)	1/31 (3%)	Not done
Failed IVF	72	10/28 (36%)	4/20 (20%)	6/24 (25%)
No previous IVF	127	8/38 (21%)	16/42 (38%)	16/47 (34%)

* From reference 6.

showed an increase in the fertilisation rate with SUZI compared with IVF when the former was used on oocytes the day after they failed to fertilise with conventional IVF. They also demonstrated an increase in fertilisation with SUZI in patients who had severe and very severe teratozoospermia. However, no pregnancies were obtained in this study. Palermo et al.[10] demonstrated a fertilisation rate of 31 per cent per oocyte with SUZI and seven pregnancies were obtained from 43 cycles of treatment. Patients had previous failure of IVF, but no sibling control oocytes were used even though their lower sperm classification was a mean density, percentage motility and per cent abnormal forms of $\leq 5 \times 10^6$/ml, 35 per cent and 17.1 per cent respectively.

In contrast to the apparently more positive results described above, van de Leu and Zeilmaker[11] reported on 25 patients with at least one previous failure of fertilisation, and found that 16 of the patients had similar results whether SUZI or IVF was used. Jean et al.[12] attempted to make precise indications of semen alterations in relation to zona breaching procedures as a result of the lack of clarity in the data of Cohen et al.[6] In 20 cases of previously failed IVF, they concluded that PZD offered no improvement for sperm samples with low counts ($< 4 \times 10^6$/ml), only with high counts; but this was associated with an unacceptably high incidence of polyspermy. In a study of 70 cycles, 67 patients, Tucker et al.[12] evaluated the use of PZD for male infertility; although the seminal parameters were not severe (mean count, motility, velocity and morphology were 30.7×10^6/ml, 45.7 per cent, 36.2 μm/sec and 39.3 per cent, respectively). One subgroup of 33 patients (35 cycles) had fertilisation and a third subgroup achieved fertilisation with PZD

and conventional IVF. None of the semen param eters measured, namely sperm density, motility velocity or morphology, were significantly differen between the subgroups. However, 35 of the 70 (5(per cent) cycles achieved fertilisation solely througl the use of PZD. But in 16 cycles in which oocyte: were fertilised after conventional IVF and PZD Tucker et al.[13] found that the use of PZD 'seemec unnecessary and possibly even disadvantagous i1 that multi-spermic penetration was very high'.

In a recent publication of Ng et al.[14] patients witl severe oligoasthenoteratozoospermia were evalu ated. The rate of monospermic fertilisation usin; SUZI was 16.6 per cent and polyspermy 2.3 pe cent. Of a total of 131 patients, 58 had embryc transfer, four had a clinical pregnancy with on(of these resulting in a delivery. This representec a clinical pregnancy rate of 3 per cent per patien of 7 per cent per embryo transfer. Concomitan IVF was performed in some patients. By grouping patients according to the density of spermatozo: in the original ejaculate – Table 2.3 – only thos(patients with a sperm density of $< 5.1 \times 10^6$/m had fertilisation with SUZI and none with IVF. A a sperm density of $> 5.1 \times 10^6$/ml, the incidence o fertilisation with SUZI and IVF was similar (Table 20.3). These authors described the use of the Ficol technique, in contrast to the use of Percoll.[15] In th(former procedure, the spermatozoa are centrifugec at 3352 for 20 minutes, compared to 300–500 fo1 ten minutes with the latter technique. Ng e al.[14] acknowledged that such prolonged centrifuga force may precipitate membrane damage and, the) suggest, may result in the leakage of adenosin(5'-triphospate.

It is clear from the above discussion that ther(

Table 20.3 SUZI versus IVF for severe oligoasthenoteratozoospermia*

Group	Oocyte fertilisation rate			
	Sperm parameters			
	< 5.1 ($\times 10^6$/ml)	5.1 – 10 ($\times 10^6$/ml)	10.1 – 20 ($\times 10^6$/ml)	> 20 ($\times 10^6$/ml)
IVF	0/7	17%	18%	17%
SUZI	13%	11%	21%	25%

* From reference 14.

s no opinion of singular perspicacity of the use of MAF. Until there is a distinct and universal accept-ance on patient evaluation, assessment of useful eminal parameters, standardised techniques and the presentation only of control studies, further data will only increase the opacity of our understanding.

Efficiency

Given that the MAF procedures offer benefit to some patients in certain circumstances, there is an urgent need to improve the efficiency and usefulness of these procedures. In particular, it is necessary to increase the incidence of fertilisation with SUZI, and to reduce the incidence of polyspermy with PZD. The former may require various techniques or safe drugs which can increase the fertilising potential of a population of spermatozoa. This might increase the fertilisation with SUZI while inserting fewer spermatozoa into the perivitelline space. Reducing the concentration of spermatozoa in the inseminating medium, perhaps in combina-tion with procedures to enhance fertilising ability, may also maintain the high incidence of fertilisa-tion with PZD while reducing the incidence of polyspermy.

How can we improve the fertilising potential of a given population of spermatozoa? One of the obvious approaches is to increase the percent-age of acrosome-reacted spermatozoa in a given population. This is likely to improve the rate of fertilisation with MAF, and possibly aid in reducing polyspermy by utilising less spermatozoa.[10,16]

For populations of spermatozoa with poor motil-ity, progressive activity can be enhanced by using pentoxifylline.[17] For populations of spermatozoa with a low incidence of acrosome-reacted sperm, this may be increased by incubation with drugs 2-deoxyadenosine has been tried[16] but appears toxic – human follicular fluid, or by electroporation (Fishel et al., unpublished),[10] for example.

As yet there is no specific sperm function test which can evaluate unequivocally the fertilising potential of a population of spermatozoa. The techniques described above represent a few options available for improving the chances of fertilisation. The efficiency of any procedure, especially the MAF techniques, would be improved dramatically if there were sperm function tests available which provided reliable data from which the practitioners could act. This will be an important area of research in the coming decade.

Safety

There are three major concerns associated with the safety of MAF procedures: abnormal fertilisation leading to the formation of abnormal embryos, the induction of parthenogenesis, and gene or chromo-some aberration in the products of conception. The first two of these concerns can be eradicated by the embryologist after careful microscopic observation of the zygote. Should mutli-pronucleate eggs arise, or if parthenogenetic activation has occurred, these can be assessed by the observance of pronuclei, more than two in the former or a single pronucleus in the latter, and these zygotes can be disposed of before cleavage. The third concern, the passage of gene or chromosome aberrations, cannot at this stage, be entirely ignored. The two major worries in this regard have been, first, the artificial crea-tion of an environment facilitating fertilisation with chromosomally abnormal sperm, which would not otherwise have been possible. Secondly, whether the techniques themselves predispose to the induc-tion of aberrant chromosomes. At this stage, the latter can be answered with much more conviction than the former. Animal research, and increasing data on the human, indicate that the techniques per se are unlikely to upset the chromosome make-up of either gamete. However, it would be unwise at this early stage to have the same degree of confidence in the quality of embryo production. Many of the com-mentators on this problem refer to the work of Kola et al.[18] who observed the karyotypes in embryos after fertilisation with SUZI. In the study, 20 cou-ples had previously failed to achieve fertilisation in multiple cycles of IVF and presented with male subfertility. The incidence of chromosomal abnor-mality in the 18 karyotypes of the 260 embryos produced after SUZI was not significantly different from those produced after conventional IVF (22 per cent versus 30 per cent, respectively). The latter group of embryos were produced from the gametes of six couples donating for the purposes of this study. Although this data provides a certain degree of confidence, 18 karyotypes observed after SUZI is a very small number. A high incidence of abnormality arises in the human embryo after conception with IVF; it would require hundreds, if not thousands, of embryos fertilised by each technique to demonstrate an effect of MAF. Confidence can be gained from the clinical work reported to date. About one hundred babies have been born by these procedures and no abnormality has yet been recorded. Whether the primary fertilisation ratio generates a high incidence of abnormality in these circumstances, such that the rate of implantation failure or miscarriage is higher than after natural conception or conventional IVF, remains to be evaluated.

Some attention should be drawn to the studies of Martin-DeLeon et al.[19] on the incidence of chromosome abnormalities in rabbit blastocysts after the spermatozoa had been aged in the male tract. Table 20.4 presents their data. They observed more

Table 20.4 Chromosome abnormalities in rabbit blastocysts resulting from spermatozoa aged in the male tract*

Period of aging (days)	Number of karyotypes analysed	% abnormalities
0 (sham operated)	20	0.8%
0 (control)	105	0.8%†
7–21 days	72	11.1%†

* From reference 19.
† $P < 0.001$.

Table 20.5 Results with direct cytoplasmic injection

	Report		
	A	B	C
Number of eggs injected	47	38	37
Number fertilised	31 (66%)	4 (10.5%)	4 (10.8%)
Pregnancies	4	0	0

Notes: A: from reference 10.
　　　　B: from reference 14.
　　　　C: from Fishel et al. (unpublished).

than a ten-fold increase in the incidence of abnormal karyotypes analysed in the blastocysts formed after conception with aged sperm compared to the blastocysts produced after conception with normal sperm. This study may be relevant to cases using epididymal aspiration for blockage or absence of the vasa deferentia.

Another area for careful observation is the use of direct injection of spermatozoa into the cytoplasm of the oocyte (see Chapter 1). Data presented by Ng et al.,[14] Palermo et al.[10] and Fishel et al. (unpublished) are shown in Table 20.5. From this limited series of data it is clear that there are considerable difficulties with the technique and successful outcome is extremely limited. Martin et al.,[20] in 1988, studied the chromosome complements of human sperm after micro-injection into the cytoplasm of hamster eggs. In this study it was noted that there was approximately a four-fold increase in the incidence of abnormal chromosomes after micro-injection compared with normal fertilisation. More recently, Ng et al.[14] stated that 'direct ooplasmic injection of sperm should not be done until a clearer picture is known'. In relation to the finding of Sathananthan (Chapter 6) that the sperm mid-piece contributes a centriole to the first mitotic spindle, it may be that the technique used by Martin et al. predisposed to their particular data. Hence, spermatozoa used for direct injection should, perhaps, remain either untreated, or be treated such that the proximal centriole next to the basal plate of the mid-piece remains intact. Goto et al.[21] have reported on the successful use of direct intracytoplasmic injection with bovine gametes.

Pre-implantation diagnosis

For couples with inherited genetic disorders, four possible options might be available: (a) not to procreate, (b) to select the healthy gametes prior to conception, (c) to have conception *in vitro* and preimplantation diagnosis by embryo biopsy, or (d) to conceive naturally, undergo prenatal diagnosis and, if necessary, terminate the afflicted pregnancy. Because the latter is not a viable option for many not least because some couples have previously had numerous pregnancies terminated, the possibility of the choice to establish a known healthy pregnancy would be an enormous advantage.

There are two approaches for preconception diagnosis, analysis of the spermatozoon or the first polar body of the oocyte; and two possible stages for pre-implantation diagnosis, cleavage stage blastomeres or the trophectoderm at the blastocyst stage.

The previous chapters on embryo micromanipulation (Chapters 15–19) described the technical possibilities and the first successes with human pre-implantation sex selection by genetic screening. For sex-linked disorders, separation of X and Y bearing spermatozoa would be the least invasive and most widely accepted option. The alternative would be to screen the pre-implantation embryo and exclude the gender that might be affected. Selection of a pure population of X or Y bearing viable spermatozoa has not yet been achieved. Although polymerase chain reaction (PCR) can identify individual Y bearing spermatozoa, they are rendered inviable during the procedure.

One currently realistic option for preconception diagnosis is analysis of the first polar body of the oocyte. This technique, applicable for the detection of maternally inherited disorders, involves analysis of the polar body DNA. In the absence of crossing over, the gene content of the oocyte of heterozygous carriers for a mutant gene would be opposite to that of the first polar body. However, complications inevitably arise as a function of heterozygosity of alleles during crossing over. Navidi and Arnheim[22] have calculated the probabilities of errors using PCR on target DNA sequences from the first polar body or blastomeres for dominant and recessive disorders. Errors can arise in PCR efficiency, contamination of apparatus or as a result of erroneous cell transfer. In only a few exceptional circumstances does first polar body analysis yield lower rates of misdiagnosis than blastomere analysis; for example, when a defective gene is recessive and isolated virtually at the centromere, or if it is dominant and lies within 25 cM of the centromere. As Navidi and Arnheim[22] point out, it is unlikely that many defective genes will be located in such close proximity to the centromere. Therefore, polar body typing will, in the majority of cases, result in an unacceptable level

of misdiagnosis. A multiple diagnosis approach, using initially the first polar body followed by blastomere biopsy in the postconception embryo, significantly increases the accuracy of typing.[23] In a recent report by Verlinksy et al.[24] PCR analysis was used for the delta-F508 mutation after the extraction of the first polar body and, subsequently, blastomeres of the oocytes and embryos, respectively. The procedures were performed on the oocytes and embryos of patients who had had children affected with cystic fibrosis, or who were heterozygous for the delta-F508 mutation. There was amplification failure in 18 per cent (4/22) of polar bodies and 14 per cent (2/14) of blastomeres assayed. Blastomeres were obtained from four- to eight-cell embryos.[24] However, one concern is that if one of the primers failed to amplify, leading to a presumption of homozygosity, the level of misdiagnosis could exceed 18 per cent. Diagnosis would be further compromised if a misdiagnosed heterozygous oocyte was fertilised by a sperm of a man who is also a carrier. This would result in an embryo homozygous for cystic fibrosis.

Amplification failure is one of the widely recognised problems of PCR. As discussed previously (Chapter 17), a failure of amplification of the Y specific DNA fragment of embryonic blastomeres has arisen. This failure to detect the Y signal resulted in 1/7 pregnancies established with a male instead of a female embryo. Handyside and Delhanty[25] have explored the possibility of co-amplification of a constant target sequence as a control for amplification failure. Success with this approach is so far limited due to the apparent independence of primers to amplify.

In the excellent article by Navidi and Arnheim,[22] they demonstrate that single cell analysis is subject to a number of errors decreasing the reliability of diagnosis. In general, and except for dominant diseases caused by genes extremely close to the centromere, blastomere analysis is subject to less misdiagnosis than polar body analysis. Taking multiple blastomeres from a single embryo, or combining polar body analysis with blastomere analysis significantly decreases the level of misdiagnosis with unacceptable consequences.

In 1989, Holding and Monk,[26] using DNA from individual mouse blastomeres, reported that 16 per cent failed to amplify when a positive amplification was expected. Li et al.,[27] using DNA from single spermatozoa, had 18 per cent of samples failing to amplify. Gomez et al.,[28] using DNA from trophectoderm biopsies of mouse blastocysts, found that 31 per cent failed to detect specific alleles and Monk and Holding[26] using DNA from the polar body of human oocytes reported failure rates of 33 per cent (4/12), 29 per cent (2/7), zero percent (0/4), 71 per cent (5/7) and 14 per cent (1/7) depending on the sample being analysed.

A recent report by Pickering et al.[25] used PCR to amplify a 680 base per fragment of the beta-globin gene. These authors had successful amplification more frequently with DNA from intact embryos, containing between one and 11 cells, and from polar bodies, than from single blastomeres. The reason for the unreliable amplification of DNA from single blastomeres was unclear, although using the nuclear chromophore diamino-pheynyl-indole showed considerable inter-blastomere variation.

Amplification of single copy genes using PCR therefore requires an additional level of stringency. It is essential that the use of this method on DNA from human polar bodies or blastomeres for pre-implantation diagnosis of single gene defects is assessed unequivocally. In certain situations, such as the case of sickle-cell anaemia, which is an autosomal recessive disease, failure to detect an amplified product would lead to a failure to type the embryo and it would not be replaced.[29] This level of misdiagnosis, in which the embryo containing the mutant allele would never be replaced but some carrying normal alleles might be mistakenly discarded, may be acceptable for clinical use. However, the utmost stringency must be applied to the technical process such that misdiagnosis did not arise due to an observed signal resulting from amplification of contaminating DNA which did not carry the defect in one or both of its alleles. This would lead to the erroneous decision to replace an embryo that had presumably contained at least one normal allele, but in reality it had none.

The encouraging aspects of this work, elegantly demonstrated by Handyside[30] and Handyside and Delhanty[25] (see Chapter 17), is that biopsy of early cleavage stage embryos does not reduce their viability. Of 22 embryos biopsied, 45 per cent implanted and seven (32 per cent) developed to clinical pregnancies. Many couples requesting pre-implantation diagnosis would be fertile and would possibly have a higher incidence of implantation and delivery than is seen in general IVF procedures. Providing up to 75 per cent of the cell mass is retained after biopsy, this would be compatible with full developmental potential.[31,32] As discussed in earlier chapters (Chapters 17 and 18) *in situ* hybridisation to identify ploidy and sex chromosomes in interphase and metaphase nuclei presents an exciting possibility for the future. Different fluorochromes could be used simultaneously to detect a number of autosomes in addition to sex chromosomes. *In situ* hybridisation might also be developed for the detection of inheritable genetic disorders. However, one of the associated problems for pre-implantation diagnosis by *in situ* hybridisation is numerical mosaicism of chromosomes, which can arise in the blastomeres of human embryos, and the presentation of aneuploidy which may be due to an artefact during the preparation of the specimen.

From the discussion above, it is apparent that preconception diagnosis is currently at higher risk of misdiagnosis than assessment of blastomeres of the cleavage stage embryo. Furthermore, continued research on pre-implantation genetic analysis is necessary before there is complete confidence in the accuracy and efficiency of these techniques for routine clinical service. However, pre-implantation diagnosis offers an exciting new development in reproductive medicine, and a hitherto unprecedented option for potential parents who are carriers of an inheritable genetic disease.

References

1. Hall JA, Fishel SB, Timson J, Faratian B. Evaluation of human sperm morphology in relation to subzonal insemination. (In preparation.)
2. Kruger TF, Acosta AA, Simmons KF. Predicted value of abnormal sperm morphology in *in vitro* fertilisation. *Fertility and Sterility.* 1988; **49**: 112–17.
3. Menkweld R, Stander FSH, Kotze TJvW, Kruger TF, van Zyl JA. The evaluation of morphological characteristics of human spermatozoa according to stricter criteria. *Human Reproduction.* 1990; **5**: 586–92.
4. Wolf JPH, Rodrigues D, Ducot B, Jouannet P. Gametes parameters influence on the post-SUZI fertilisation rate for patients with previous unexplained IVF failures. *Human Reproduction.* Abstracts of the VIIIth annual meeting of ESHRE, abstract 255. 1992; 139.
5. Aitken RJ. Evaluation of human sperm function. *British Medical Bulletin.* 1990; **46**: 654–74.
6. Cohen J, Alikani M, Malter HE, Adler A, Talansky BE, Rosenwaks Z. Partial zona dissection or subzonal sperm insertion: microsurgical fertilisation alternatives based on evaluation of sperm and embryo morphology. *Fertility and Sterility.* 1991; **56**: 696–706.
7. Fishel SB, Timson J, Lisi F, Rinaldi R. The use of microdrop IVF and high insemination concentrations increase the incidence of fertilisation in male infertility. (In preparation.)
8. Payne D, McLaughlin KJ, Depypere HT, Kirby CA, Warnes GM, Matthews CD. Experience with zona drilling and zona cutting to improve fertilisation rates of human oocytes in vitro. *Human Reproduction.* 1991; **6**: 423–31.
9. Schmutzler AG, Al-Hasani S, Casper AN, Thiebold A, Diedrich K, Krebs D. Assisted fertilisation: SZI and PZD with mostly severe and very severe teratozoospermia. *Human Reproduction.* Abstracts from the VIIIth meeting of ESHRE, abstract 256. 1992; 115.
10. Palermo G, Joris H, Devroey P, van Steirteghem AC. Induction of acrosome reaction in human spermatozoa used for subzonal insemination. *Human Reproduction.* 1992; **7**: 248–54.
11. Van de Leur JJCM, Zeilmaker GH. Microinsemination compared with IVF in the same patients. *Human Reproduction.* Abstracts from the VIIIth meeting of ESHRE, abstract 252. 1992; 137–8.
12. Jean M, Barriere P, Sagot P, L'Hermite A, Lopes P. Utility of zona pellucida drilling in cases of severe and very severe teratozoospermia. *Human Reproduction.* Abstracts from the VIIIth meeting of ESHRE, abstract 256. 1992; 115.
13. Tucker MJ, Bishop FM, Cohen J, Wiker SR, Wright G. Routine application of partial zona dissection for male factor infertility. *Human Reproduction.* 1991; **6**: 676–81.
14. Ng S–C, Bongso A, Ratnam SS. Microinjection of human oocytes: a technique for severe oligoasthenoteratozoospermia. *Fertility and Sterility.* 1991; **56**: 1117–23.
15. Fishel S, Timson J, Lisi F, Rinaldi L. Evaluation of 225 patients undergoing subzonal insemination for the procurement of fertilisation *in vitro. Fertility and Sterility.* 1992; **57**: 840–9.
16. Sjögren A, Hamberger L, Lundin K, Soderlund B. Avoidance of polyspermia in microsurgical fertilisation techniques. *Human Reproduction.* Abstract from the VIIIth meeting of ESHRE, abstract 253. 1992; 138.
17. Yovich JM, Edirisinghe WR, Collins JM. Yovich JL. Influence of pentoxifylline in severe male factor infertility. *Fertility and Sterility.* 1990; **53**: 715–22.
18. Kola I, Lacham O, Jansen RPS, Turner N, Trounson A. Chromosomal analysis of human oocytes fertilised by micro-injection of spermatozoa into the perivitelline space. *Human Reproduction.* 1990; **5**: 575–7.
19. Martin-DeLeon PA, Shaver EL, Gammal EB. Chromosome abnormalities in rabbit blastocysts resulting from spermatozoa aged in the male tract. *Fertility and Sterility.* 1973; **24**: 212–19.
20. Martin RH, Ko E, Rademaker A. Human sperm chromosome complements after microinjection of hamster eggs. *Journal of Reproduction and Fertility.* 1988; **84**: 179–86.
21. Goto K, Kinoshita A, Takuma Y, Ogawa K. Fertilisation of bovine oocytes by the injection of immobilised, killed spermatozoa. *The Veterinary Record.* 1990; **127**: 517–20.
22. Navidi W, Arnheim N. Using PCR in preimplantation genetic disease diagnosis. *Human Reproduction.* 1991; **6**: 836–49.
23. Verlinsky Y, Cieslak J, Esikov S, Milayeva A, Strom C, White M, Lifchez A, Valle J, Moise J, Ginsburg N, Applebaum M. Effect of subsequent oocyte and blastomere biopsy on pre-implantation development. VIIth World Conference on IVF and Assisted Procreations (abstract). *Human Reproduction* 1991; 136.
24. Verlinsky Y, Rechitsky S, Evsikov S, White M, Cieslak J, Lifchez A, Valle J, Moise J, Strom CM. Preconception and pre-implantation diagnosis for cystic fibrosis. *Prenatal Diagnosis.* 1992; **12**: 103–10.
25. Handyside AH, Delhanty DA. Cleavage stage biopsy of human embryos and diagnosis of X-linked recessive disease. In: Edwards RG (ed.) *Pre-Implantation Diagnosis of Human Genetic Disease.* Cambridge: Cambridge University Press, 1992. (in press.)
26. Holding C, Monk M. Diagnosis of beta-thalassaemia

by DNA amplification in single blastomeres from mouse pre-implantation embryos. *Lancet.* 1989; **ii**: 532–5.

27. Li H, Cui X, Arnheim N. Direct electrophoretic detection of the allelic state of single DNA molecules in human sperm by using the polymerase chain reaction. *Proceedings of the National Academy of Sciences, USA* 1990; **87**: 4580–4.

28. Gomez CM, Muggleton-Harris AL, Whittingham D, Hood L, Readhead C. Rapid pre-implantation detection of mutant (shiverer) and normal alleles of the mouse myelin basic protein gene allowing selective implantation and birth of live young. *Proceedings of the National Academy of Sciences, USA.* 1990; **87**: 4481–4.

29. Pickering SJ, McConnell JM, Johnson MH, Braude PR. Reliability of detection by polymerase chain reaction of the sickle cell-containing region of the β-globin gene in single human blastomeres. *Human Reproduction.* 1992; **7**: 630–6.

30. Handyside AH, Kontogianni EH, Hardy K, Winston RML. Pregnancies from human pre implantation embryos sexed by Y-specific DNA amplification. *Nature.* 1990; **344**: 768–70.

31. Wilton L, Shaw JM, Trounson AO. Successful single-cell biopsy and cryopreservation of pre implantation mouse embryos. *Fertility and Sterility* 1989; **51**: 513–17.

32. Somers GR, Trounson AO, Wilton LJ. Allocation of cells to the inner cell mass and trophectoderm of 3– mouse embryos. *Reproduction Fertility and Development* 1990; **2**: 51–9.

Section VII
Legal and ethical debate

Chapter 21

Legal implications raised by micromanipulation techniques

Judge C Byk

Introduction

DIPI, DIFI, FREDI, GIFT, GIPT, IVI, ITI, IVF-ET, IVTPF, OPT, POST, PROST, SHIFT, SUZI, TET, TOAST, TU-GIFT, TV-TEST, US-GIFT, US-TET, VITI, ZIFT, US-ZIFT.[1] This selection of the impressive enumeration of English acronyms shows that medical science and the technology surrounding *in vitro* fertilization (IVF) never ceases to offer a dazzling array of techniques to respond to the numerous specific indications suffered by infertile couples. Such 'developments' have been called the capernaum of human reproductive technology.[2] At the 1989 Milazzo Group Conference on Reproductive Medicine, R. Scott considered that 'the proper role (of the law) in relation to Human Artificial Procreation is by no means clear, and is likely to remain obscure for some time to come'.[3]

However, the British Parliament has recently placed their Human Fertilisation and Embryology Act, 1990, on the statute books from 1 August 1991. This is the first European country to make a clear and comprehensive legal statement concerning the contemporary reproductive technologies.

Still, most countries worldwide are undecided on the appropriate ethical and legal approach to the problems raised by the increasing development of reproductive technologies.

The legal debate

It is axiomatic that the law must first consider and then respond to new developments; it cannot pre-empt technological innovation. Can the law prejudge the appropriate technology and the type of scientific research? The law should only intervene to define a balanced position between the different interests concerned in the major issues raised by the new biology: that is, the societal issues. Simply, who should have access to the techniques and what are the rights and duties of the different parties in terms of human rights, civil law and public health law? Beyond this is the matter of professional ethics, relying upon the individual professional bodies in accordance with the conscience of physicians and scientists themselves.

There often exist conflicting apprehensions. On the one hand, lawyers who believe the law has no role to play in relation to these new technologies; on the other scientists groping within a legislative vacuum at the birth of a new technology.

The micro-assisted fertilisation techniques are a good example to illustrate such difficulties and must be considered an extension of the protracted debates on human assisted reproduction during the decade of the 1980s. The polemic during this period defined some trends in the law policy approach of these issues.[4]

Gamete and embryo micromanipulation in the human poses two major issues: the first is related to the fact that they are still experimental technologies. The second issue is the tentation of embryo biopsy and genetic selection, which could derive from the use of micromanipulation techniques for pre-implantation diagnosis.

I will try to demonstrate that the legal framework we dispose in the field of human reproduction could also apply to these two issues.

The experimental aspects of MAF techniques

The international context

The use of MAF techniques clinically has recently been authorised in a number of countries. Prior to this, various authorities had to consider the use of MAF for research only. In debating the question 'should the use of micromanipulation techniques in fertilisation be authorised?', the issue of using embryos not intended to be implanted was paramount. Many countries do not permit embryo research. It could be argued that it is merely research on oocytes. But taking into account that the objective of this experiment is to obtain the fertilisation of the egg, it would consequently result in the creation of an embryo. Although the embryo is not a priori the subject of research, it is the potential outcome of the procedure. Moreover, the resulting embryo may be affected by the process of micro-assisted fertility.

Therefore these techniques would be qualified as procedures involving research on embryos.

Denmark voted in 1987 a moratorium on embryo research[5] which will be kept effective until Par-

liament will approve the proposals of the Danish National Ethics Council.[6]

Norway passed a legislation in 1987[7] to prohibit all embryo research. In the USA, no federal funding for research has been provided since 1975[8] and some states explicitly put a ban on embryo research.[9] In the Netherlands, there are no legal restrictions, but no research is undertaken.[10]

This restrictive approach will probably extend to other countries as demonstrated by the German bill adopted by the Bundestag in November 1990.[11]

A number of countries/states do authorise experiments on spare embryos (those surplus to treatment and not subject to cryopreservation for the patients). This is the case in South Australia,[12] Spain,[13] Sweden[14] and France.[15]

The proposed guidelines prepared by the Committee on Bioethics of the Council of Europe (CAHBI) made the same suggestion.[16] Only the Warnock Report and the subsequent British Bill[17], the Ontario Law Reform Commission Report[18], the amended Victoria legislation (up to syngamy) and the New South Wales Report[19] in Australia accepted that embryos could be created uniquely for research purposes. However, in the State of Victoria (Australia) until 1987, the Infertility (Medical Procedures) Act (1984) prohibited the creation of embryos for research purposes.

A project involving the micro-injection of a single human sperm into human ova to determine whether this technique could safely be used in the treatment of male infertility was submitted to the standing Review and Advisory Committee on Infertility.

Given the high reported incidence of male infertility, the Committee came to the view that the proposed research was most desirable and recommended that an appropriate amendment to the Act be made.[20] This was effected in 1987:[21] experimentation on human eggs with a sperm already inside is allowed until 22 hours after the sperm has penetrated the egg, that is before syngamy, subject to the approval of the Victorian Standing Review and Advisory Committee. Then the mentioned research was approved by the Committee.

Because of the specific nature of this type of research an embryo is going to be created. Therefore the use of micro-assisted (MAF) techniques is limited either to states where the social context makes it difficult to have legislation (for example, Italy) or to states which explicitly permit the creation of embryos only for research purposes.

But even in this last case, as an experimental procedure, MAF will have to follow the conditions applying to embryo research and to research in general.

MAF and research regulations

Concerning the specific conditions related to embryo research, generally all the regulations in this field were prohibiting the transfer to the uterus of an embryo which has been submitted to experimental procedures.[22] However, since the introduction of the Human Fertilisation and Embryology Act, 1990, of the British Parliament on 1 August 1991, and the concomitant dissolution of the Interim Licensing Authority, MAF techniques have been introduced for clinical use in only a few specific centres in England. Britain's first pregnancies with the zona breaching techniques and subzonal insemination have been achieved.[23]:

Some practitioners argued that the experimentation is beneficial to the patients, and perhaps the embryo itself, as it has been created to provide an infertile couple with a future child. However, to admit this argument it is necessary to demonstrate that the intended child has some chance to come to life through an efficient and safe procedure.

In recommending that the Victorian 1984 Act be suitably amended to allow the experimentation of the micro-injection technique, the Standing Review and Advisory Committee based its proposal on the following conditions and intentions:

'Pre-syngamy embryos should be allowed to be formed for the purposes of *destructive*, non-therapeutic experimentation in research projects designed to assist in the alleviation of infertility.'[24]

It is clear then that the Committee came to the view that the proposed research was most desirable but 'the research would determine whether this technique could *safely* be used in the treatment of male infertility'.

The technique, developed by Professor C. Wood and Dr A. Trounson at Monash University, was first used clinically in March 1988 where an unsuc-cessful attempt was made to implant embryos into the uterus of a patient at the Monash Medical Centre in Melbourne.[25]

In April 1988, the Victorian Minister for Health ordered IVF scientists to stop using this new technique to create embryos in laboratory before transferring them to mothers.

The Victorian Standing Review Committee then approved in July 1988 research on 80 pre-syngamy embryos in order to assure the safety of the technique before any clinical application.[26] This resulted in the publication of the first assessment of the chromosome status of embryos conceived by SUZI.[27]

In declining in 1989 one project whose applicants 'wished to transfer the resulting pre-embryos to the uterus without having first established that the chromosomal content was normal', the UK Voluntary Licensing Authority, then renamed Independent, clearly expressed that such a project contravened Principle 4 of its guidelines which prohibits the transfer to the uterus of 'pre-embryos resulting or used in clinical research'.[28]

As we have seen, the situation is changing rapidly in a few countries, including Britain. However, the precautions taken by the various authorities remind us of the general guidelines applying to research on human beings and in particular the necessity to perform research on animals before going ahead with similar research on man.

Nevertheless, differences do exist between the results of research on animals and research on human beings. Animal research data cannot always be extrapolated directly to the human. The French National Bioethics Consultative Committee in its advise on embryo research stated that 'the differences that could be observed in the diverse mammalian species and in the human species, concerning the first stages of the development are subsidiary in regard to the common mechanisms concerned ...'. The Committee also remarked that we still know very little about these first steps of the development in animals. Therefore research on animals, in particular with those species permitting the use of numerous embryos (mouse, hamster, rat and rabbit), should be increased and 'no scientific team should consider practising fundamental research only with human embryos'.[29]

One could answer to such an objection to the use of human embryos that the research related to MAF procedures does not concern fundamental research but research intended to improve the use of reproductive technology. I do not know what would be the position of the French Committee in regard to the nature of this kind of research. The Committee has no overt equivalent opinion of non-fundamental research. The Committee noted that 'in general the medical teams working in the field of reproductive technologies have no scientific approach based on animal research. They compensate this absence of project in submitting protocols which are only aimed to improve reproductive procedures'. And the Committee concluded: 'this useless instrumentalisation of the human embryo is in the long term detrimental to embryo research ... [because] it will raise protests in the public [against new technological discoveries, such as nuclear transfer] when these new techniques could raise fundamental questions with a more efficient approach'.[30]

The 1989 ILA report concerning the rejection of a project involving the micro-injection of a single spermatozoon recognised the importance of progressive research involving in the first instance animal studies, before research on human gametes: 'It is important that where animal experiments have shown a technique to be promising it should not be translated immediately into clinical practice without prior work, using human pre-embryos to demonstrate its safety and efficacy.'[31]

This statement clearly implies that research on animals should take place prior to research on man and that this research should be promising enough to consider further research on human embryos.

As the French biologist J. Testart observed, research on animals already shows that 'among the diversity of existing micro-assisted fertilisation techniques, some of them could not be used for human therapeutical purposes, either because they suppress the zona pellucida (depellucidation) which protects the embryo, or they imply a high percentage of polyspermy (zona drilling)'.[32]

Research on the technique of sperm drilling,[33] which was reported successful in animals, proved to be deleterious to the human zygote and ineffective in producing pregnancies.

MAF techniques after clinical application

Currently the MAF techniques are not utilised clinically in a number of countries/states.

Clinical applications have finally been permitted in 1989 in Australia (Victoria) and in 1991 in the United Kingdom and France, but have been ongoing in countries without specific regulations (Italy and some states of America). However, the results of such applications are still insufficient to conclude that the MAF technologies have progressed beyond the experimental stage.

As quoted by the Interim Licensing Authority when giving its approval to a clinical application, it is still a trial which implies some legal and ethical consequences. The most important is certainly that legislation governing experimentation on human beings could probably apply to such a practice when realised to alleviate infertility. It means that the protocol for clinical application will need the approval of an ethics committee and that informed consent of the patient should be fully respected. But also indications for such a practice should also be better known and controlled groups of patients should be set up to evaluate these technologies.

Micromanipulation is also a technique which implies or permits the selection of spermatozoa. Preceeding chapters of this book address these issues in relation to the particular problems concerning the quality of the conceptus. However, the clinical data herein indicate that these procedures will offer a viable option to patients with no alternative for a child of their own.

MAF procedures and embryo biopsy

Reproductive technologies are usually facing two main risks concerning the health and well being of the child: the creation of abnormalities, and the use (or abuse) of sex/genetic selection techniques.

The risk of creating abnormalities

The handling, the micromanipulation and the cryopreservation of gametes and embryos could result in some unknown damage which could affect the resulting child. An understanding of the nature of the risks and the improvement in the technical process as well as the expertise of the practitioner, would in general allay these fears. It is already a matter of fact that, although more triploids were obtained through MAF techniques, these triploids could be detected and eliminated. Alternatively, to 'solve' the problems raised by polyspermy some biologists have even proposed to 'repair' the triploid in eliminating a nucleus (see Chapter 8).[34]

It has also been reported that the percentage of grave abnormalities in children born through IVF in some countries is higher than in children born without the help of reproductive medicine.[35] However, more data is needed for verification. It may be that with MAF techniques, the question is even more acute, not least because of the already recognised high incidence of abnormal fertilisations. This will need close inspection in the years ahead.

The risk of selection

The second risk in reproductive technologies is related to the fact that the infertile couples do not only wish to have a child, but that they are generally preferring to have a normal child. This attitude explains the widely supported technique of prenatal diagnosis as it is applied to high risk parents. But it also opens the possibility for deviation in the medical practice which permits the choice of the sex of the embryo or which simply allows prenatal diagnosis when it is not medically indicated.

Although mainly developed to detect single genetic defects, techniques such as polymerase chain reaction (see Chapter 14) raise issues concerning the potential selection of embryos for personal but non-clinical reasons. In France, the National Bioethics Consultative Committee condemned the use of prenatal diagnosis before implantation[36] but in Spain, in the summer of 1990, a first instance court authorised a woman who wished very strongly to have a girl to use a sex

selection technique:[37] however this was overruled by the Court of Appeals.

Conclusions

Micro-assisted fertilisations are remarkable tools with which to study gametic interaction, the chronology of fertilisation and to determine the fertilising power of a single spermatozoon. Some of them also offer new perspectives for the treatment of male infertility and for pre-implantation diagnosis.

But only after the beginning of their application in the human species, MAF techniques will probably remain in the realm of 'experimental' or clinical trials. As for IVF and other associated artificial insemination procedures, it will probably be many years before we can conclude that the risk physicians accept as normal are of no consequence to the resulting children.

In view of the necessary expertise of the clinical and scientific practitioners, and the high degrees of responsibility, licensing procedures for clinics and research centres are urgently needed.

It is the duty and the honour of physicians and biologists to establish their own framework for micromanipulation procedures which will not require any specific legislation but the recognition of existing ones, associated with professional ethics and the exercise of individual conscience.

Acknowledgements

I would like to acknowledge the following for the information they kindly gave me: The Interim Licensing Authority (London, UK), Professor P. Jouannet (Kremlin-Bicetre Hospital, Paris, France), Ms M. Plachot (U 173 INSERM, Paris, France), Professor L. Roche (Medical School, Lyons, France), Professor L. Wallers, Chairman, Standing Review and Advisory Committee on Infertility (Victoria, Australia).

References

1. DIPI : direct intraperitoneal insemination (1986)
   DIFI : direct intrafollicular insemination
   FREDI : fallopian replacement of eggs with delayed insemination 1989)
   GIFT : gametes intrafallopian transfer (1984) (1988)
   GIPT : gametes intraperitoneal transfer (1989)
   ITI : intratubal insemination (1987)
   IVTPF : *in vivo* transperitoneal fertilisation (1989)
   OPT : ovum pick up and transfer chamber (1989)
   POST : peritoneal oocyte and sperm transfer (1987)
   PROST : pronuclear stage tubal transfer (1987)
   SHIFT :synchronised hysteroscopic insemination of the fallopian tube (1987)
   SUZI : subzonal insemination
   TET : tubal embryo transfer (1989)
   TOAST : transcervical oocyte and sperm transfer (1982) (1989)
   TV-GIFT : transvaginal GIFT (1989)
   TV-TEST : transvaginal tubal embryo stage transfer (1989)
   US-GIFT : ultrasonically guided GIFT (1989)
   US-TET : ultrasonically guided TET (1989)
   VITI : vaginal intratubal insemination (1989)
   ZIFT : zygote intrafallopian transfer (1986)
   US-ZIFT : ultrasound guided ZIFT (1989)
   IVI : intra-uterine insemination
   IVF-ET : *in vitro* fertilisation and embryo transfer
2. Testart, J. Le caphernaüm des fécondations artificielles. *Le Monde, Sciences Medecine*, 3 January 1990, p. 22.
3. Scott, R. Regulations of artificial procreation: law, ethics and other options. *International Journal of Bioethics*. 1990; 1.
4. For an overview of international developments in this field, see OTA, Infertility Medical and Social Choices, Washington DC, 1988, p. 329.
5. Law N353 of 3 June 1987, Act on Establishment of an Ethical Council and Regulation of Certain Forms of Biomedical Experiments.
6. The Danish Council of Ethics Second Annual Report, 1989, Protection of Human Gametes, Fertilised Ova, Embryos and Fetuses, Copenhagen, 1990.
7. Act No. 628, 1987, relating to artificial procreation.
8. Fletcher JC. US federally supported research in reproductive genetics and fetal tissue: restriction and suppression, 1974–1988. In Byk C, *Artificial Procreation, the Present State of Ethics and Law*. Ed. Lacassagne, Lyon, 1989, p. 261.
9. OTA, Infertility, op. cit., p. 251.
10. Gunning J. *Human IVF, Embryo Research, Fetal Tissue for Research and Treatment, and Abortion*. International Information, Department of Health, 1990, London, HMSO, p. 32.
11. Entwuft eines Gesetzes zum Schutz von Embryonen, 22 September 1989.
12. South Australia Reproductive Technology Act.
13. Law 35/1988 – Health: Assisted Reproduction Techniques.
14. In Vitro Fertilisation Act, 1988.
15. Comite Consultatif National D'Éthique, Recomendation concerning research on embryos in vitro and their use for medical and scientific purposes, 15 December 1986.
16. CAHBI, Principles on Human Artificial Procreation, 1987.
17. Report of the Committee of Injury into Human Fertilisation and Embryology, London, HMSO, 1984.
18. Ontario Law Reform Commission, Report on Human Artificial Reproduction and Related Matters, Toronto, 1985.
19. New South Wales Law Reform Commission, In Vitro Fertilisation, Sydney, 1988.
20. Standing Review and Advisory Committee on Infertility, Review of Embryo Experimentation 'Post Syngamy', An Information Paper, Melbourne, 1989, p. 8.
21. The amending Bill was introduced into the Parliament on 30 April 1987.
22. For example, see article 4 of the UK ILA guidelines, and Principle 18 of the Council of Europe draft recommendation.
23. Fishel SB, personal communication.
24. Standing Review and Advisory Committee on Infertility, op. cit., p. 13 (see note 20).
25. Bioethics News, July 1988, p. 6.
26. The Age, 14 July 1988.
27. Kola I, Lacham O, Jansen RPS, Turner M, Trounson A. Chromosomal analysis of human oocytes fertilized by micro-injection of spermatozoa into the perivitelline space. *Human Reproduction*. 1990; **5**: 575–7.
28. The Fourth Report of the VLA for Human In Vitro Fertilisation and Embryology, London, 1989, p. 14.
29. Comité consultatif National D'Éthique, Report on embryo research under moratorium since 1986, Paris, 18th July 1990, p. 4.
30. Ibid., p. 5.
31. The Fourth Report of the VLA, op. cit., p. 14.
32. Testart J, Lassalle, B. La fécondation assistée, op. cit., p. 250.
33. Gordon JW, Talansky BE. Assisted fertilisation by zona drilling; a mouse model for correction of oligospermia. *Journal of Experimental Zoology*. 1988; **239**: 347–54.
34. Malter M, Cohen J. Cleavage and blastocyst formation following microsurgical repair of polyspermic human zygotes. VIth World Conference on IVF. Jerusalem, 1989.

35. See IVF and GIFT Pregnancies, Australia and New Zealand, 1988. Perinatal Statistics Unit, Sydney, 1990, p. 2.

36. Comité Consultatif National D'Éthique, avis sur les recherches sur l'embryon soumises à moratoire depuis 1986, et qui visent à permettre la réalisation d'un diagnostic génétique avant transplantation, 18 July 1990.

37. Juzgado de Premera Instancia de Mataro, 2 August 1990, and Audiencia de Barcelona, 2 November 1990.

Chapter 22

Ethics of gamete and embryo micromanipulation in human reproduction

Gordon Dunstan

Introduction

A commentator on the ethics of a medical practice must ask himself two questions. May or should it be done at all? And, if so, how should it be done? Doing, and the manner of the doing.

Doing

Logic is a fierce leader. Logic can drive philosophers on to absurdity, theologians to heresy, politicians to disaster. To what point has the logic of treatment for the infertile now brought us? Is there a point beyond which we ought not to go in the application of new scientific discovery and mastery of new techniques? And, if so, have we reached it?

The desire for children is natural. The search for remedies for childlessness seems to be as old as recorded time. The observation and scientific study – accelerated in this half century – of gametes, ovulation, spermatogenesis and embryology has led to *in vitro* fertilisation and other related means of medically assisted conception. Involuntary infertil-

ity still remains. Researchers point away from the earlier focus of interest, the woman, to the failed process of fertilisation itself, and to the sperm, the product of the man. Micromanipulation of sperm into ovum is the next logical step. This volume describes various ways of doing it. But should it be done? Or is the venture the product of arrogance, a taking advantage of exploitable human desire in demonstration of brilliant technique?

Scientists sometimes can appear to be arrogant without intending to. Tadir, in Chapter 11, tell us that 'mammalian fertilisation is an inefficient process in which only one sperm, of millions initially deposited in the female reproductive tract, penetrates the egg'. Zona drilling can do it more efficiently. No doubt, if his model is the ratio between tons of coal shovelled into a steam engine and the output of motive energy, and if his concern is limited to the fertilisation of one woman with the seed of one man, then 'inefficiency' is a possible description. (Dr Fishel and colleagues, incidentally, in Chapter 7, rank the efficiency of micromanipulation as 'relatively low'.) But if the profusion of sperm, as of frog spawn and beech mast and thistledown, is measured in relation to the need for randomness and variety on which the health of evolution itself depends, then natural mammalian fertilisation may not be so 'inefficient' after all. Rather, the scientist has to show that, improve on it as he may in certain cases of infertility, he does not thereby cause more harm than may result from the mass spermatic assault. Should he attempt to?

He has a ready defence: he is meeting a demand from would-be parents who can conceive a child by no other means known. Parenthood is a 'right', some would even say, in their desperation to achieve it; and he is but trying to give them what they want.

But couples also, or one partner in them, may be driven on by a perverse logic into making these demands, inordinate demands, perhaps. The parallel is close: the 'we know we can, therefore we will' of the scientist is matched by the 'we know it can be done, therefore we are going to have it' of the couple. The scientist need have no fear of 'exploiting' such patients in the furtherance of his research, for they are willing: *volenti non fit injuria* – no wrong is done to one who wills what is done; and they will pay for the service. The logic is collusive. But does it justify the practice?

Risk comes to be considered. Risks are of two sorts. There are risks arising from practice, and these will be considered in their turn. There is also risk inherent in the enterprise itself: a risk relevant, therefore, to the question of undertaking. Micromanipulation is undertaken when there is oligozoospermia or asthenozoospermia, sperm too few or two weak in motive power to penetrate the zona pellucida of the egg. Is it possible that the injection of enfeebled sperm might engender enfeebled progeny? Television presents vivid pictures of might, struggles between males for dominance, for mates, in the wild – trials of strength, horn interlocked with horn, until the weaker yields. Thus is assured the perpetuation of the strongest in the herd. When micromanipulation enables sperm, otherwise incapable, to fertilise an ovum, what quality of genes is being transmitted to the child, to the family, to posterity? Animal aggression is by no means the highest human endowment – 'the meek shall inherit the earth'; but a manipulation which appears to go against the natural selection of the strong requires some defence.

There are hints in the papers that this may not be a groundless fear. Sathananthan and colleagues (Chapter 6), writing of the micro-injection of immotile sperm, state that 'abnormal sperm were also encountered within the ooplasm and if a single sperm is injected, which is usually the case, the chance of selecting an abnormal sperm is quite high, considering the quality of sperm used for MI'. In particular they draw attention to the ethical concerns in treating patients with Kartagener syndrome, an autosomal recessive condition, with immotile sperm. Mettler and Kuranty (Chapter 3), writing from experience of subzonal insemination in mouse and cow, states that 'the problem of selecting spermatozoa is not the selection of only one sperm but how to select one fraction that contains "good spermatozoa".' He quotes Markert to the effect that 'the phenotype of the sperm does not reflect the genotype in terms of fertilising ability after micro-injection, and immotile and grossly defective sperm produce the same results that are produced by healthy, robust sperm'. (The reference here is to 'fertilising ability', not to the eventual product of fertilisation.) It is true that, by postponing the transfer of embryos to the uterus until the two- to four-cell stage, tests can be made, when chromosomal patterns can be identified or markers exist for known major genetic defects. But, those apart, what more is known, or can be known, of the all-round constitution of offspring from the micro-injection of weak human sperm? Is it proper to proceed until this question has been addressed?

Further, scientists in their zeal and couples in their intense desire for a child may be colluding, not only to transmit a genome which, left to itself, would never have come into existence, but also to add to the world's population precisely when the need is to arrest its accelerating growth. Our resources, ingenuity and science would be put to better use, it is said, in restricting population growth rather than in adding to it.

These are examples of arguments advanced against micromanipulation in human fertilisation: arguments why it should not be done. Can they be refuted?

It would be folly to protest too much: to claim that such arguments could have no substance. Heads might be found to fit the caps. An ethical defence does not rest on the supposed perfection of scientists, doctors or patients. It must rest on the inherent value of the work attempted as judged by the criteria normally applicable to medical advances of a comparable nature. The first allegation, of a ruthless logic driving scientists and doctors on in unending pursuit, is sometimes urged in other terms, 'the technological imperative'. It is made regularly against medical innovations which stagger the imagination and arouse fear: in renal medicine and dialysis; in cardiac and thoracic surgery; in organ transplantation; intensive care, especially neonatal intensive care. Reflection on these other areas of practice shows how the pursuit of logic has in fact been faced and checked. The 'logical' conclusion of the notion that the overriding duty of medicine is to save life was leading to the unnatural prolongation of dying by persistence in intrusive intervention. The profession has been persuaded, morally obliged, to withdraw from this course: to recognise when to change the management, and to heighten skills in palliative medicine, in order that life at its ending may take its natural course. The logic of 'the sanctity of life' seeks still to impose a duty to keep every baby alive, however premature, however handicapped – because the technical skills have been developed to do so. In fact the common conscience prevails over that logic: with the authority of the law as declared in the Courts, management must be decided by what serves best the interest of the child, whether in living longer or in being allowed peacefully to die.

Advances in the treatment of infertility are subject to the same imperatives and controls. The imperative to which the scientist properly responds is to pursue knowledge where it may be found, by apt and proportionate means. When that knowledge gives the physician a therapeutic opportunity his profession obliges him to apply it in the interest of patients. But that interest is paramount: it may not be sacrificed either to the pursuit of knowledge or to the advance of technical skills. In recent decades two defences have been raised against the 'logic' of the 'technological imperative'. The first is an enhanced doctrine of personal consent. Consent is such a shibboleth now that it is commonly forgotten how new is the intensity of our interest in

it.[1] The second defence is the establishment of research ethics committees to scrutinise and oversee projects for research involving human – and, increasingly, animal – subjects; these are to assure social, corporate consent, as well as personal, to what is done. Since *in vitro* fertilisation and embryo implantation first proved itself as a remedy for some forms of infertility, the development of both science and practice, including the micromanipulation of human gametes, has been subjected to this sort of ethical control: first by the Voluntary, Interim, Licensing Authority; and then, since 1991, by the Human Fertilisation and Embryology Authority set up by Act of Parliament in 1990.

If this is society's protection against aggressive medical science and technology, where lies the doctor's protection against the logic of demand – 'if it is there, I have a right to have it'? His professional duty, made explicit in the Act of 1990, is to have regard to the would-be patient and to the interest of any child which might be born as a result of the medical intervention. There is thus laid upon him the obligation of assessment, not only of patients' anatomical and physiological indications, but also of their personalities and of the emotional and other pressures under which they may come to him. It is his duty to inform, to discern, to counsel, and finally to decide whether to provide the treatment sought or not. It may be his duty to dissuade: to tell the patient when further pursuit of what might be technically possible would not be in her interest, or in the potential interest of a child if born; and to maintain his professional opinion and liberty, if need be, against strong pressure to provide. When there is financial pressure also, the knowledge that fees will accrue for every treatment undertaken, the duty of professional integrity is the more to be recalled. The false imperatives of logic remain a possibility; but that possibility, recognised for the hazard that it is, is not sufficient to invalidate ethical practice.

The capacity for parenthood is a natural endowment of men and women, and one reinforced by strong personal desire as well as social expectation – varying in different cultures but present in all. But only in a limited sense can this desire be called a 'right'. It is one only in the sense that the law will normally protect the capacity to procreate, and the liberty of a committed couple to do so, against external restriction or infringement, as by enforced sterilisation. Patients in the British National Health Service have a statutory right to medical advice and to available treatment to enable them to fulfil that capacity. But the right is not absolute: it cannot oblige a doctor to provide whatever treatment a patient might choose, particularly if it is still in an experimental or innovative stage of development. The decision normally rests with both of them as responsible (but not autonomous) persons; but ultimately, if they cannot agree, the responsible practitioner must remain free not to treat.

But should he treat at all with micro-injected human sperm? If that expedient is required to help enfeebled sperm into the ovum, what risk is there, it has been asked, of enfeebled progeny? There is, in fact, no known correlation in any animals studied between the vigour of the sperm and the vigour of the organism resulting from its conception.[2] There appears to be very, very little competition between sperm from the same male. It is theoretically possible that a male resulting from micro-injected feeble sperm might himself have poor sperm; he might be oligozoospermic or asthenozoospermic. But in that unlikely event it may be assumed that a new generation of infertility specialists would help him to deal with it. (There is an analogy here in medical genetics: selective non-implantation or abortion of a defective embryo still leaves the gene to express again in a future generation; but the practice is ethical nevertheless.) There is insufficient scientific plausibility for this objection to micro-assisted fertilisation to be sustained. Nevertheless, the fear exists; it is right that it should have been addressed by Dr Fishel in his chapter on 'Gamete and Embryo Micromanipulation in Human Reproduction: Perspicacity or Opacity?' (Chapter 20).

The last count against micro-assisted fertilisation is that it adds to the world's population at a time when it ought to be diminished. The argument fails first for lack of proportion. The number of children ever likely to be conceived in this way is infinitesimal in comparison with the rate of natural increase; and the resources devoted to it are minute in comparison with the cost of combating the imbalance of population with food production. It fails secondly because one of the fruits of gamete and embryo research is likely to be the development of new contraceptive methods, some of which may be more acceptable and applicable in over-populated regions than the methods now available.[3]

If, then, these are the substantial arguments why micro-assisted fertilisation should not be undertaken, they do not convince. If the practice itself is permissible, we may go on to ask how ethically it should be conducted.

The manner of doing

The question dominant in the mind of any clinician contemplating a new treatment concerns risk: will he, while trying to benefit the patient, inadvertently cause harm? Before he may ethically begin treatment he has to assure himself and others, either that he has eliminated predictable risk, or, if he cannot, that the risk is minor or minimal in relation to the benefit predictably conferred. Risk may be low or high in relation both to the likelihood of incidence and to the severity of the impairment should it occur. Permission to advance to clinical application of micromanipulation was withheld in Britain by the Interim Licensing Authority until these conditions had been met.

It is normal for the results of *in vitro* studies to be tested in animal models before clinical application in human patients. Examples appear in several chapters of this book, and particularly in those by Godke (Chapter 15), Mettler and Kuranty (Chapter 3) and Wilton (Chapter 19). The ethics of using animals in this way are widely debated and cannot be analysed here. Reference may be made to a recent thorough study, *Lives in the Balance*, edited by Smith and Boyd.[4] Experimental work with animals is itself under strict ethical control and must meet the requirements of the Animals (Scientific Procedures) Act 1986 as administered by the Home Office and its Inspectorate. Some medical organisations, like the Royal College of Surgeons and the Imperial Cancer Research Fund, have also their own ethics committees to supervise their own animal work.

Awareness of risk, and evidence of adverse events, occur throughout the scientific chapters of this volume. Malter et al. (Chapter 8) have a summary list of them. Calderon and Veiga (Chapter 10) report a high incidence of polyspermia in partial zona dissection; and Fishel (Chapter 14), while expressing surprise at this, relates his own efforts to reduce it by regulating the number of spermatozoa inserted by micro-injection. Calderon adds to this the occurrence of aneuploidies and the establishment of molar pregnancies. Iatrogenic damage, in sperm preparation, in embryonic infection through the split zona pellucida, and in embryonic biopsy are reported by Mortimer (Chapter 4) and Malter (Chapter 8), though without evidence of resulting fetal abnormality. The main loss from such events is in the reduction of embryos suitable for transfer to the uterus. Chromosomal defect has been reported by Jouannet and by Kola et al,.[5] but occurring no more with subzonal micro-injection than in the practice of IVF; and evidence so far indicates no higher incidence of this in IVF treatment than occurs in nature.

Micromanipulation techniques share with other treatments for infertility the serious risk of multi-pregnancies, some unacceptably high in that they threaten fetuses or children with early death or congenital impairment and perhaps social deprivation. The risk is inherent in the uncertainties surrounding conception, but can be reduced. More seriously it is connected also with clinical management offered in relation to these uncertainties. As experience grows in the monitoring of folliculation and ovulation, and in the selecting and implanting of IVF embryos, the duty of care increases to reduce the number of embryos replaced to the minimum thought necessary to establish a pregnancy. The Interim Licensing Authority set a normal limit of three, with permission to go to four only in exceptional circumstances; but what was 'exceptional' was undefined. Winston (Chapter 16) draws attention to the injustice inflicted on a woman who has already a demanding handicapped child if unguarded clinical management leaves her with a new triplet pregnancy. He would set a normal maximum of two embryos replaced. Clearly he regrets what he calls an 'unhappy decision' when twice he submitted to parental persuasion to replace three embryos simultaneously, with serious obstetric results. Ethically that regret must be shared by

anyone who affirms – as tradition has affirmed – that the final responsibility for decision in such matters must lie with the clinician, even against the wish of the patient. Confidence in ethical practice is strengthened by this clinician's own admission of misjudgement.

The practice of reducing a high multiple pregnancy by selective feticide early in pregnancy may have its clinical justification in that, by killing some, the remnant may have a better chance to live. But it is an unfortunate remedy for a condition brought about by medical intervention. It confirms the worst suspicions of those who are hostile to 'high technology' treatment for infertility *a priori*; it offers gratuitous ammunition to groups who denounce feticide in any circumstances as a violation of an absolute 'right to life'. Thereby it threatens the public perception of legitimate practice with the shadow of disrepute.

Risks, then, are identified and admitted; and the duty is accepted of trying to eliminate or reduce them by pre-clinical experiment, by persistent observation and reporting, and by practice disciplined by experience and expectation. Such risks as remain are accepted, by patients as well as clinicians, because they are incidental to the pursuit of benefits sought and judged reasonably attainable. The duty to advise patients of these risks, and of the limited expectations of success, and to enable them to make the choice for themselves, is common to medical practice. The duty is of a higher order in micro-assisted fertilisation because of the innovative and still experimental stage of the procedure. The first direct benefit sought is, of course, the enabling of conception from sperm too few or too weak to penetrate the ovum unassisted. But there are other substantial benefits as well.

Micromanipulation is a new addition to the techniques which make pre-implantation embryonic cells available for biopsy, and so for the identification of single gene or chromosomal disorders. The purpose of this is not 'eugenic', part of a grand scheme to improve the genetic quality of the human race. It is to utilise the new understanding of genetic disease in the treatment of particular patients: to offer a woman liable to conceive a child bearing some serious genetic handicap a better alternative to abortion; the liberty to choose whether to have a compromised embryo replaced or not. The chapters by Wilton, Delhanty and Handyside report progress in this.

The stage at which the biopsy is taken – oocyte, pronucleus, early cleavage, or blastocyst – is a matter for scientific decision, depending on the knowledge sought in relation to the timing of gene expression, the number of cells and amount of DNA available, and the risk of harm to the developing embryo. There is still a risk of error in the interpretation of the biopsy, as Winston and Handyside admit. Winston demonstrates the value of sex determination in the detection of sex-linked deleterious genes, like that for the Lesch-Nyhan syndrome: the option of replacing only female embryos eliminates the risk of bearing a handicapped child at least in this generation, for the gene expresses adversely only in males. Ethical questions arise. Logic, again, followed too far, would lead to the discarding of embryos in which the congenital defect, if predictable, might be trivial. The question to be faced in counselling is, what degree of handicap justifies non-replacement? What reasons are serious enough to justify the determining and disclosure of the sex of the embryo? It is not in the human interest to replace (if that were possible) the ethics of care by sliding into a too easy acceptance of disposal. It is not in the interest of society in having a balanced population to facilitate individual choice of sex for reasons other than the avoidance of sex-linked genetic disease, particularly in cultures which strongly value one sex, generally male, more than the other. And these cultures are no longer isolated in particular and distant regions of the globe; immigration has brought them into the midst of Western societies.

These questions take us into the heart of the ethical relationship of practitioner and patient. Given an adverse prognosis from the biopsy, the choice, whether to have the embryo replaced or not, must lie with the potential mother. The doctor owes her a duty of sufficient, accurate information, clearly given and with the time and help for assimilation, to enable her to make that choice.[6] But if some choices are not to be open to the mother, for instance the option to reject an embryo simply because it is not of the sex desired, exclusions of this sort should be explained and accepted early in the consultation, before the biopsy is performed. It is as important for the patient to respect the ethical position of the practitioner as it is for him to respect hers. An ethical relationship rests on mutual obligation.

Handyside (Chapter 17) considers ways of respecting the scruple of a patient who feels bound to refuse biopsy of an embryo (perhaps because of a belief that all 'embryo experimentation' violates 'the sanctity of human life') but would accept biopsy of the first polar body removed from a gamete, the oocyte. But the gain in terms of intention proves to be superficial in terms of consequence. Knowledge gained from the gamete lacks the completeness of that gained from the embryonic genes; its predictive value is limited. The investigation itself, for reasons explained, leaves fewer embryos for implanting, and so reduces the chances of the desired pregnancy. Avoidance of embryonic biopsy, similarly, by taking cells from the trophectoderm of the developed blastocyst – which are not from the embryo – offers no better remedy; the pregnancy rate following this intervention is low. Respect for the scruple results in embryonic wastage, loss *in utero*, and this is what the scruple was alleged to avoid. When assertions of 'absolute' value or obligation surface in a clinical relationship they are to be faced openly and with honesty on both sides; and the earlier they are faced, the fewer conflicts of conscience or of will there are likely to be.

It has been assumed throughout this discussion of the ethics of practice that guardianship of the ethics lies with the moral agents themselves: the scientist, the clinician and the patient. The clinician in particular may have to hold a delicate balance between the interest of a patient whom he wishes to serve and a legitimate social interest which may pull in another direction. This is a common feature in professional ethics – in law or accountancy, for instance, as much as in experimental science and medicine. Professional ethics are society's first line of defence against malpractice. Byk's survey (Chapter 21) of legislation and legislative tendency shows that this primacy is not relied on everywhere. Recent legislation in Britain indicates a shift of balance here also.

The Interim Licensing Authority regulated developing practice in centres where IVF was offered and embryo research was conducted. The Authority was consensual; it had no statutory or coercive power. It succeeded because practitioners wanted it to, and the public seemed to be content with it, as a determined interim measure. It was established and funded by the Medical Research Council and the Royal College of Obstetricians and Gynaecologists jointly; regulation in accordance with the Authority's guidelines was accepted voluntarily. Only seldom was a licence withdrawn or renewal deferred. In August 1991 the Authority was superseded by the Human Fertilisation and Embryology Authority, created by Statute. Research or practice contrary to the terms of the Act are criminal offences. Law and guidelines are more far-reaching and the powers of the new Authority are wider than those of the voluntary body, and they are coercive. The bureaucracy of control is heavier and licence fees – unknown before – are high. Rehoboam's scorpions bite more deeply than Solomon's whips.[7] But the new Authority has inherited from the interim one, first, a set of procedures – inspection, licensing, practice directed by published guidelines, consultation, scrutiny of research protocols, published reports on centres and procedures licensed. More valuably it has inherited the confidence and co-operation of the professions involved. The new powers were taken

by Parliament, not in reaction to any scandal or instance of malpractice (as happened with the Human Organ Transplants Act, 1989) but because of public uncertainty about the moral status of embryonic cells in cleavage and the protection due to them, and a consequent fear that 'the sanctity of human life' would be infringed by embryo manipulation.

Among groups which opposed in Parliament the permissions enshrined in the Act that fear is a settled conviction; for some it has dogmatic ecclesiastical warrant. Micromanipulation of the human embryo will be subject to their scrutiny. To the first question addressed in this chapter, 'May it be done at all?', their answer would be 'No'. In practice doctors and counsellors may encounter patients inwardly divided between at least a half belief in that absolutist rejection and a strong personal desire for the service offered. To those patients is owed respect for their scruple and delicate help in resolving their inner conflict.

Sensitive control by the statutory Authority may give the public at large the assurance that it needs. It will do so the more easily as it finds its own assurance in the professional integrity of the embryologists, doctors, nurses, counsellors and medical secretaries whose work it oversees.

References

1. Dunstan GR, Seller MJ. *Consent in Medicine: Convergence and Divergence in Tradition*. London: King Edward's Hospital Fund, 1983.
2. Dame Anne McLaren FRS, personal communication.
3. Aitken RJ, Irvine DS. Molecular mechanisms that control sperm function. In: Asch RH, Balmaceda JP, Johnston I (eds.) *Gamete Physiology*. Norwell, Massachusetts: Serono Symposia, 1990, pp. 69.
4. Smith JA, Boyd KM. *Lives in the Balance: The Ethics of Using Animals in Biomedical Research*. Oxford: Oxford University Press, 1991.
5. Kola I, Lacham O, Jansen RPS, Turner M Trounson A. Chromosomal analysis of human oocytes fertilized by micro-injection of spermatozoa into the perivitelline space. *Human Reproduction*. 1990 **5**: 575–7.
6. Ferguson-Smith MA, Ferguson-Smith ME. Relationships between patient, clinician and scientist in prenatal diagnosis. In: Dunstan GR, Shinebourne EA (eds.) *Doctors' Decisions: Ethical Conflicts in Medical Practice*. Oxford: Oxford University Press, 1989, pp 18–34.
7. I Kings 12:11.

Index